Hematologic Malignancies

Series Editor

Martin Dreyling
Großhadern Hospital,Medicine III
Ludwig Maximilians University of Munich
München
Germany

More information about this series at http://www.springer.com/series/5416

Oliver A. Cornely · Martin Hoenigl
Editors

Infection Management in Hematology

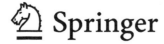 Springer

Editors
Oliver A. Cornely
Department I for Internal Medicine
CECAD Translational Research Institute
University Hospital of Cologne
Cologne
Germany

Martin Hoenigl
Department of Internal Medicine
Medical University of Graz
Graz
Steiermark
Austria

Department of Medicine
University of California San Diego
San Diego
California
USA

ISSN 2197-9766   ISSN 2197-9774   (electronic)
Hematologic Malignancies
ISBN 978-3-030-57316-4   ISBN 978-3-030-57317-1   (eBook)
https://doi.org/10.1007/978-3-030-57317-1

This Springer imprint is published by the registered company Springer Nature Switzerland AG
The registered company address is: Gewerbestrasse 11, 6330 Cham, Switzerland

Preface

Infections are major causes of morbidity and mortality in patients with hematological malignancies, particularly in those with prolonged neutropenia and recipients of hematopoietic stem cell transplantation (HSCT). Successful management of infectious diseases in this setting often necessitates not only expert knowledge in infectious diseases but also expertise in diagnosis and treatment of the underlying hematologic diseases.

In the hematologic setting differential diagnosis of presumed infection always includes multiple different pathogens, as bacterial, fungal, viral, and parasitic infections occur. In addition, the underlying hematologic disease can sometimes mimic an infectious disease process, with similar radiological and clinical findings. Recently, a swiftly increasing number of drugs target and modify immune response and may result into previously unknown inflammatory syndromes simulating signs and symptoms of infection. Diagnosis of the underlying infectious cause is demanding and requires broad knowledge in the field of infectious diseases.

The high risk of developing infectious complications has resulted in approaches of antibacterial, antifungal, antiviral, and antiparasitic prophylaxis in patient groups at highest risk for infections. Patients with hematological malignancies are also at risk for infections that are potentially preventable by vaccination. However, many vaccines have not been used to their full potential, because immune response may be attenuated by antineoplastic treatment. Outside of the HSCT setting, clinical vaccine trials are mostly missing, although many patients receive treatments that interfere with vaccine efficacy, for example, B cell-directed strategies. Even less is known about such interference of the many new treatment options in hematology. Ideally, patients would be vaccinated prior initiation of immunosuppressive therapy, but this is not always possible.

Once infection establishes, rapid action is essential. Management relies on early diagnosis and anti-infective treatment, frequently before a pathogen is identified. While the use of broad-spectrum antibacterial drugs has reduced the mortality in febrile neutropenia, it may have contributed to the emergence of drug resistant pathogens. To balance the most effective treatment of the individual versus the risk of promoting resistance, antimicrobial stewardship has established a firm place at hematology departments and hospitals.

Hematologic patients are also particularly vulnerable to pandemics and outbreaks, including the current outbreak of SARS-CoV-2 and coronavirus disease 2019 (COVID-19), which has resulted in delays of necessary treatment for underlying hematological malignancies, and devastating infection related mortality rates, particularly in older or comorbid patients.

Infection management in hematology is a prime example of modern medicine where complexity of diagnostics and therapies needs to be addressed by a multidisciplinary team to achieve the best possible outcome for our patients.

This book summarizes the current understanding in patient management, where hematology and infectious diseases intersect.

Cologne, Germany   Oliver A. Cornely
Graz, Austria   Martin Hoenigl

Contents

Epidemiology and Risk Factors of Invasive Fungal Infections

1

Frédéric Lamoth

1.1 Introduction

Invasive fungal infections (IFI) are well-known and feared infectious complications among patients with hematologic malignancies. The prolonged immunosuppressive state resulting from deep and long-lasting neutropenia following myeloablative chemotherapies or long-term anti-rejection therapies post hematopoietic stem cell transplantation (HSCT) represents the highest risk for the development of such infections.

The epidemiology of IFI is difficult to assess, as their diagnosis often relies on a scale of probability (proven, probable, possible) according to the definitions of the European Organization for Research and Treatment of Cancer (EORTC) and Mycoses Study Group (MSG) (De Pauw et al. 2008). Given the limited sensitivity of culture, most IFIs nowadays are diagnosed in the absence of positive cultures and species identification.

Multiple studies have assessed the incidence, distribution of fungal pathogens and risk factors of IFI among patients with hematologic malignancies. The epidemiology of IFI can be influenced by several factors, such as the geographical situation (temperate versus tropical regions), environmental conditions (e.g., building renovation works), diagnostic procedures (e.g., use of serological or molecular diagnostic tests), definition and classification of IFI (inclusion or not of probable and possible cases) or use of antifungal prophylaxis.

This chapter aims to provide an overview of the epidemiology of IFI according to the different categories of onco-hematological patients and the type of fungal pathogens.

1.2 Hematopoietic Stem Cell Transplantation (HSCT)

The cumulative incidence of IFI was estimated at 3.4% per year among a large cohort of HSCT recipients in the United States with molds accounting for about two-thirds of cases (Kontoyiannis et al. 2010). Among allogeneic HSCT recipients, the risk was higher among recipients from mismatched related or matched unrelated donors (8.1% and 7.7% per year, respectively) compared to matched related donors (5.8%). IFI were rarely observed among autologous HSCT recipients (1.2% per year), who experience shorter duration of neutropenia (usually less than 10 days) and a predominant cellular-mediated immune depression in follow-up. Data from the European continent show a similar epidemiological picture as illustrated by a large Italian cohort reporting an overall incidence of IFI of 3.7% over 5 years

F. Lamoth (✉)
Infectious Diseases Service, Department of Medicine, Lausanne University Hospital and University of Lausanne, Lausanne, Switzerland

Institute of Microbiology, Lausanne University Hospital and University of Lausanne, Lausanne, Switzerland

© Springer Nature Switzerland AG 2021
O. A. Cornely, M. Hoenigl (eds.), *Infection Management in Hematology*, Hematologic Malignancies, https://doi.org/10.1007/978-3-030-57317-1_1

among all HSCT recipients (7.8% among allo-geneic HSCT recipients) with the difference that recipients of matched related donors were more frequently affected (Pagano et al. 2007). Results from these two recent cohorts can be compared to epidemiological data before the year 2005 showing an overall incidence of IFI of about 10–15% among HSCT recipients (Baddley et al. 2001; Cornet et al. 2002; Fukuda et al. 2003; Garcia-Vidal et al. 2008; Martino et al. 2002). A large study conducted at the Fred Hutchinson Cancer Research Center (Seattle, WA) showed an increased annual incidence of invasive mold infections from 1990 to 1998 (Marr et al. 2002). However, it is difficult to assess the impact of the advent of azole prophy-laxis and the improvements in diagnostic approaches on epidemiological trends of IFI from 2000.

Epidemiological reports from the pediatric HSCT population account for an overall inci-dence of about 5%, similar to the adult popula-tion (Cesaro et al. 2017; Dvorak et al. 2005).

IFI among HSCT usually occur at a median of 2–4 months post-transplantation and are rarely observed (<15% cases) beyond one year (Kontoyiannis et al. 2010). The risk is particu-larly high after bone marrow recovery among patients with severe graft-versus-host disease (GVHD) and intensive immunosuppressive regi-mens. Despite antifungal prophylaxis, the inci-dence of IFI among patients with acute (grade II to IV) or chronic extensive GVHD remains around 5–10% (Ullmann et al. 2007).

Distinct risk factors have been identified according to the timing of IFI after HSCT (Garcia-Vidal et al. 2008). Early IFI (<40 days post HSCT) was found to be associated with transplant variables (unrelated donor or HLA mismatch), type of immunosuppression regimen (receipt of anti-thymocyte globulin or corticoste-roids), lymphopenia, hyperglycemia, iron over-load, cytomegalovirus (CMV) disease, and blood transfusions. Factors associated with late IFI (>40 days post HSCT) were advanced age, female sex, acute GVHD, CMV disease, cortico-steroids, and blood transfusions.

1.3 Acute Leukemia

Induction or consolidation chemotherapies of acute leukemia are usually associated with pro-longed periods (>14 days) of profound neutrope-nia. A multicenter Italian study reported an incidence of IFI of 12% among patients with acute myeloid leukemia (AML) and 6.5% among those with acute lymphoid leukemia (ALL) with a predominance of mold infections (64%) (Pagano et al. 2006). Similar incidence was reported from other countries (Barreto et al. 2013; Koehler et al. 2017; Mariette et al. 2017). IFIs are more rarely observed among patients with acute promyelo-cytic leukemia who are treated with different che-motherapeutic regimens and usually experience shorter period of neutropenia (Pagano et al. 2015). Chemotherapeutic regimens with azacitidine, a hypomethylating agent, have also been associated with a lower incidence of IFI (1.6% per patient) (Pomares et al. 2016). Among children with acute leukemia, incidence rates of 3–7% have been reported (Cesaro et al. 2017; Ducassou et al. 2015; Zaoutis et al. 2006).

The use of systemic antifungal prophylaxis during the neutropenic phase has an important impact on the incidence of IFI in patients with acute leukemia. IFI rates as high as 35–50% have been reported among AML patients who did not receive any antifungal prophylaxis following induction chemotherapy (Neofytos et al. 2013; Tang et al. 2015). A multicenter randomized study conducted among hematologic cancer patients with chemotherapy-induced neutropenia has demonstrated the efficacy of posaconazole prophylaxis in reducing the incidence of IFI to 2% compared to 8% in patients receiving flucon-azole or itraconazole prophylaxis (Cornely et al. 2007).

While prolonged neutropenia resulting from intensive chemotherapy is the main risk factor in this population, other factors predisposing to invasive mold infections have been identified in multivariate analysis, such as performance status ≥2, low body weight, chronic obstructive pulmo-nary disease and environmental conditions (building renovation or professional activities, such as farmer, gardener, and construction worker) (Caira et al. 2015). Post-chemotherapy esophagitis grade > 2 was also an independent risk factor of both invasive yeast and mold infections (Caira et al. 2015).

1.4 Other Hematologic Diseases

Out of the context of HSCT, IFI rarely affect patients with other hematologic malignancies, such as chronic leukemia, multiple myeloma, Hodgkin disease, or non-Hodgkin lymphoma, because chemotherapies used for the treatment of these cancers are usually associated with neutropenia of short duration (<10 days). The overall incidence of IFI in these patients ranges from 0.5 to 2.5% (Pagano et al. 2006). Mold infections are predominant among patients with chronic leukemia, while molds and yeasts equally contribute to IFI in the others categories.

Patients with myelodysplastic syndromes who also undergo intensive myeloablative chemotherapies and prolonged neutropenia exhibit the same risk and incidence of IFI as those with acute leukemia (Barreto et al. 2013; Cornely et al. 2007).

Patients with aplastic anemia, who may experience prolonged leucopenia and receive immunosuppressive therapies are at high risk of developing invasive fungal infections, in particular, mold infections, with a reported incidence of 5–10% (Quarello et al. 2012; Torres et al. 2003).

1.5 Invasive Candidiasis

Invasive candidiasis (IC) can be divided in two categories in hematologic cancers patients: candidemia and chronic disseminated (or hepatosplenic) candidiasis. Central venous catheters that remain in place for long duration following chemotherapies may be a source of infection. However, chemotherapy-induced enterocolitis is often the origin of translocation. *Candida* spp. are commensal yeasts of the gastrointestinal tract and skin. While *Candida albicans* is the predom-

inant pathogen, the proportion of non-*albicans Candida* spp. has increased during the last decade and currently exceeds 50% (Lamoth et al. 2018). IC represents 25–30% of IFI among hematologic cancer patients; its incidence has decreased as azole prophylaxis has become common practice (Kontoyiannis et al. 2010; Pagano et al. 2007; Pagano et al. 2006; Neofytos et al. 2009). As a consequence, non-*albicans Candida* spp. with intrinsic level of azole resistance are now predominant in many regions of the world. *Candida glabrata* is the most frequent yeast pathogen among US HSCT recipients and *Candida krusei* infections are more commonly observed among neutropenic patients with hematologic malignancies compared to other populations (Kontoyiannis et al. 2010; Neofytos et al. 2009; Horn et al. 2009; Schuster et al. 2013). However, the epidemiology of *Candida* spp. may differ from one hospital to another. For instance, *Candida parapsilosis* and *Candida tropicalis* are more prevalent in Spain and Greece (Gamaletsou et al. 2014; Puig-Asensio et al. 2015). *Candida auris* is an emerging pathogen that has appeared simultaneously on different continents since 2009 (Lockhart et al. 2017). Its ability to rapidly develop resistance to all antifungal drug classes and cause hospital outbreaks by nosocomial transmission is particularly concerning. While this yeast was mainly associated with IC outbreaks in intensive care units (Schelenz et al. 2016), it could also affect oncohematology units in the future.

While candidemia is the most frequent form of IC, chronic disseminated candidiasis (CDC) is a rare disease occurring mainly in acute leukemia patients at the stage of neutrophil recovery, which has been considered as a kind of immune reconstitution inflammatory syndrome (IRIS) (Rammaert et al. 2012). Before the era of azole prophylaxis, CDC was estimated to affect 3–6% of patients with acute leukemia and chemotherapy-induced neutropenia (Sallah et al. 1999), but it is now considered as a rare disease (<3%) (Rammaert et al. 2012).

CDC can be missed because of non-specific clinical signs (persistent fever, abdominal symptoms, and hepatic tests disturbances) and lack of sensitivity of blood cultures that recover yeasts in only 20% cases (Rammaert et al. 2012; De Castro et al. 2012). The diagnosis usually relies on imaging showing nodular lesions in the liver and spleen and positive serological markers (1,3-beta-d-glucan, mannan/anti-mannan). Other organs, such as the lungs or kidneys, can be affected.

Risk factors for IC in hematologic cancer patients are overall similar to those reported in non-neutropenic patients and include the presence of central venous catheters, gastrointestinal tract mucositis, and colonization with *Candida* spp. (Caira et al. 2015; Pagano et al. 1999).

1.6 Other Invasive Yeast Infections

Invasive fungal infections due to yeasts other than *Candida* spp. are rare (<2% of IFI) (Kontoyiannis et al. 2010; Fernandez-Ruiz et al. 2017; Richardson and Lass-Florl 2008). Cryptococcosis is not common among patients with hematologic malignancies accounting for less than 1% of IFI in this population (Kontoyiannis et al. 2010). Other yeast pathogens are commensals of the skin, and central venous catheters are supposed to be the major source of infection. *Trichosporon* spp. is a cause of fungemia affecting mainly hematologic cancer patients (de Almeida Junior and Hennequin 2016). It has also been reported as a cause of disseminated disease with hepatosplenic lesions, similar to chronic disseminated candidiasis (Alby-Laurent et al. 2017). *Rhodotorula* spp. (*Rhodotorula mucilaginosa* and *Rhodotorula glutinis*) and *Saprochaete* spp. (*Saprochaete capitata* and *Saprochaete clavata*) can occasionally cause fungemia (Fernandez-Ruiz et al. 2017; Del Principe et al. 2016; Duran Graeff et al. 2017; Garcia-Suarez et al. 2011). *Geotrichum candidum* often colonizes the stools of hematologic cancer patients, but is a very rare cause of fungemia (Duran Graeff et al. 2017; Henrich et al. 2009).

1.7 Invasive Aspergillosis

Invasive aspergillosis (IA) is the most frequent IFI in hematologic cancer (40–60% of all IFI cases) (Kontoyiannis et al. 2010; Pagano et al. 2007; Pagano et al. 2006; Neofytos et al. 2009). The lung is the primary site of infection in most cases with dissemination to other organs in about 10% of patients (Steinbach et al. 2012). Primary extrapulmonary infections usually originate from the tracheobronchial tree, sinuses, skin, or brain (Steinbach et al. 2012). *Aspergillus fumigatus* is the cause of 60–80% cases, followed by *Aspergillus flavus*, *Aspergillus niger* and *Aspergillus terreus* (Kontoyiannis et al. 2010; Neofytos et al. 2009; Steinbach et al. 2012; Pagano et al. 2010). *Aspergillus calidoustus* is an emerging pathogen, which deserves mention because of its intrinsic pan-azole resistance and its association with breakthrough IA in patients receiving azole prophylaxis (Lamoth et al. 2017; Seroy et al. 2017). Other rare pathogenic *Aspergillus* spp. include *A. versicolor*, *A. nidulans* and *A. glaucus* (Steinbach et al. 2012). It is important to note that the diagnosis of IA only relies on a positive galactomannan test without species identification in up to half of cases (Neofytos et al. 2009; Steinbach et al. 2012; Maertens et al. 2016a).

Patients with acute leukemia (in particular acute myeloid leukemia) are at highest risk for IA during the neutropenic phase of intensive chemotherapy with 70% cases occurring beyond 10 days of neutropenia (Steinbach et al. 2012; Pagano et al. 2010; Lortholary et al. 2011). Allogeneic HSCT recipients represent the second group at risk (Steinbach et al. 2012). In one French cohort, an important proportion of IA cases (22%) occurred in patients with chronic lymphoproliferative disorders, which may represent another important and underestimated group at risk (Lortholary et al. 2011).

Other predisposing factors of IA were identified among allogeneic HSCT recipients, such as active malignancy at HSCT, CMV reactivation and delayed lymphocyte engraftment for early IA and chronic extensive GVHD, steroid therapy, secondary neutropenia, and relapse after HSCT for late IA (Mikulska et al. 2009).

Genetic factors have been found to play an important role with some single-nucleotide polymorphisms (SNPs) associated with increased risk of IA (Lamoth et al. 2011). Some pattern recognition receptors (PRRs) of the toll-like receptors (TLRs) or C-type lectin receptors (CLRs) are crucial for the innate immune response against *Aspergillus* spp. A large matched control study identified a TLR4 donor haplotype (D299G and T399I) that increased the risk of IA among unrelated HSCT recipients (Bochud et al. 2008). An SNP in Dectin-1 (Y238X present in either the donor or recipient), a PRR of the fungal cell wall component 1,3-beta-d-glucan, has also been associated with an increased risk of IA (Cunha et al. 2010). Currently, the most promising approach for a future clinical application focuses on pentraxin 3 (PTX3), a soluble PRR binding to conidia and facilitating their phagocytosis by human macrophages. A homozygous haplotype (h2/h2) with reduced PTX3 production was associated with an increased risk of IA if present in the donor for HSCT recipients or in the recipients of solid-organ transplantation (Cunha et al. 2014; Wojtowicz et al. 2015).

1.8   Mucormycosis

Filamentous fungi of the order *Mucorales* are responsible for this severe infection usually affecting the sinuses or lungs with local extension to adjacent structures (e.g., orbit, brain) or hematogenous dissemination (Roden et al. 2005). Primary intestinal infection or wound infection are also described. Increasing incidence of mucormycosis in the general population has been reported worldwide, especially since 2000, which is associated with the increasing number of immunocompromised patients at risk, such as HSCT or solid organ transplant recipients (Roden et al. 2005; Abidi et al. 2014; Bitar et al. 2009; Saegeman et al. 2010). Mucormycosis is the second most frequent invasive mold infection accounting for 5–10% of all IFI cases in hemato-

logic cancer patients (Kontoyiannis et al. 2010; Neofytos et al. 2009). In North America and Europe, *Rhizopus* spp. (e.g., *R. oryzae, R. microsporus*) is responsible of about 30–50% cases, followed by *Mucor* spp. (e.g., *M. circinelloides*), *Lichtheimia* spp. (e.g., *L. corymbifera, L. ramosa*), *Rhizomucor* spp. (e.g., *R. pusillus*) and *Cunninghamella* spp. (e.g., *C. bertholletiae*) (Roden et al. 2005; Kontoyiannis et al. 2014; Pagano et al. 2009; Skiada et al. 2011; Xhaard et al. 2012). Local epidemiology may differ according to regions/countries: for instance, *Lichtheimia* spp. is frequently observed in Europe, but rarely in the US (Kontoyiannis et al. 2014; Skiada et al. 2011; Xhaard et al. 2012; Guinea et al. 2017). In addition to neutropenia, uncontrolled diabetes, corticosteroid therapy, and iron overload are considered as risk factors for mucormycosis (Roden et al. 2005; Skiada et al. 2011; Xhaard et al. 2012; Maertens et al. 1999).

1.9   Fusariosis

The importance of *Fusarium* spp. as causal agents of IFI varies from one region to another. In Brazil, disseminated fusariosis was reported to be the most frequent IFI among HSCT recipients (Nucci et al. 2013a), while it accounts for only ≤3% of cases in US and Europe (Kontoyiannis et al. 2010; Pagano et al. 2007; Pagano et al. 2006; Neofytos et al. 2009). Disseminated fusariosis occurs mainly in hematologic cancer patients with neutropenia (Nucci et al. 2014). Contrarily to most IFI, the primary focus of infection is the skin (e.g., onychomycosis or intertrigo) in two-thirds of cases, and not the lung (one-third of cases) (Nucci et al. 2013b). Fungemia can be documented by blood cultures in up to 40% cases and secondary embolic skin lesions are common features (Nucci and Anaissie 2007). The most frequent pathogenic species are *Fusarium solani* complex, followed by *Fusarium oxysporum* complex (Nucci et al. 2014; Lortholary et al. 2010). Other relevant pathogenic species include *Fusarium proliferatum*, *Fusarium moniliforme*, *Fusarium dimerum*, *Fusarium verticilloides*, and

Fusarium incarnatum. Profound neutropenia represents the major condition predisposing to disseminated fusariosis. Other risk factors were analyzed in a Brazilian cohort (Garnica et al. 2015). An association with active smoking was found among patients with acute leukemia. Disseminated fusariosis was also associated with hyperglycemia, receipt of anti-thymocyte globulin, and acute myeloid leukemia in the early phase post HSCT, while nonmyeloablative conditioning regimen, severe graft-versus-host disease, and previous mold infection were identified as risk factors in the late phase.

1.10 Other Invasive Mold Infections

Mold invasive infections other than the above-mentioned diseases are rare (<1% of cases), but may be due to a large variety of opportunistic pathogenic fungi, such as black molds (e.g., *Exophiala* spp., *Alternaria* spp., *Bipolaris* spp.) or hyaline molds (e.g., *Scedosporium* spp., *Lomentospora* spp., *Paecilomyces* spp., *Acremonium* spp.) (Richardson and Lass-Florl 2008; Chowdhary et al. 2014). A shift in the epidemiology of invasive mold infections has been reported in the setting of azole or echinocandin treatment with an increasing proportion of rare and intrinsically azole-resistant molds, such as *Scopulariopsis* spp., *Lomentospora prolificans* (formerly known as *Scedosporium prolificans*) and *Hormographiella aspergillata* (Lamoth et al. 2017; Conen et al. 2011; Grenouillet et al. 2009; Pang et al. 2012). These infections may become more prevalent in the era of systematic azole prophylaxis. A recent report also found an association between inherited CARD9 deficiency and *Exophiala* invasive infections (Lanternier et al. 2015).

1.11 Pneumocystosis

Formerly considered as a protozoan, *Pneumocystis jirovecii*, the causal agent of pneumocystosis (a severe form of pneumonia) has been recently reclassified as a fungus. *P. jirovecii* mainly affects patients with HIV or other T-lymphocyte-mediated immune defect (especially low CD4 count). The incidence of pneumocystosis among patients with HSCT or hematologic malignancies has decreased with the use of co-trimoxazole prophylaxis and is currently estimated to be lower than 0.5%, representing only 2% of all IFI (Kontoyiannis et al. 2010; Fillatre et al. 2014; Pagano et al. 2002). However, increasing overall incidence has been reported in some countries (Maini et al. 2013), which can be related to the expanding population of immunosuppressed patients, but also to improvements in diagnostic approaches with the advent of molecular methods. The risk of pneumocystosis is related to the type of underlying disease and anti-cancer therapy, and their impact on lymphocyte count and function. For instance, chemotherapeutic regimens used against ALL, including corticosteroids, vincristine, methotrexate, and cyclophosphamide, are associated with a high risk of pneumocystosis, while the disease is rare among AML patients (Cordonnier et al. 2016). Lymphoproliferative disorders (chronic lymphocytic leukemia, non-Hodgkin lymphoma, and multiple myeloma) and recipients of allogeneic or autologous HSCT represent the other groups at risk (Cordonnier et al. 2016). Most hematologic cancer patients developing pneumocystosis have received corticoid therapy within the previous month, which represents the major predisposing factor (Cordonnier et al. 2016). Monoclonal antibodies, such as rituximab, inducing B-cell defect, also increase the risk of pneumocystosis with often severe and fulminant courses (Martin-Garrido et al. 2013).

The authors of a French retrospective study conducted between 1990 and 2010 proposed to classify the risk of pneumocystosis among hematologic cancer patients as follows: (1) high-risk (incidence rates >45 cases/100'000 patient-year): acute leukemia, chronic lymphocytic leukemia and non-Hodgkin lymphoma, (2) intermediate-risk (25–45 cases/100'000 patient-year): hematopoietic stem cell transplantation, multiple myeloma, Waldenström macroglobulinemia, and

(3) low-risk (<25 cases/100'000 patient-year): Hodgkin lymphoma (Fillatre et al. 2014). Concomitant chronic lung disease (e.g., asthma, chronic obstructive pulmonary disease) also increases the risk of pneumocystosis (Maini et al. 2013; Cordonnier et al. 2016).

1.12 Endemic Mycoses

These infections due to dimorphic fungi, such as *Histoplasma capsulatum* (the agent of histoplasmosis), *Blastomyces dermatitidis* (blastomycosis), *Coccidioides immitis/posadasii* (coccidioidomycosis), *Paracoccidioides brasiliensis/lutzii* (paracoccidioidomycosis) and *Talaromyces marneffei* (Penicilliosis), are rarely observed among hematologic cancer patients. Their incidence among HSCT recipients in US was estimated to be less than 0.1% (Kauffman et al. 2014). In Europe, these fungal infections are very rare, affecting mainly patients who have traveled in endemic regions in the past (with possible reactivation after decades) and exceptional autochthonous cases (e.g., Italy) (Ashbee et al. 2008). Endemic mycoses manifest as severe and usually disseminated diseases (in about two-thirds of cases) in this population of deeply immunocompromised patients (Kauffman et al. 2014). They should be suspected in patients coming from regions with significant prevalence. Histoplasmosis is particularly endemic in Central-East United States, in parts of Central and South America (*H. capsulatum var capsulatum*), and in West Africa (*H. capsulatum var. duboisii*) with sporadic cases occurring in South Africa, China, and South East Asia (Bahr et al. 2015). Coccidioidomycosis is mainly observed in arid regions of Southwestern United States and parts of Central and South America, causing occasional outbreaks (Freedman et al. 2018). Blastomycosis is widespread in North America with sporadic cases reported from South Africa and Asia (Saccente and Woods 2010). Paracoccidioidomycosis is limited to some regions of Central and South America and Penicilliosis to South East Asia.

1.13 Risk Stratification and Preventive Strategies

Because IFI represents a life-threatening complication, which can compromise the success of anti-cancer therapies and HSCT, it is important to assess the risk factors of IFI and to select the appropriate preventive approach. These strategies should consider the local epidemiology of IFI, the type of hematologic malignancy and chemotherapy, as well as other individual predisposing conditions, which are summarized in Fig. 1.1. Overall, three different approaches may be considered according to the estimated risk of developing IFI. In high-risk patients, antifungal prophylaxis with an anti-mold active agent with broad activity against *Aspergillus* spp. and *Mucorales*, such as posaconazole, may be warranted. An alternative is the monitoring (once or twice weekly) of a fungal marker in serum, such as galactomannan, 1,3-beta-d-glucan, or *Aspergillus* PCR. For low-risk patients, a clinically driven approach with punctual testing of fungal markers and CT-scan in case of clinical suspicion is sufficient. For patients at high risk of pneumocystosis, co-trimoxazole administered three times weekly is the recommended approach, with daily atovaquone as an alternative in case of intolerance or toxicity concerns (Maertens et al. 2016b).

Systematic antifungal prophylaxis has been shown to decrease the incidence of IFI in selected group at risk (Ullmann et al. 2007; Cornely et al. 2007), but is also associated with significant costs, toxicity, and potential interactions with anti-cancer chemotherapies. Moreover, the management of confirmed or possible IFI cases in this subgroup is difficult because of emerging multiresistant fungi and limited therapeutic options (Lamoth et al. 2017). Therefore, it is important to limit the use of antifungals whenever possible. A personalized medicine approach using systematic screening for high-risk genetic polymorphisms, in particular PTX3, appears as the most promising strategy to target patients who may best benefit from antifungal prophylaxis in the future.

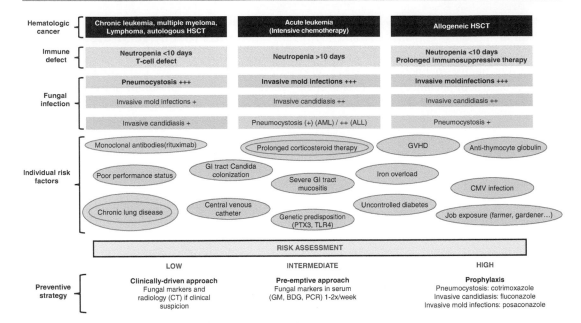

Fig. 1.1 Assessment of the risk of invasive fungal infections and choice of preventive strategy. HSCT: hematopoietic stem cell transplantation, GVHD: graft-versus-host disease, CT: computed tomography, GM: galactomannan, BDG: 1,3-beta-d-glucan, PCR: *Aspergillus* polymerase chain reaction. The colors link the type of invasive fungal infections with the risk factors (red: invasive candidiasis, blue: invasive mold infections, green: pneumocystosis)

References

Abidi MZ, Sohail MR, Cummins N, Wilhelm M, Wengenack N, Brumble L et al (2014) Stability in the cumulative incidence, severity and mortality of 101 cases of invasive mucormycosis in high-risk patients from 1995 to 2011: a comparison of eras immediately before and after the availability of voriconazole and echinocandin-amphotericin combination therapies. Mycoses 57:687–698

Alby-Laurent F, Dollfus C, Ait-Oufella H, Rambaud J, Legrand O, Tabone MD et al (2017) Trichosporon: another yeast-like organism responsible for immune reconstitution inflammatory syndrome in patients with hematological malignancy. Hematol Oncol 35:900–904

de Almeida Junior JN, Hennequin C (2016) Invasive Trichosporon infection: a systematic review on a re-emerging fungal pathogen. Front Microbiol 7:1629

Ashbee HR, Evans EG, Viviani MA, Dupont B, Chryssanthou E, Surmont I et al (2008) Histoplasmosis in Europe: report on an epidemiological survey from the European Confederation of Medical Mycology Working Group. Med Mycol 46:57–65

Baddley JW, Stroud TP, Salzman D, Pappas PG (2001) Invasive mold infections in allogeneic bone marrow transplant recipients. Clin Infect Dis 32:1319–1324

Bahr NC, Antinori S, Wheat LJ, Sarosi GA (2015) Histoplasmosis infections worldwide: thinking outside of the Ohio River valley. Curr Trop Med Rep 2:70–80

Barreto JN, Beach CL, Wolf RC, Merten JA, Tosh PK, Wilson JW et al (2013) The incidence of invasive fungal infections in neutropenic patients with acute leukemia and myelodysplastic syndromes receiving primary antifungal prophylaxis with voriconazole. Am J Hematol 88:283–288

Bitar D, Van Cauteren D, Lanternier F, Dannaoui E, Che D, Dromer F et al (2009) Increasing incidence of zygomycosis (mucormycosis), France, 1997-2006. Emerg Infect Dis 15:1395–1401

Bochud PY, Chien JW, Marr KA, Leisenring WM, Upton A, Janer M et al (2008) Toll-like receptor 4 polymorphisms and aspergillosis in stem-cell transplantation. N Engl J Med 359:1766–1777

Caira M, Candoni A, Verga L, Busca A, Delia M, Nosari A et al (2015) Pre-chemotherapy risk factors for invasive fungal diseases: prospective analysis of 1,192 patients with newly diagnosed acute myeloid leukemia (SEIFEM 2010-a multicenter study). Haematologica 100:284–292

Cesaro S, Tridello G, Castagnola E, Calore E, Carraro F, Mariotti I et al (2017) Retrospective study on the incidence and outcome of proven and probable invasive fungal infections in high-risk pediatric onco-hematological patients. Eur J Haematol 99:240–248

Chowdhary A, Meis JF, Guarro J, de Hoog GS, Kathuria S, Arendrup MC et al (2014) ESCMID and ECMM joint clinical guidelines for the diagnosis and management of systemic phaeohyphomycosis: diseases caused by black fungi. Clin Microbiol Infect 20(Suppl 3):47–75

Conen A, Weisser M, Hohler D, Frei R, Stern M (2011) Hormographiella aspergillata: an emerging mould in acute leukaemia patients? Clin Microbiol Infect 17:273–277

Cordonnier C, Cesaro S, Maschmeyer G, Einsele H, Donnelly JP, Alanio A et al (2016) Pneumocystis jirovecii pneumonia: still a concern in patients with haematological malignancies and stem cell transplant recipients. J Antimicrob Chemother 71:2379–2385

Cornely OA, Maertens J, Winston DJ, Perfect J, Ullmann AJ, Walsh TJ et al (2007) Posaconazole vs. fluconazole or itraconazole prophylaxis in patients with neutropenia. N Engl J Med 356:348–359

Cornet M, Fleury L, Maslo C, Bernard JF, Brucker G (2002) Epidemiology of invasive aspergillosis in France: a six-year multicentric survey in the greater Paris area. J Hosp Infect 51:288–296

Cunha C, Di Ianni M, Bozza S, Giovannini G, Zagarella S, Zelante T et al (2010) Dectin-1 Y238X polymorphism associates with susceptibility to invasive aspergillosis in hematopoietic transplantation through impairment of both recipient- and donor-dependent mechanisms of antifungal immunity. Blood 116:5394–5402

Cunha C, Aversa F, Lacerda JF, Busca A, Kurzai O, Grube M et al (2014) Genetic PTX3 deficiency and aspergillosis in stem-cell transplantation. N Engl J Med 370:421–432

De Castro N, Mazoyer E, Porcher R, Raffoux E, Suarez F, Ribaud P et al (2012) Hepatosplenic candidiasis in the era of new antifungal drugs: a study in Paris 2000-2007. Clin Microbiol Infect 18:E185–E187

De Pauw B, Walsh TJ, Donnelly JP, Stevens DA, Edwards JE, Calandra T et al (2008) Revised definitions of invasive fungal disease from the European Organization for Research and Treatment of Cancer/invasive fungal infections cooperative group and the National Institute of Allergy and Infectious Diseases mycoses study group (EORTC/MSG) consensus group. Clin Infect Dis 46:1813–1821

Del Principe MI, Sarmati L, Cefalo M, Fontana C, De Santis G, Buccisano F et al (2016) A cluster of Geotrichum clavatum (Saprochaete clavata) infection in haematological patients: a first Italian report and review of literature. Mycoses 59:594–601

Ducassou S, Rivaud D, Auvrignon A, Verite C, Bertrand Y, Gandemer V et al (2015) Invasive fungal infections in pediatric acute myelogenous leukemia. Pediatr Infect Dis J 34:1262–1264

Duran Graeff L, Seidel D, Vehreschild MJ, Hamprecht A, Kindo A, Racil Z et al (2017) Invasive infections due to Saprochaete and Geotrichum species: report of 23 cases from the FungiScope registry. Mycoses 60:273–279

Dvorak CC, Steinbach WJ, Brown JM, Agarwal R (2005) Risks and outcomes of invasive fungal infections in pediatric patients undergoing allogeneic hematopoietic cell transplantation. Bone Marrow Transplant 36:621–629

Fernandez-Ruiz M, Guinea J, Puig-Asensio M, Zaragoza O, Almirante B, Cuenca-Estrella M et al (2017) Fungemia due to rare opportunistic yeasts: data from a population-based surveillance in Spain. Med Mycol 55:125–136

Fillatre P, Decaux O, Jouneau S, Revest M, Gacouin A, Robert Gangneux F et al (2014) Incidence of Pneumocystis jiroveci pneumonia among groups at risk in HIV-negative patients. Am J Med 127:1242 e1211–1247

Freedman M, Jackson BR, McCotter O, Benedict K (2018) Coccidioidomycosis outbreaks, United States and worldwide, 1940-2015. Emerg Infect Dis 24:417–423

Fukuda T, Boeckh M, Carter RA, Sandmaier BM, Maris MB, Maloney DG et al (2003) Risks and outcomes of invasive fungal infections in recipients of allogeneic hematopoietic stem cell transplants after nonmyeloablative conditioning. Blood 102:827–833

Gamaletsou MN, Walsh TJ, Zaoutis T, Pagoni M, Kotsopoulou M, Voulgarelis M et al (2014) A prospective, cohort, multicentre study of candidaemia in hospitalized adult patients with haematological malignancies. Clin Microbiol Infect 20:O50–O57

Garcia-Suarez J, Gomez-Herruz P, Cuadros JA, Burgaleta C (2011) Epidemiology and outcome of Rhodotorula infection in haematological patients. Mycoses 54:318–324

Garcia-Vidal C, Upton A, Kirby KA, Marr KA (2008) Epidemiology of invasive mold infections in allogeneic stem cell transplant recipients: biological risk factors for infection according to time after transplantation. Clin Infect Dis 47:1041–1050

Garnica M, da Cunha MO, Portugal R, Maiolino A, Colombo AL, Nucci M (2015) Risk factors for invasive fusariosis in patients with acute myeloid leukemia and in hematopoietic cell transplant recipients. Clin Infect Dis 60:875–880

Grenouillet F, Botterel F, Crouzet J, Larosa F, Hicheri Y, Forel JM et al (2009) Scedosporium prolificans: an emerging pathogen in France? Med Mycol 47:343–350

Guinea J, Escribano P, Vena A, Munoz P, Martinez-Jimenez MDC, Padilla B et al (2017) Increasing incidence of mucormycosis in a large Spanish hospital from 2007 to 2015: epidemiology and microbiological characterization of the isolates. PLoS One 12:e0179136

Henrich TJ, Marty FM, Milner DA Jr, Thorner AR (2009) Disseminated Geotrichum candidum infection in a patient with relapsed acute myelogenous leukemia following allogeneic stem cell transplantation and review of the literature. Transpl Infect Dis 11:458–462

Horn DL, Neofytos D, Anaissie EJ, Fishman JA, Steinbach WJ, Olyaei AJ et al (2009) Epidemiology and outcomes of candidemia in 2019 patients: data from the prospective antifungal therapy alliance registry. Clin Infect Dis 48:1695–1703

Kauffman CA, Freifeld AG, Andes DR, Baddley JW, Herwaldt L, Walker RC et al (2014) Endemic fungal infections in solid organ and hematopoietic cell transplant recipients enrolled in the transplant-associated infection surveillance network (TRANSNET). Transpl Infect Dis 16:213–224

Koehler P, Hamprecht A, Bader O, Bekeredjian-Ding I, Buchheidt D, Doelken G et al (2017) Epidemiology of invasive aspergillosis and azole resistance in patients with acute leukaemia: the SEPIA study. Int J Antimicrob Agents 49:218–223

Kontoyiannis DP, Marr KA, Park BJ, Alexander BD, Anaissie EJ, Walsh TJ et al (2010) Prospective surveillance for invasive fungal infections in hematopoietic stem cell transplant recipients, 2001-2006: overview of the transplant-associated infection surveillance network (TRANSNET) database. Clin Infect Dis 50:1091–1100

Kontoyiannis DP, Azie N, Franks B, Horn DL (2014) Prospective antifungal therapy (PATH) alliance((R)) : focus on mucormycosis. Mycoses 57:240–246

Lamoth F, Rubino I, Bochud PY (2011) Immunogenetics of invasive aspergillosis. Med Mycol 49(Suppl 1):S125–S136

Lamoth F, Chung SJ, Damonti L, Alexander BD (2017) Changing epidemiology of invasive Mold infections in patients receiving azole prophylaxis. Clin Infect Dis 64:1619–1621

Lamoth F, Lockhart SR, Berkow EL, Calandra T (2018) Changes in the epidemiological landscape of invasive candidiasis. J Antimicrob Chemother 73:i4–i13

Lanternier F, Barbati E, Meinzer U, Liu L, Pedergnana V, Migaud M et al (2015) Inherited CARD9 deficiency in 2 unrelated patients with invasive Exophiala infection. J Infect Dis 211:1241–1250

Lockhart SR, Etienne KA, Vallabhaneni S, Farooqi J, Chowdhary A, Govender NP et al (2017) Simultaneous emergence of multidrug-resistant Candida auris on 3 continents confirmed by whole-genome sequencing and epidemiological analyses. Clin Infect Dis 64:134–140

Lortholary O, Obenga G, Biswas P, Caillot D, Chachaty E, Bienvenu AL et al (2010) International retrospective analysis of 73 cases of invasive fusariosis treated with voriconazole. Antimicrob Agents Chemother 54:4446–4450

Lortholary O, Gangneux JP, Sitbon K, Lebeau B, de Monbrison F, Le Strat Y et al (2011) Epidemiological trends in invasive aspergillosis in France: the SAIF network (2005-2007). Clin Microbiol Infect 17:1882–1889

Maertens J, Demuynck H, Verbeken EK, Zachee P, Verhoef GE, Vandenberghe P et al (1999) Mucormycosis in allogeneic bone marrow transplant recipients: report of five cases and review of the role of iron overload in the pathogenesis. Bone Marrow Transplant 24:307–312

Maertens JA, Raad II, Marr KA, Patterson TF, Kontoyiannis DP, Cornely OA et al (2016a) Isavuconazole versus voriconazole for primary treatment of invasive mould disease caused by Aspergillus and other filamentous fungi (SECURE): a phase 3, randomised-controlled, non-inferiority trial. Lancet 387:760–769

Maertens J, Cesaro S, Maschmeyer G, Einsele H, Donnelly JP, Alanio A et al (2016b) ECIL guidelines for preventing Pneumocystis jirovecii pneumonia in patients with haematological malignancies and stem cell transplant recipients. J Antimicrob Chemother 71:2397–2404

Maini R, Henderson KL, Sheridan EA, Lamagni T, Nichols G, Delpech V et al (2013) Increasing Pneumocystis pneumonia, England, UK, 2000-2010. Emerg Infect Dis 19:386–392

Mariette C, Tavernier E, Hocquet D, Huynh A, Isnard F, Legrand F et al (2017) Epidemiology of invasive fungal infections during induction therapy in adults with acute lymphoblastic leukemia: a GRAALL-2005 study. Leuk Lymphoma 58:586–593

Marr KA, Carter RA, Crippa F, Wald A, Corey L (2002) Epidemiology and outcome of mould infections in hematopoietic stem cell transplant recipients. Clin Infect Dis 34:909–917

Martin-Garrido I, Carmona EM, Specks U, Limper AH (2013) Pneumocystis pneumonia in patients treated with rituximab. Chest 144:258–265

Martino R, Subira M, Rovira M, Solano C, Vazquez L, Sanz GF et al (2002) Invasive fungal infections after allogeneic peripheral blood stem cell transplantation: incidence and risk factors in 395 patients. Br J Haematol 116:475–482

Mikulska M, Raiola AM, Bruno B, Furfaro E, Van Lint MT, Bregante S et al (2009) Risk factors for invasive aspergillosis and related mortality in recipients of allogeneic SCT from alternative donors: an analysis of 306 patients. Bone Marrow Transplant 44:361–370

Neofytos D, Horn D, Anaissie E, Steinbach W, Olyaei A, Fishman J et al (2009) Epidemiology and outcome of invasive fungal infection in adult hematopoietic stem cell transplant recipients: analysis of Multicenter Prospective Antifungal Therapy (PATH) Alliance registry. Clin Infect Dis 48:265–273

Neofytos D, Lu K, Hatfield-Seung A, Blackford A, Marr KA, Treadway S et al (2013) Epidemiology, outcomes, and risk factors of invasive fungal infections in adult patients with acute myelogenous leukemia after induction chemotherapy. Diagn Microbiol Infect Dis 75:144–149

Nucci M, Anaissie E (2007) Fusarium infections in immunocompromised patients. Clin Microbiol Rev 20:695–704

Nucci M, Garnica M, Gloria AB, Lehugeur DS, Dias VC, Palma LC et al (2013a) Invasive fungal diseases in haematopoietic cell transplant recipients and in patients with acute myeloid leukaemia or myelodysplasia in Brazil. Clin Microbiol Infect 19:745–751

Nucci M, Varon AG, Garnica M, Akiti T, Barreiros G, Trope BM et al (2013b) Increased incidence of invasive fusariosis with cutaneous portal of entry. Brazil Emerg Infect Dis 19:1567–1572

Nucci M, Marr KA, Vehreschild MJ, de Souza CA, Velasco E, Cappellano P et al (2014) Improvement in the outcome of invasive fusariosis in the last decade. Clin Microbiol Infect 20:580–585

Pagano L, Antinori A, Ammassari A, Mele L, Nosari A, Melillo L et al (1999) Retrospective study of candidemia in patients with hematological malignancies. Clinical features, risk factors and outcome of 76 episodes. Eur J Haematol 63:77–85

Pagano L, Fianchi L, Mele L, Girmenia C, Offidani M, Ricci P et al (2002) Pneumocystis carinii pneumonia in patients with malignant haematological diseases: 10 years' experience of infection in GIMEMA centres. Br J Haematol 117:379–386

Pagano L, Caira M, Candoni A, Offidani M, Fianchi L, Martino B et al (2006) The epidemiology of fungal infections in patients with hematologic malignancies: the SEIFEM-2004 study. Haematologica 91:1068–1075

Pagano L, Caira M, Nosari A, Van Lint MT, Candoni A, Offidani M et al (2007) Fungal infections in recipients of hematopoietic stem cell transplants: results of the SEIFEM B-2004 study--Sorveglianza Epidemiologica Infezioni Fungine Nelle Emopatie Maligne. Clin Infect Dis 45:1161–1170

Pagano L, Valentini CG, Posteraro B, Girmenia C, Ossi C, Pan A et al (2009) Zygomycosis in Italy: a survey of FIMUA-ECMM (Federazione Italiana di Micopatologia Umana ed Animale and European Confederation of Medical Mycology). J Chemother 21:322–329

Pagano L, Caira M, Candoni A, Offidani M, Martino B, Specchia G et al (2010) Invasive aspergillosis in patients with acute myeloid leukemia: a SEIFEM-2008 registry study. Haematologica 95:644–650

Pagano L, Stamouli M, Tumbarello M, Verga L, Candoni A, Cattaneo C et al (2015) Risk of invasive fungal infection in patients affected by acute promyelocytic leukaemia. A report by the SEIFEM-D registry. Br J Haematol 170:434–439

Pang KA, Godet C, Fekkar A, Scholler J, Nivoix Y, Letscher-Bru V et al (2012) Breakthrough invasive mould infections in patients treated with caspofungin. J Infect 64:424–429

Pomares H, Arnan M, Sanchez-Ortega I, Sureda A, Duarte RF (2016) Invasive fungal infections in AML/MDS patients treated with azacitidine: a risk worth considering antifungal prophylaxis? Mycoses 59:516–519

Puig-Asensio M, Ruiz-Camps I, Fernandez-Ruiz M, Aguado JM, Munoz P, Valerio M et al (2015) Epidemiology and outcome of candidaemia in patients with oncological and haematological malignancies: results from a population-based surveillance in Spain. Clin Microbiol Infect 21:491 e491–410

Quarello P, Saracco P, Giacchino M, Caselli D, Caviglia I, Longoni D et al (2012) Epidemiology of infections in children with acquired aplastic anaemia: a retrospective multicenter study in Italy. Eur J Haematol 88:526–534

Rammaert B, Desjardins A, Lortholary O (2012) New insights into hepatosplenic candidosis, a manifestation of chronic disseminated candidosis. Mycoses 55:e74–e84

Richardson M, Lass-Florl C (2008) Changing epidemiology of systemic fungal infections. Clin Microbiol Infect 14(Suppl 4):5–24

Roden MM, Zaoutis TE, Buchanan WL, Knudsen TA, Sarkisova TA, Schaufele RL et al (2005) Epidemiology and outcome of zygomycosis: a review of 929 reported cases. Clin Infect Dis 41:634–653

Saccente M, Woods GL (2010) Clinical and laboratory update on blastomycosis. Clin Microbiol Rev 23:367–381

Saegeman V, Maertens J, Meersseman W, Spriet I, Verbeken E, Lagrou K (2010) Increasing incidence of mucormycosis in university hospital. Belgium Emerg Infect Dis 16:1456–1458

Sallah S, Semelka RC, Wehbie R, Sallah W, Nguyen NP, Vos P (1999) Hepatosplenic candidiasis in patients with acute leukaemia. Br J Haematol 106:697–701

Schelenz S, Hagen F, Rhodes JL, Abdolrasouli A, Chowdhary A, Hall A et al (2016) First hospital outbreak of the globally emerging Candida auris in a European hospital. Antimicrob Resist Infect Control 5:35

Schuster MG, Meibohm A, Lloyd L, Strom B (2013) Risk factors and outcomes of Candida krusei bloodstream infection: a matched, case-control study. J Infect 66:278–284

Seroy J, Antiporta P, Grim SA, Proia LA, Singh K, Clark NM (2017) Aspergillus calidoustus case series and review of the literature. Transpl Infect Dis 19

Skiada A, Pagano L, Groll A, Zimmerli S, Dupont B, Lagrou K et al (2011) Zygomycosis in Europe: analysis of 230 cases accrued by the registry of the European Confederation of Medical Mycology (ECMM) working group on Zygomycosis between 2005 and 2007. Clin Microbiol Infect 17:1859–1867

Steinbach WJ, Marr KA, Anaissie EJ, Azie N, Quan SP, Meier-Kriesche HU et al (2012) Clinical epidemiology of 960 patients with invasive aspergillosis from the PATH Alliance registry. J Infect 65:453–464

Tang JL, Kung HC, Lei WC, Yao M, Wu UI, Hsu SC et al (2015) High incidences of invasive fungal infections in acute myeloid leukemia patients receiving induction chemotherapy without systemic antifungal prophylaxis: a prospective observational study in Taiwan. PLoS One 10:e0128410

Torres HA, Bodey GP, Rolston KV, Kantarjian HM, Raad II, Kontoyiannis DP (2003) Infections in patients with aplastic anemia: experience at a tertiary care cancer center. Cancer 98:86–93

Ullmann AJ, Lipton JH, Vesole DH, Chandrasekar P, Langston A, Tarantolo SR et al (2007) Posaconazole or fluconazole for prophylaxis in severe graft-versus-host disease. N Engl J Med 356:335–347

Wojtowicz A, Lecompte TD, Bibert S, Manuel O, Rueger S, Berger C et al (2015) PTX3 polymorphisms and invasive Mold infections after solid organ transplant. Clin Infect Dis 61:619–622

Xhaard A, Lanternier F, Porcher R, Dannaoui E, Bergeron A, Clement L et al (2012) Mucormycosis after allogeneic haematopoietic stem cell transplantation: a French multicentre cohort study (2003-2008). Clin Microbiol Infect 18:E396–E400

Zaoutis TE, Heydon K, Chu JH, Walsh TJ, Steinbach WJ (2006) Epidemiology, outcomes, and costs of invasive aspergillosis in immunocompromised children in the United States, 2000. Pediatrics 117:e711–e716

Antibacterial and Antiparasitic Prophylaxis

2

Mohammed Alsaeed and Shahid Husain

2.1 Introduction

Patients with hematological malignancies are at increased risk for infections caused by disease-related and therapy-induced immunosuppression. (Akova et al. 2005; Crawford et al. 2008) With the change in practice over the last five decades, a significant improvement in the outcome of hematological malignancies with serious infections has been noted. The expected mortality rate was higher than 60% in neutropenic patients in the 1960s.(Hersh et al. 1965) The incidence has dropped to less than 5% with current practice. (Homsi et al. 2000) Antimicrobial prophylaxis is one of the most successful strategies in reducing infection-associated morbidity and mortality in hematological malignancy patients.(Verhoef 1993) Antimicrobial prophylaxis aims to prevent infectious morbidity and all its consequences, including hospitalization, quality of life, cost of treatment, treatment-related adverse events, and death.

M. Alsaeed (✉)
Division of Infectious Disease, Department of Medicine, Prince Sultan Military Medical City, Riyadh, Saudi Arabia

S. Husain (✉)
Division of Infectious Disease, Multi-Organ Transplant Program, Department of Medicine, University of Toronto, University Health Network, Toronto, ON, Canada
e-mail: shahid.husain@uhn.ca

2.2 Antibacterial Prophylaxis

2.2.1 Who Is at Risk?

The key to prophylactic strategy is to identify those patients at high risk for infection. Patients with hematological malignancies are subject to infections because of several factors, notably breakdown of healthy skin and mucosal barriers, obstruction related to the tumor, alteration of host defenses secondary to infiltration of bone marrow, reduced or altered immunoglobulin or cytokine production, or neutropenia related to chemotherapy.(Apostolopoulou et al. 2010) Neutrophils are critical for providing host defense against infections.(Hubel et al. 1999; Kuderer et al. 2006) Bacteria are by far the most infectious pathogens during neutropenia.(Bodey et al. 1966; Bodey 1986; Viscoli et al. 2005) The risk of bacterial infection is directly related to the severity and duration of neutropenia. Bacterial infections occur more frequently when the neutrophil count is $<100/\mu L$ and for 7 days or longer. (Lyman et al. 2005) Several factors contribute to the risk of infection by interfering with neutrophil homeostasis; including patient characteristics, underlying malignancy, and treatment regimens (Fig. 2.1).(Pettengell et al. 2008; Lyman et al. 2004; Intragumtornchai et al. 2000; Ray-Coquard et al. 2003)

Seven guidelines have been published between 2010 and 2016, all recommending

© Springer Nature Switzerland AG 2021
O. A. Cornely, M. Hoenig (eds.), *Infection Management in Hematology*, Hematologic Malignancies, https://doi.org/10.1007/978-3-030-57317-1_2

Risk Factors for Neutropenic Fever		
Patient Related Predictors	**Disease Related Predictors**	**Treatment Related Predictors**
Age 65 years or more	Elevated lactate dehydrogenase in patients with lymphoreticular diseases.	High-dose chemotherapy regimens
Female sex	Monocytopenia	Failure to administer prophylactic hematopoietic growth factor support
High body surface area	Lymphopenia	
Poor performance status	Advanced stage of the underlying malignancy.	
Comorbidities		
Poor nutritional status		

Fig. 2.1 Summary of risk factors for the development of neutropenia

Table 2.1 Summary of the guidelines for antibacterial prophylaxis in hematological malignancies

Guideline	Year	Recommendation
European Society for Medical Oncology	2016	**Never**: the use of antimicrobials, including fluoroquinolones, should be discouraged.
National Comprehensive Cancer Network	2016	**High risk**: expected neutrophil count <1000/microL for 7 days or more
German Society of Hematology and Oncology	2013	**High risk**: neutropenia ≥7 days; **some low risk** (first chemo, aggressive chemo with high infections rate, elderly)
American Society of Clinical Oncology	2013	**High risk**: neutropenia for >7 days, unless other factors which increase risks for complications or mortality
National Institute for Health and Care Excellence	2012	Adult patients (aged ≥18 years) with acute leukemia, HSCT, or solid tumors
Australian Consensus Guidelines	2011	**Consider** in outpatient HSCT and palliative patients with bone marrow failure
Infectious Disease Society of America	2011	**High risk**: neutropenia ≥7 days

fluoroquinolone prophylaxis in high-risk patients. However, the Australian guidelines gave a low-level recommendation for high-risk patients except for outpatient stem cell recipients and patients on palliative management with bone marrow failure, while the European Society for Medical Oncology (ESMO) disgorged any antimicrobial prophylaxis (Table 2.1).(Taplitz et al. 2018; Klastersky et al. 2016; Freifeld et al. 2011; Slavin et al. 2011; Phillips et al. 2012; Flowers et al. 2013; Neumann et al. 2013; Baden et al. 2016; Averbuch et al. 2013)

Although several randomized controlled trials have demonstrated the protective effect of antibacterial prophylaxis in low-risk patients, the number of patients is high to prevent one infection. Other drawbacks of antibacterial prophylaxis in low-risk patients include lack of cost-effectiveness, drug-related adverse effects, susceptibility to superinfections, and selection for antimicrobial resistance.(Eleutherakis-Papaiakovou et al. 2010; Cullen et al. 2005)

A useful scoring system from the Multinational Association for Supportive Care in Cancer

Table 2.2 Multinational Association for Supportive Care in Cancer (MASCC) score for identifying the patients with low risk of febrile neutropenia

Prognostic Factor	Weight
Burden of febrile neutropenia (no or mild symptoms)	5
No hypotension (systolic BP >90 mmHg)	5
No chronic obstructive pulmonary disease	4
Solid tumor or hematological malignancy with no previous fungal infection	3
No dehydration requiring parenteral fluids	3
Burden of febrile neutropenia (moderate symptoms)	3
Outpatient status	3
Age < 60 years	2

(MASCC) has been developed to identify low-risk patients. The MASCC risk-index score is based on seven independent factors present at the onset of febrile neutropenia. Patients with a score of ≥21 are regarded as low risk; patients with a score of <21 are considered as high risk. This has been validated by Uys and colleagues with a positive predictive value of 98.3% in low-risk patients (Table 2.2).(Uys et al. 2004; Klastersky et al. 2000)

2.2.2 Antibacterial Prevention Strategies in Neutropenic Patients: Past and Present

The epidemiology of bacterial infections in neutropenic patients is dynamic and depends on multiple factors: the severity and duration of neutropenia, the nature and intensity of antineoplastic therapy, host-related factors, selection pressures created using chemoprophylaxis and/or empirical antibiotic therapy, the use of central venous catheters and other external medical devices, environmental and geographic factors, and the duration of the hospital stay.(Rolston 2005; Bodey et al. 1988; Rolston et al. 1996; Jacobson et al. 1999; Jones 1999) Most infections in neutropenic patients originate from the microflora that colonizes the skin and mucosal surface. Theoretically, suppression of patients' endogenous flora should protect the host against infections.(Schimpff et al. 1972) Two strategies

have been evaluated to prevent bacterial infections during neutropenia by antibiotics: intestinal decontamination by oral non-absorbable antibiotics (such as gentamicin, vancomycin, and colistin in various combinations) and oral absorbable antibiotics that act systemically (such as trimethoprim/sulfamethoxazole (TMP-SMX) and fluoroquinolones).

Early studies with oral non-absorbable antibiotics have shown a reduction in infection rates in neutropenic patients. However, regimens were poorly tolerated, making compliance a problem. Failure to take oral non-absorbable antibiotics has resulted in rapid gut re-population with aggressive and opportunistic organisms and subsequent infection. The use of oral non-absorbable antibiotics has also been associated with colonization by resistant Gram-negative strains and selective intestinal decontamination.(Levi et al. 1973; Hahn et al. 1978; Bender et al. 1979; King 1980; Funada et al. 1983)

With disappointing outcome of oral non-absorbable antibiotics, orally absorbable antibiotics were evaluated. The first orally absorbed antibiotic evaluated as an antibacterial prophylactic in neutropenic patients was TMP/SMX. Although most of the earlier studies suggested benefit from TMP/SMX prophylaxis, several additional trials have led to negative results. Resistance turned out to be an essential problem when using TMP/SMX. In a large EORTC study, the rate of blood isolates resistant to TMP/SMX was significantly higher in TMP/SMX recipients in comparison with placebo recipients (80 vs. 26%, respectively). Other drawbacks included its myelosuppressive effect and prolongation of neutropenia.(Watson et al. 1982; Dekker et al. 1981; Gualtier et al. 1983; Wade et al. 1983; Wilson and Guiney 1982; No authors listed 1984)

In the 1980s, fluoroquinolones were introduced as a new class of antimicrobials. They were attractive in many ways; they have systemic bactericidal activity and broad antimicrobial spectrum, including Gram-negative bacteria such as *Pseudomonas* spp., and some Gram-positive organisms. Most fluoroquinolones are well absorbed orally and are excreted in high concentration in feces. They lacked a myelosuppressive effect and were well tolerated by patients. (Wolfson and Hooper 1985; Hooper and Wolfson 1985) Several studies from the last two decades of the past century showed a reduction in the number of infectious episodes, particularly by Gram-negative pathogens, but failed to demonstrate a reduction in mortality.

In 2005, two multicenter large controlled trials conducted in Europe evaluating the role of antibacterial prophylaxis in neutropenic cancer patients were published. The Italian GIMEMA group conducted the first study. It was a double-blind, placebo-controlled trial of 760 hospitalized adult patients in whom chemotherapy-induced neutropenia (<1000 neutrophils/μL) was expected for more than 7 days. They were randomized to receive oral levofloxacin 500 mg once daily or placebo from the start of chemotherapy until the resolution of neutropenia. The trial included solid tumor, lymphoma, and acute leukemia patients. The study demonstrated a statistically significant reduction in the incidence of fever in patients receiving levofloxacin compared to placebo (65 vs. 85%, P < 0.001) but did not show any significant reduction in mortality. (Bucaneve et al. 2005)

The second study was the British SIGNIFICANT trial. One thousand five hundred sixty-five patients receiving cyclic chemotherapy for solid tumors or lymphoma who were at risk for chemotherapy-induced neutropenia (<500 neutrophils/μL) were randomized to receive either levofloxacin 500 mg once daily or placebo for 7 days during the expected neutropenic period of up to six cycles of chemotherapy. A significant reduction in febrile episodes was documented in the levofloxacin group during the first cycle of chemotherapy (3.5 vs. 7.9%, P < 0.001) and all cycles of treatment (10.8 vs. 15.2%, P = 0.01), but no effect on documented infections was observed.(Cullen et al. 2005)

Gafter-Gvili and colleagues undertook a meta-analysis of trials comparing prophylactic antibiotic therapy with placebo, no intervention, or another antibiotic regimen in patients receiving chemotherapy. They analyzed 95 randomized controlled trials conducted between 1973 and 2004 involving 9283 patients. The primary out-come was all-cause mortality, and secondary outcomes included infection-related death, febrile episodes, bacteremia, adverse events, and emergence of bacterial resistance. The meta-analysis demonstrated a statistically significant reduction in all-cause mortality of 34% in patients receiving prophylaxis compared with placebo or no intervention and a 45% reduction in mortality in those receiving fluoroquinolone prophylaxis. The meta-analysis was updated in 2006 to include the GIMEMA and SIGNIFICANT trial data. Among acute leukemia and bone marrow transplantation patients, the relative risk of death with quinolone prophylaxis was 0.67 (0.55–0.83) compared to control. For solid tumors and lymphomas, there was also a significant impact of fluoroquinolone prophylaxis on all-cause mortality during the first cycle of chemotherapy with a relative risk of 0.48 (0.26–0.88) compared with controls.(Gafter-Gvili et al. 2005; Gafter-Gvili et al. 2012)

Mikulska and colleagues undertook another meta-analysis to evaluate whether the rates of fluoroquinolone resistance in community and hospital settings influenced the efficacy of fluoroquinolone prophylaxis. They analyzed 2 randomized controlled trials and 12 observational studies conducted between 2006 and 2014. The meta-analysis demonstrated that fluoroquinolones did not have any effect on mortality (pooled OR 1.01, 95%CI 0.73–1.41), but were associated with a lower rate of bloodstream infections (pooled OR 0.57, 95%CI 0.43–0.74) and fewer episodes of fever during neutropenia (pooled OR 0.32, 95%CI 0.20–0.05).(Mikulska et al. 2018)

As outlined earlier, the use of prophylactic antibiotics in adult patients with neutropenia secondary to cancer therapy is supported by meta-analyses of randomized trials, demonstrating a decreased risk of infection confirmed by blood cultures and death. Data describing prophylactic antibiotics in children with cancer are limited, and this could be due to concerns of fluoroquinolone adverse events. Alexander and colleagues looked into the risk and efficacy of levofloxacin prophylaxis among children receiving intensive chemotherapy or HSCT. In a multicenter randomized trial, 624 patients, 200 with acute leukemia and 424 undergoing hematopoietic stem cell transplantation (HSCT), were randomized to receive levofloxacin prophylaxis or not. In the acute leukemia group, the likelihood of bacteremia was significantly lower in the levofloxacin prophylaxis group than in the control group (21.9% vs. 43.4%), whereas among patients undergoing HSCT, the risk of bacteremia was not significantly lower in the levofloxacin prophylaxis group (11.0% vs. 17.3%).(Alexander et al. 2018)

Data regarding other fluoroquinolones, such as moxifloxacin, as an alternative to levofloxacin/ciprofloxacin as primary prophylaxis in febrile neutropenia are limited. Przybylski and colleagues retrospectively compared moxifloxacin to levofloxacin/ciprofloxacin. They found the incidence of febrile neutropenia and of documented infections was similar between those receiving moxifloxacin and levofloxacin/ciprofloxacin, respectively. Hospital readmission for infection within 30 days of hospital discharge was also similar between groups as was the incidence of *Clostridioides difficile*. (Przybylski and Reeves 2017) In a controlled before and after prospective observational study, von Baum and colleagues also assessed the efficacy of moxifloxacin as primary prophylaxis in neutropenic patients. They found similar survival rates as compared with levofloxacin. The rate of Gram-negative bacteremia was higher during prophylaxis with moxifloxacin (11%) when compared with levofloxacin (6%). Additionally, they observed a marked increase in diarrhea associated with *C. difficile* after a change from levofloxacin to moxifloxacin (attack rate 6% vs. 33%).(von Baum et al. 2006)

Despite guidelines recommend fluoroquinolone use as prophylaxis for preventing infection in neutropenic patients, it has been associated with adverse events that range from common gastrointestinal disturbances and hypersensitivity reactions to rare but life-threatening abnormalities in glucose homeostasis and QT prolongation. In addition to drug-related adverse events, fluoroquinolone use has been associated with an increased rate of resistance in Gram-negative infections, *C. difficile* infection, and colonization with vancomycin-resistant *Enterococcus* spp.

(Liu 2010; Rangaraj et al. 2010; Kern et al. 2005a; Muto et al. 2005; Paterson 2004) An alternative agent for prophylaxis in neutropenic patients will eventually be needed. Yemm and colleagues retrospectively compared the clinical and microbiological outcomes in acute leukemia patients receiving fluoroquinolones and oral third-generation cephalosporins as antibacterial prophylaxis after chemotherapy. One hundred and twenty patients were included and matched. They demonstrated a comparable rate of febrile neutropenia and culture positivity in both groups. (Yemm et al. 2018)

2.3   Concerns About Antibiotic Prophylaxis

2.3.1   Treatment Cost

Kawatkar and colleagues looked into the cost of cancer-related neutropenia or fever hospitalization in the United States. They found the mean length of stay for cancer-related neutropenia hospitalization was 7.9 days, with a mean cost of US$ 37.555 per stay.(Kawatkar et al. 2017) The cost of a 7-day course of levofloxacin in the United States is US$82. The GIMEMA study showed that five patients undergoing chemotherapy for cancer needed to be treated with oral levofloxacin to prevent one episode of febrile neutropenia. Taking into consideration the cost of managing one episode of febrile neutropenia, antibiotic prophylaxis is cost-effective in these patient groups.

2.3.2   Antibiotic Resistance

The major drawback of routine prophylaxis of neutropenic patients with fluoroquinolones is the emergence of antibiotic resistance.(Kern et al. 2005b; Kara et al. 2015; Trecarichi et al. 2015) Variable outcomes from various studies were reported. The International Antimicrobial Therapy Group of the European Organization for Research and Treatment of Cancer (IATG-EORTC) retrospectively analyzed studies for

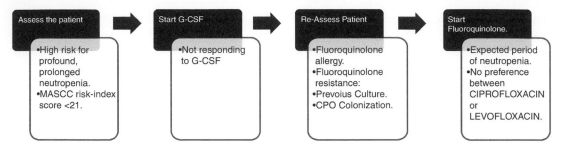

Fig. 2.2 Approach to antibacterial prophylaxis in chemotherapy-induced neutropenia patients

empiric antibacterial therapy in neutropenic patients conducted between 1983 and 1993. During this period, the proportion of neutropenic patients who received fluoroquinolone prophylaxis increased from 1.4 to 45%, and an increase in strains of *Escherichia coli* resistant to fluoroquinolones from 0 to 27% was observed. (Gudiol et al. 2013) In the European cohort, Kern and colleagues had a similar observation where patients receiving fluoroquinolones had significantly more bloodstream infections due to ESBL-positive Enterobacteriaceae (0.8% vs. 0.3%, RR 2.2).(Kern et al. 2005c)

On the other hand, the GIMEMA study did not show any significant increase in the incidence of levofloxacin-resistant Gram-negative bacteremia among patients receiving levofloxacin. Gafter-Gvili in her meta-analysis also did not observe any risk of developing fluoroquinolone resistance secondary to prophylaxis. This was also the observation in the Mikulska meta-analysis.

Although studies show mixed outcomes for the risk of fluoroquinolone resistance secondary to prophylaxis; the appearance of carbapenems and colistin, for empiric treatment of febrile neutropenia in the new ECIL guidelines, is a direct reflection of escalating antibiotic resistance. Fluoroquinolone prophylaxis during afebrile neutropenia may have shown a survival benefit in certain high-risk groups in the past; its current role must be questioned. Attention should now be directed toward reducing unnecessary antibiotic exposure in an attempt to preserve the increasing limited agents available for the treatment of established infections. Widespread use of antibacterial agents of one class can encourage multiclass drug

resistance, which reduces prophylaxis and treatment efficacy in neutropenic cancer patients.

Based on previous evidence we recommend the approach presented in Fig. 2.2.

2.4 Antiparasitic Prophylaxis

2.4.1 Introduction

Parasitic infections in hematological malignancy patients are uncommon.(Hughes 1976) With the dramatic increase in tourism and international migration, physicians should be aware of particular geographically restricted infections. Currently, there are no specific recommendations for antiparasitic prophylaxis in this unique high-risk group. Health promotion and education are essential and advice for this group of travelers should be tailored according to individual needs and should be planned well in advance, preferably at least 2 months before departure and at specialized clinics. Hematological malignancy patients during the immediate post-radiotherapy or chemotherapy period should be advised not to travel to specific areas in the world.

2.4.2 Recommendations for Prevention of Specific Infections

2.4.2.1 Enteric Pathogens

Diarrhea caused by parasites (*Giardia intestinalis, Entamoeba histolytica, Cryptosporidium parvum,* and *Cyclospora cayetanensis*) is less frequent in travelers and tends to be chronic, affecting long-term travelers visiting developing countries. Although no antiparasitic prophylaxis is recommended, patients should be educated about food and water handling.

2.4.2.2 Infections Transmitted by Arthropod Bites

Mosquitoes, ticks, and flies are the primary vectors for transmission of tropical or geographically restricted infections such as malaria, leishmaniasis, trypanosomiasis, filariasis, and borreliosis. Malaria is the most frequent infection transmitted by arthropods in travelers. (Leder et al. 2004) However, the risk of acquiring malaria in hematological malignancies is unknown. Splenectomized patients do have an increased risk of severe malaria. The choice of malaria prophylaxis will depend, among other factors, on destination and specific itinerary. Chloroquine would be the first choice in areas of the world with chloroquine-sensitive malaria (mainly in Central America and the Caribbean). For areas with chloroquine-resistant malaria, the options are atovaquone-proguanil, mefloquine, and doxycycline. The latter two drugs interact with some of the common immunosuppressant drugs, and drug levels should be mea-sured. Co-medication commonly used by travelers, such as antidiarrheals, cardiovascular drugs, and analgesics, does not appear to have a significant clinical impact on the safety and effectiveness of mefloquine and chloroquine prophylaxis. Caution is advised in diabetic travelers using mefloquine due to the possibility of hypoglycemia in certain situations. Folic acid supplements should be given to patients taking proguanil who are on other antifolate medications such as trimethoprim-sulfamethoxazole. Before initiating malaria prophylaxis, significant side effects such as the possibility of cardiac toxicity associated with chloroquine and mefloquine use in patients with chronic cardiac disease should also be considered, bearing in mind that these may be particularly harmful in patients with underlying disease.(Freedman 2008)

2.4.2.3 Infections Transmitted Through Skin and Mucous Membranes

Patients should be advised to avoid swimming in freshwater and walking barefoot due to the risk of infections like schistosomiasis and strongyloidiasis.

Figure 2.3 summarizes antiparasitic recommendations in neutropenic patients.

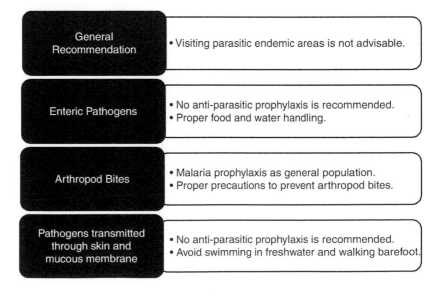

Fig. 2.3 General recommendation for antiparasitic prophylaxis in chemotherapy-induced neutropenia

General Recommendation	• Visiting parasitic endemic areas is not advisable.
Enteric Pathogens	• No anti-parasitic prophylaxis is recommended. • Proper food and water handling.
Arthropod Bites	• Malaria prophylaxis as general population. • Proper precautions to prevent arthropod bites.
Pathogens transmitted through skin and mucous membrane	• No anti-parasitic prophylaxis is recommended. • Avoid swimming in freshwater and walking barefoot.

References

Akova M, Paesmans M, Calandra T, Viscoli C, International Antimicrobial Therapy Group of the European Organization for Research and Treatment of Cancer (2005) A European Organization for Research and Treatment of Cancer-International Antimicrobial Therapy Group Study of secondary infections in febrile, neutropenic patients with cancer. Clin Infect Dis 40(2):239–245. Epub 2004 Dec 20

Alexander S, Fisher BT, Gaur AH, Dvorak CC, Villa Luna D, Dang H, Chen L, Green M, Nieder ML, Fisher B, Bailey LC, Wiernikowski J, Sung L, Children's Oncology Group (2018) Effect of levofloxacin prophylaxis on bacteremia in children with acute leukemia or undergoing hematopoietic stem cell transplantation: a randomized clinical trial. JAMA 320(10):995–1004

Apostolopoulou E, Raftopoulos V, Terzis K et al (2010) Infection probability score, APACHE II and KARNOFSKY scoring systems as predictors of bloodstream infection onset in hematology oncology patients. BMC Infect Dis 10:135

Averbuch D, Orasch C, Cordonnier C, Livermore DM, Mikulska M, Viscoli C, Gyssens IC, Kern WV, Klyasova G, Marchetti O, Engelhard D, Akova M, ECIL4, a joint venture of EBMT, EORTC, ICHS, ESGICH/ESCMID and ELN (2013) European guidelines for empirical antibacterial therapy for febrile neutropenic patients in the era of growing resistance: summary of the 2011 4th European Conference on Infections in Leukemia. Haematologica 98(12):1826–1835

Baden LR, Swaminathan S, Angarone M, Blouin G, Camins BC, Casper C, Cooper B, Dubberke ER, Engemann AM, Freifeld AG, Greene JN, Ito JI, Kaul DR, Lustberg ME, Montoya JG, Rolston K, Satyanarayana G, Segal B, Seo SK, Shoham S, Taplitz R, Topal J, Wilson JW, Hoffmann KG, Smith C (2016) Prevention and treatment of cancer-related infections, version 2.2016, NCCN clinical practice guidelines in oncology. J Natl Compr Cancer Netw 14(7):882–913

von Baum H, Sigge A, Bommer M, Kern WV, Marre R, Döhner H, Kern P, Reuter S (2006) Moxifloxacin prophylaxis in neutropenic patients. J Antimicrob Chemother 58(4):891–894

Bender JF, Schimpff SC, Young VM, Fortner CL, Brouillet MD, Love LJ, Wiernik PH (1979 Mar) Role of vancomycin as a component of oral nonabsorbable antibiotics for microbial suppression in leukemic patients. Antimicrob Agents Chemother 15(3):455–460

Bodey GP (1986) Infection in cancer patients: a continuing association. Am J Med 81(Suppl 1A):11–26

Bodey GP, Buckley M, Sathe YS, Freireich EJ (1966) Quantitative relationships between circulating leukocytes and infection in patients with acute leukemia. Ann Intern Med 64:328–340

Bodey GP, Ho DH, Elting L (1988) Survey of antibiotic susceptibility among gram-negative bacilli at a cancer hospital. Am J Med 85(Suppl 1A):49–51

Bucaneve G, Micozzi A, Menichetti F, Martino P, Dionisi MS, Martinelli G, Allione B, D'Antonio D, Buelli M, Nosari AM, Cilloni D, Zuffa E, Cantaffa R, Specchia G, Amadori S, Fabbiano F, Deliliers GL, Lauria F, Foà R, Del Favero A, Gruppo Italiano Malattie Ematologiche dell'Adulto (GIMEMA) Infection Program (2005) Levofloxacin to prevent bacterial infection in patients with cancer and neutropenia. N Engl J Med 353(10):977–987

Crawford J, Dale DC, Kuderer NM, Culakova E, Poniewierski MS, Wolff D, Lyman GH (2008) Risk and timing of neutropenic events in adult cancer patients receiving chemotherapy: the results of a prospective nationwide study of oncology practice. J Natl Compr Cancer Netw 6(2):109–118

Cullen M, Steven N, Billingham L, Gaunt C, Hastings M, Simmonds P, Stuart N, Rea D, Bower M, Fernando I, Huddart R, Gollins S, Stanley A, Simple Investigation in Neutropenic Individuals of the Frequency of Infection after Chemotherapy +/− Antibiotic in a Number of Tumours (SIGNIFICANT) Trial Group (2005) Antibacterial prophylaxis after chemotherapy for solid tumors and lymphomas. N Engl J Med 353(10):988–998

Dekker AM, Rozenberg-Arska M, Sixma J, Verhoef J (1981) Prevention of infection by trimethoprim-sulfamethoxazole plus amphotericin B in patients with acute nonlymphocytic leukemia. Ann Intern Med 95:555–559

Eleutherakis-Papaiakovou E, Kostis E, Migkou M, Christoulas D, Terpos E, Gavriatopoulou M, Roussou M, Kastritis E, Efstathiou E, Dimopoulos MA, Papadimitriou CA (2010) Prophylactic antibiotics for the prevention of neutropenic fever in patients undergoing autologous stem-cell transplantation: results of a single institution, randomized phase 2 trial. Am J Hematol 85(11):863–867

Flowers CR, Seidenfeld J, Bow EJ, Karten C, Gleason C, Hawley DK, Kuderer NM, Langston AA, Marr KA, Rolston KV, Ramsey SD (2013) Antimicrobial prophylaxis and outpatient management of fever and neutropenia in adults treated for malignancy: American Society of Clinical Oncology clinical practice guideline. J Clin Oncol. 31(6):794–810

Freedman DO (2008) Clinical practice. Malaria prevention in short-term travelers. N Engl J Med 359(6):603–601

Freifeld AG, Bow EJ, Sepkowitz KA, Boeckh MJ, Ito JI, Mullen CA, Raad II, Rolston KV, Young JA, Wingard JR, Infectious Diseases Society of America (2011) Clinical practice guideline for the use of antimicrobial agents in neutropenic patients with cancer: 2010 update by the infectious diseases society of America. Clin Infect Dis. 52(4):e56–e93

Funada H, Teshima H, Hattori K (1983) Total intestinal decontamination for prevention of infection in bone marrow transplantation. J Clin Oncol 13(Suppl 1):111–126

Gafter-Gvili A, Fraser A, Paul M, Leibovici L (2005) Meta-analysis: antibiotic prophylaxis reduces mortality in neutropenic patients. Ann Intern Med 142:979–995

Gafter-Gvili A, Fraser A, Paul M, Vidal L, Lawrie TA, van de Wetering MD, Kremer LC, Leibovici L (2012) Antibiotic prophylaxis for bacterial infections in afebrile neutropenic patients following chemotherapy. Cochrane Database Syst Rev 1:CD004386

Gualtier RJ, Donowitz GR, Kaiser DL, Hess CE, Sande MA (1983) Double-blind randomized study of prophylactic trimethoprim-sulfamethoxazole in granulocytopenic patients with hematologic malignancies. Am J Med 74:934–940

Gudiol C, Boron M, Simonetti A, Tubau F, González-Barca E, Cisnal M, Domingo-Domenech E, Jiménez L, Carratalà J (2013) Changing etiology, clinical features, antimicrobial resistance, and outcomes of bloodstream infection in neutropenic cancer patients. Clin Microbiol Infect 19(5):474–479

Hubel K, Hegener K, Schnell R et al (1999) Suppressed neutrophil function as a risk factor for severe infection after cytotoxic chemotherapy in patients with acute non-lymphocytic leukemia. Ann Hematol 78(2):73–77

Hahn DM, Schimpff SC, Fortner CL, Smyth AC, Young VM, Wiernik PH (1978) Infection in acute leukemia patients receiving oral nonabsorable antibiotics. Antimicrob Agents Chemother 13(6):958–964

Hersh EM et al (1965) Causes of death in acute leukemia: a ten-year study of 414 patients from 1954–1963. JAMA 193:105–109

Homsi J et al (2000) Infectious complications of advanced cancer. Support Care Cancer 8(6):487–492

Hooper DC, Wolfson JS (1985) The fluoroquinolones: pharmacology, clinical uses, and toxicities in humans. Antimicrob Agents Chemother 28:716–721

Hughes WT (1976) Protozoan infections in hematological diseases. Clint Haematol 5(2):329–345

Intragumtornchai T, Sutheesophon J, Sutcharitchan P, Swasdikul D (2000) A predictive model for life-threatening neutropenia and febrile neutropenia after the first course of CHOP chemotherapy in patients with aggressive non-Hodgkin's lymphoma. Leuk Lymphoma 37(3–4):351–360

Jacobson K, Rolston K, Elting L, LeBlanc B, Whimbey E, Ho DH (1999) Susceptibility surveillance among gram-negative bacilli at a cancer center. Chemotherapy 45:325–334

Jones RN (1999) Contemporary antimicrobial susceptibility patterns of bacterial pathogens commonly associated with febrile patients with neutropenia. Clin Infect Dis 29:495–502

Kara Ö, Zarakolu P, Aşçioğlu S, Etgül S, Uz B, Büyükaşik Y, Akova M (2015) Epidemiology and emerging resistance in bacterial bloodstream infections in patients with hematologic malignancies. Infect Dis (Lond). 47(10):686–693

Kawatkar AA, Farias AJ, Chao C, Chen W, Barron R, Vogl FD, Chandler DB (2017) Hospitalizations, outcomes, and management costs of febrile neutropenia in patients from a managed care population. Support Care Cancer 25(9):2787–2795

Kern WV, Klose K, Jellen-Ritter AS, Oethinger M, Bohnert J, Kern P et al (2005a) Fluoroquinolone resistance of Escherichia coli at a cancer center: epidemiologic evolution and effects of discontinuing prophylactic fluoroquinolone use in neutropenic patients with leukemia. Eur J Clin Microbiol Infect Dis 24(2):111–118

Kern WV, Steib-Bauert M, de With K, Reuter S, Bertz H, Frank U et al (2005b) Fluoroquinolone consumption and resistance in hematology-oncology patients: ecological analysis in two university hospitals 1999-2002. J Antimicrob Chemother 55:57–60

Kern WV, Klose K, Jellen-Ritter AS, Oethinger M, Bohnert J, Kern P, Reuter S, von Baum H, Marre R (2005c) Fluoroquinolone resistance of Escherichia coli at a cancer center: epidemiologic evolution and effects of discontinuing prophylactic fluoroquinolone use in neutropenic patients with leukemia. Eur J Clin Microbiol Infect Dis 24(2):111–118

King K (1980) Prophylactic non-absorbable antibiotics in leukaemic patients. J Hyg (Lond) 85(1):141–151

Klastersky J, Paesmans M, Rubenstein EB et al (2000) The multinational Association for Supportive Care in Cancer risk index: a multinational scoring system for identifying low-risk febrile neutropenic cancer patients. J Clin Oncol 18(16):3038–3051

Klastersky J, de Naurois J, Rolston K, Rapoport B, Maschmeyer G, Aapro M, Herrstedt J, ESMO Guidelines Committee (2016) Management of febrile neutropenia: ESMO clinical practice guidelines. Ann Oncol 27(suppl 5):v111–v118

Kuderer NM, Dale DC, Crawford J, Cosler LE, Lyman GH (2006) Mortality, morbidity, and cost associated with febrile neutropenia in adult cancer patients. Cancer 106(10):2258–2266

Leder K, Black J, O'Brien D, Greenwood Z, Kain KC, Schwartz E, Brown G, Torresi J (2004) Malaria in travelers: a review of the GeoSentinel surveillance network. Clin Infect Dis 39(8):1104–1112

Levi JA, Vincent PC, Jennis F, Lind DE, Gunz FW (1973) Prophylactic oral antibiotics in the management of acute leukaemia. Med J Aust 1(21):1025–1029

Liu HH (2010) Safety profile of the fluoroquinolones: focus on levofloxacin. Drug Saf 33(5):353–369

Lyman GH, Dale DC, Friedberg J, Crawford J, Fisher RI (2004) Incidence and predictors of low chemotherapy dose-intensity in aggressive non-Hodgkin's lymphoma: a nationwide study. J Clin Oncol 22(21):4302–4311

Lyman GH, Lyman CH, Agboola O (2005) Risk models for predicting chemotherapy-induced neutropenia. Oncologist 10(6):427–437

Mikulska M, Averbuch D, Tissot F, Cordonnier C, Akova M, Calandra T, Ceppi M, Bruzzi P, Viscoli C, European Conference on Infections in Leukemia (ECIL) (2018) Fluoroquinolone prophylaxis in hematological cancer patients with neutropenia: ECIL critical appraisal of previous guidelines. J Infect 76(1):20–37

Muto CA, Pokrywka M, Shutt K, Mendelsohn AB, Nouri K, Posey K et al (2005) A large outbreak of Clostridium difficile-associated disease with an unexpected proportion of deaths and colectomies at a teaching hospital following increased fluoroquinolone use. Infect Contr Hosp Epidemiol 26(3):273–280

Neumann S, Krause SW, Maschmeyer G, Schiel X, von Lilienfeld-Toal M, Infectious Diseases Working Party (AGIHO); German Society of Hematology and Oncology (DGHO) (2013) Primary prophylaxis of bacterial infections and Pneumocystis jirovecii pneumonia in patients with hematological malignancies and solid tumors: guidelines of the Infectious Diseases Working Party (AGIHO) of the German Society of Hematology and Oncology (DGHO). Ann Hematol. 92(4):433–442

No authors listed (1984) Trimethoprim-sulfamethoxazole in the prevention of infection in neutropenic patients. EORTC International Antimicrobial Therapy Project Group. J Infect Dis 150(3):372–379

Paterson DL (2004) Collateral damage from cephalosporin or quinolone antibiotic therapy. Clint Infect Dis 38(Suppl 4):S341–S345

Pettengell R, Schwenkglenks M, Leonard R, Bosly A, Paridaens R, Constenla M, Szucs TD, Jackisch C, Impact of Neutropenia in Chemotherapy-European Study Group (INC-EU) (2008) Neutropenia occurrence and predictors of reduced chemotherapy delivery: results from the INC-EU prospective observational European neutropenia study. Support Care Cancer 16(11):1299–1309

Phillips R, Hancock B, Graham J, Bromham N, Jin H, Berendse S (2012) Prevention and management of neutropenic sepsis in patients with cancer: summary of NICE guidance. BMJ. 345:e5368

Przybylski DJ, Reeves DJ (2017) Moxifloxacin versus levofloxacin or ciprofloxacin prophylaxis in acute myeloid leukemia patients receiving chemotherapy. Support Care Cancer 25(12):3715–3721

Rangaraj G, Granwehr BP, Jiang Y, Hachem R, Raad I (2010) Perils of quinolone exposure in cancer patients: breakthrough bacteremia with multidrug-resistant organisms. Cancer 116(4):967–973

Ray-Coquard I, Borg C, Bachelot T, Sebban C, Philip I, Clapisson G, Le Cesne A, Biron P, Chauvin F, Blay JY, ELYPSE study group (2003) Baseline and early lymphopenia predict for the risk of febrile neutropenia after chemotherapy. Br J Cancer 88(2):181–186

Rolston KV (2005) Challenges in the treatment of infections caused by gram-positive and gram-negative bacteria in patients with cancer and neutropenia. Clin Infect Dis 40(Suppl 4):S246–S252

Rolston KVI, Elting L, Waguespack S, Ho DH, LeBlanc B, Bodey GP (1996) Survey of antibiotic susceptibility among gram-negative bacilli at a cancer center. Chemotherapy 42:348–353

Schimpff SC, Young VM, Greene WH, Vermeulen GD, Moody MR, Wiernik PH (1972) Origin of infection in acute nonlymphocytic leukemia. Significance of hospital acquisition of potential pathogens. Ann Intern Med 77(5):707–714

Slavin MA, Lingaratnam S, Mileshkin L, Booth DL, Cain MJ, Ritchie DS, Wei A, Thursky KA, Australian consensus guidelines 2011 steering committee (2011) Use of antibacterial prophylaxis for patients with neutropenia. Australian Consensus Guidelines 2011 Steering Committee. Intern Med J 41(1b):102–109

Taplitz RA, Kennedy EB, Bow EJ, Crews J, Gleason C, Hawley DK, Langston AA, Nastoupil LJ, Rajotte M, Rolston KV, Strasfeld L, Flowers CR (2018) Antimicrobial Prophylaxis for Adult Patients With Cancer-Related Immunosuppression: ASCO and IDSA Clinical Practice Guideline Update. J Clin Oncol:JCO1800374

Trecarichi EM, Pagano L, Candoni A, Pastore D, Cattaneo C, Fanci R, Nosari A, Caira M, Spadea A, Busca A, Vianelli N, Tumbarello M, HeMABIS Registry—SEIFEM Group, Italy (2015) Current epidemiology and antimicrobial resistance data for bacterial bloodstream infections in patients with hematologic malignancies: an Italian multicenter prospective survey. Clin Microbiol Infect 21(4):337–343

Uys A, Rapoport BL, Anderson R (2004) Febrile neutropenia: a prospective study to validate the multinational Association of Supportive Care of Cancer (MASCC) risk-index score. Support Care Cancer 12(8):555–560

Verhoef J (1993) Prevention of infections in the neutropenic patient. Clin Infect Dis 17(Suppl 2):S359–S367

Viscoli C, Varnier O, Machetti M (2005) Infections in patients with febrile neutropenia: epidemiology, microbiology, and risk stratification. Clin Infect Dis 40(Suppl 4):S240–S245

Wade JC, DeJongh CA, Newman KA, Crowley J, Wiernik PH, Schimpff SC (1983) Selective antimicrobial modulation as prophylaxis against infection during granulocytopenia: trimethoprim-sulfamethoxazole vs. nalidixic acid. J Infect Dis 147:624–634

Watson JG, Jameson B, Powles RL, McElwain TJ, Lawson DN, Judson I, Morgenstern GR, Lumley H, Kay HE (1982) Co-trimoxazole versus non-absorbable antibiotics in acute leukaemia. Lancet 1(8262):6–9

Wilson JM, Guiney DG (1982) Failure of oral trimethoprim-sulfamethoxazole prophylaxis in acute leukemia. Isolation of resistant plasmids from strains of Enterobacteriaceae causing bacteremia. N Engl J Med 306:16–20

Wolfson JS, Hooper DC (1985) The fluoroquinolones: structures, mechanism of action and resistance, and spectra of activity in vitro. Antimicrob Agents Chemother 28:581–586

Yemm KE, Barreto JN, Mara KC, Dierkhising RA, Gangat N, Tosh PK (2018) A comparison of levofloxacin and oral third-generation cephalosporins as antibacterial prophylaxis in acute leukaemia patients during chemotherapy-induced neutropenia. J Antimicrob Chemother 73(1):204–211

Antifungal Prophylaxis

3

Rafael F. Duarte, Isabel Sánchez-Ortega, and Donald C. Sheppard

3.1 Introduction

Invasive fungal infections (IFI) remain a serious threat for patients with haematological malignancies. There is broad consensus that early antifungal therapy is a critical strategy to improve outcomes. However, controversy still remains about how early is early enough to optimise patient management and survival. For nearly three decades, since the establishment of the use of fluconazole to prevent candida infections, primary prophylaxis has been a key component of antifungal management in haematology patients. More recently, with the advent of newer triazoles, there has also been a recognition of the role of antifungal prophylaxis in the prevention of IFI caused by moulds. In addition to this longstanding experience and the general medical principle that 'prevention is better than cure', three key factors have led to the emergence of primary antifungal prophylaxis as a standard of care for high-risk haematology patients.

R. F. Duarte (✉)
Hospital Universitario Puerta de Hierro
Majadahonda, Madrid, Spain

I. Sánchez-Ortega (✉)
European Society for Blood and Marrow Transplantation, Barcelona, Spain
e-mail: isabel.sanchez-ortega@ebmt.org

D. C. Sheppard (✉)
McGill University, Montreal, QC, Canada
e-mail: don.sheppard@mcgill.ca

First, overall reported rates of IFI in haematology patients are high. In high-risk haematology patients, about one-third of IFI are due to *Candida* and other yeasts, and two-thirds to *Aspergillus* and other moulds. The largest European prospective audit of invasive mould disease in haematology, with over 1200 patients, reported a rate of invasive mould disease of 14% in all patients, 9% in allogeneic haematopoietic stem cell transplant (HSCT) recipients and 18% in acute myeloid leukaemia and myelodysplastic syndromes (AML/MDS) patients receiving intensive chemotherapy (www.pimda.eu). However, these figures likely underestimate the real incidence of mould infections, given the limitations of current diagnostic tools. Indeed, autopsy studies have reported that between half and two-thirds of IFI in haemato-oncology patients are only diagnosed post-mortem (Chamilos et al. 2006; Lewis et al. 2013). Thus, infection rates reported pre-mortem in most epidemiologic studies may represent only a small fraction of the real burden of disease. Not only are IFI rates high in haematology patients, but these infections remain associated with very high mortality rates. Despite the use of modern antifungal therapy, IFI mortality estimates range from 20% to 50% overall, and are particularly high in allogeneic HSCT recipients (Baddley et al. 2010; Pagano et al. 2010). Finally, and perhaps most importantly, randomised controlled trials have shown that effective primary antifungal prophylaxis can reduce the incidence of IFI and their associated

© Springer Nature Switzerland AG 2021
O. A. Cornely, M. Hoenigl (eds.), *Infection Management in Hematology*, Hematologic Malignancies, https://doi.org/10.1007/978-3-030-57317-1_3

mortality, leading to improved patient outcomes (Cornely et al. 2007; Goodman et al. 1992; Robenshtok et al. 2007; Slavin et al. 1995; Ullmann et al. 2007). Collectively, these observations have led to the conclusion that antifungal prophylaxis of high-risk patients is an effective strategy to improve outcomes in patients with haematological malignancies, and should be standard of care for these patients.

Traditionally, recommendations for prophylaxis have focused on patients with prolonged neutropenia, particularly AML/MDS after remission induction chemotherapy, and HSCT recipients pre-engraftment, as the population at highest risk. More recently, the increasing availability of novel agents in haematological malignancies, including many that modulate and target immune responses, has expanded the range of haematology patients at significant risk to develop IFI. Guidelines from multiple societies and working groups, with different approaches, have provided the medical community with guidance to implement the evidence coming from scientific studies into clinical practice. In this chapter, we will use guidelines from the following groups (Table 3.1): the European

Table 3.1 Quality of evidence and strength of recommendations on antifungal prophylaxis according to international guidelines

Quality of evidence		Strength of recommendation	
ECIL6 and IDSA			
I	Evidence from at least one properly designed, randomised controlled trial.	A	Good evidence to support a recommendation for or against use.
II	Evidence from at least one well-designed clinical trial without randomisation; from cohort or case-controlled analytic studies (preferably from more than one Centre); multiple time-series studies; or from dramatic results from uncontrolled experiments.	B	Moderate evidence to support a recommendation for or against use.
		C	Poor evidence to support a recommendation.
III	Evidence from opinions of respected authorities based on clinical experience, descriptive studies or reports from expert committees.		
ESCMID-ECMM-ERS and AGIHO-DGHO			
I	As in IDSA/ECIL-6 (above).	A	Strong support of a recommendation for use.
II	As in IDSA/ECIL-6 (above), with an index for source of evidence: a: Published abstract (presented at an international symposium or meeting). h: Comparator group is a historical control. r: Meta-analysis or systematic review of randomised controlled trials. t: Transferred evidence, that is, results from different patients' cohorts, or similar immune-status situation. u: Uncontrolled trial.	B	Moderate support of a recommendation for use.
		C	Marginal support of a recommendation for use.
		D	Support of a recommendation against use.
III	As in IDSA/ECIL-6 (above).		
NCCN			
1	High-level evidence.	1	There is uniform consensus that the intervention is appropriate.
2A	Lower-level evidence.	2A	There is uniform consensus that the intervention is appropriate.
2B	Lower-level evidence.	2B	There is consensus that the intervention is appropriate.
C	Any level of evidence.	3	There is major disagreement that the intervention is appropriate.

AGIHO-DGHO: Infectious Diseases Working Party of the German Society for Haematology and Medical Oncology; ECIL: European Conference on Infections in Leukaemia; ECMM: European Confederation of Medical Mycology; ERS: European Respiratory Society; ESCMID: European Society of Clinical Microbiology and Infectious Diseases; IDSA: Infectious Diseases Society of America; note: by default all NCCN recommendations are category 2A unless otherwise indicated

Conference on Infections in Leukaemia (ECIL) (Maertens et al. 2018; Marschmeyer et al. 2019), which brings together the European Society for Blood and Marrow Transplantation (EBMT), the European Organization for Research and Treatment of Cancer (EORTC), the European Leukemia Net (ELN) and the International Immunocompromised Host Society (ICHS); the European Society for Clinical Microbiology and Infectious Diseases (ESCMID), European Confederation of Medical Mycology (ECMM) and European Respiratory Society (ERS) Joint Clinical Guidelines (Ullmann et al. 2018); the Infectious Diseases Working Group of the German Society for Haematology and Medical Oncology (AGIHO-DGHO) (Mellinghoff et al. 2018; Ullmann et al. 2016); the Infectious Diseases Society of America (IDSA) and the American Society of Medical Oncology (ASCO) (Taplitz et al. 2018); and the National Comprehensive Cancer Network (NCCN) (available at www.nccn.org/professionals/physician_gls/pdf/infections.pdf). Beyond the guidelines, a number of additional factors should also be taken into consideration in the process of implementation of antifungal prophylaxis into practice. These include the analysis of local fungal epidemiology to inform antifungal policies, the identification of novel risk factors for IFI which may allow better patient IFI-risk stratification (reviewed in Chap. 2), the prevalence and risk of promotion of resistance through a broader use of antifungals in the target population, as well as the impact of prophylaxis on other aspects of antifungal and chemotherapy management in haematology patients.

3.2 General Measures for Prevention of Invasive Fungal Infections

General hygiene measures, housing of patients and environmental exposure to airborne conidia are key elements of infection-control that may impact the risk of IFI and potentially outweigh the benefit of antifungal prophylaxis. Regrettably, in the absence of randomised studies in this field, infection-control recommendations remain debat-able and primarily based on expert opinion and observational case series.

Available studies suggest a benefit of air filtration and positive pressure to prevent IFI in high-risk haematology patients, although the main gain is on reduction of conidia air concentration rather than on the incidence of infection or patient outcome (Eckmanns et al. 2006; Hayes-Lattin et al. 2005; Kruger et al. 2003; Nihtinen et al. 2007; Oren et al. 2001; Schlesinger et al. 2009). International quality standards for HSCT (JACIE—Joint Accreditation Committee of the International Society for Cellular Therapy and the EBMT) have established that HSCT recipients should be nursed in rooms of "adequate space and design that minimises airborne microbial contamination" (seventh Edition JACIE Standards: standard B2.1; available at www.jacie.org). While these standards do not require that every unit has laminar flow availability, standard recommendations for high-risk patients such as allogeneic HSCT recipients would be for isolation in a single hospital room equipped with high-efficiency particulate air (HEPA) filtration with positive pressure (>12 exchanges per hour). Beyond allogeneic HSCT, novel risk factors may help indicate how allocation of rooms should be prioritised for other haematology patients who may also benefit from air filtration and positive pressure.

Face masks are used for protection of immunocompromised high-risk patients, but neither surgical nor well-fitting masks have been demonstrated to result in the reduction of mould infections (Marschmeyer et al. 2009). While specific settings may justify the use of well-fitting face masks (e.g. during hospital construction or patient transport outside the isolation units), routine use is not recommended (Raad et al. 2015). In the hospital environment, renovation and construction activities should be kept to a minimum, and if required, the appropriate environmental controls must be present. Out of the hospital, the ubiquitous nature of airborne fungal spores makes environmental question a challenge; however, patients at risk of mould IFI should avoid prolonged contact with environments that have high concentrations of airborne fungal spores (e.g. construction and demolition sites, intensive exposure to soil through gardening or digging, or household renovation) (Taplitz et al. 2018). There is no evidence of reduction of IFI with germ-reduced diets, including the so-called neutropenic diets, or with other infection-control measures normally used to prevent other nosocomial infections. Appropriate hand disinfection may be also of use, as hands can be vectors in the transmission of yeasts, as has been documented with *Candida auris* outbreaks (Schelenz et al. 2016).

3.3 Acute Myeloid Leukaemia and Myelodysplastic Syndromes

Patients with AML/MDS undergoing myelosuppressive chemotherapy for remission-induction, relapse-salvage or similar courses of chemotherapy associated with prolonged and profound neu-

tropenia are at high risk for IFI. Despite the limitations of diagnostic tools and the lack of autopsy information, the incidence of mould disease reported in these patients is as high as 15%-20%, as best illustrated by the PIMDA prospective study mentioned above (www.pimda.eu). Given this high rate of disease, primary prophylaxis is strongly supported by all major guidelines. Posaconazole prophylaxis in this population has demonstrated a marked reduction of the rates of proven and probable IFI, invasive aspergillosis, and all-cause mortality (Cornely et al. 2007), leading to the universal recommendation for this agent as the drug of choice for antifungal chemoprophylaxis in this setting (Table 3.2). Since then, the original formulation of posaconazole as an oral suspension has been improved with an oral gastro-resistant tablet (Cornely et al. 2016; Duarte et al. 2014a) and an intravenous formulation (Cornely et al. 2017a; Maertens et al. 2014). Greater bioavailability, higher and more predict-

Table 3.2 Guidelines recommendations on primary antifungal prophylaxis in adult patients with AML/MDS undergoing intensive remission-induction chemotherapy or similar chemotherapies with prolonged and profound neutropenia

Antifungal agent	ECIL-6	ESCMID-ECMM-ERS	NCCN	AGIHO-DGHO	IDSA-ASCO
Fluconazole	B-I[a]	–	2B	C-I	–
Itraconazole OS	B-I	D-II	–	C-I	Mould-active triazole[b]
Posaconazole	A-I	A-I	1	A-I	
Voriconazole	B-II	C-IIt	2B	C-II	
Isavuconazole	–	–	–	C-IIu	–
Echinocandins	C-II (all echinocandins)	C-IIt (micafungin)	2B (micafungin)	C-IIh (micafungin) C-I (caspofungin)	–
Liposomal AmB	C-II	C-IIu	2B (AmB products)	C-I	–
Lipid-associated AmB	C-II	C-IIh		–	–
Aerosolised liposomal AmB	B-I (plus fluconazole)	B-I (plus fluconazole)	–	B-II (plus fluconazole)	–
AmB deoxycholate	A-II against/A-I against (aerosolised)	–	–	D-I	–

AGIHO-DGHO: Infectious Diseases Working Party of the German Society for Haematology and Medical Oncology; AML/MDS: acute myeloid leukaemia/myelodysplastic syndromes; AmB: amphotericin B; ECIL: European Conference on Infections in Leukaemia; ASCO: American Society of Clinical Oncology; ECMM: European Confederation of Medical Mycology; ERS: European Respiratory Society; ESCMID: European Society of Clinical Microbiology and Infectious Diseases; IDSA: Infectious Diseases Society of America; OS: oral solution
[a]Only recommended if the incidence of mould infections is low. Fluconazole may be part of an integrated care strategy together with a mould-directed diagnostic approach
[b]Risk of invasive aspergillosis >6% (type: evidence-based, benefits outweigh harms; evidence quality: intermediate; strength of recommendation: moderate)

able serum concentrations, and once-daily administration with no clinically relevant food effect make the gastro-resistant tablet the preferred formulation for the majority of cases. Of note, although there is not a formal contraindication for the concomitant administration of posaconazole in patients receiving anthracyclines, given its potential inhibition of anthracyclines transport kinetics, a washout period of 24 hours before starting posaconazole prophylaxis in these patients is prudent (Maertens et al. 2018). Most authorities agree that posaconazole prophylaxis should be continued until neutrophil recovery.

Azoles other than posaconazole have limitations, inconsistent evaluations in the guidelines, and should not be recommended for prophylaxis in these patients. Fluconazole has no clinically relevant activity against moulds and is therefore only of use if the incidence of mould IFI is low, which is rare in this population. Itraconazole is poorly tolerated, erratically absorbed and associated with significant drug–drug interactions. Use of this agent therefore requires monitoring serum levels for both efficacy and toxicity. The evidence for the efficacy for voriconazole in antifungal prophylaxis in this population is poor as there are no large comparative trials with this triazole in prophylaxis in AML/MDS. Extrapolation from trials of voriconazole use during the pre-engraftment neutropenic phase after allogeneic HSCT suggests that, as compared to fluconazole (Wingard et al. 2010) and to itraconazole (Marks et al. 2011), voriconazole prophylaxis neither reduces the incidence of IFI nor its associated mortality. These findings in two pivotal trials seem at odds with the use of voriconazole as a standard of care for treatment of invasive aspergillosis. Beyond potential issues of trial design and patient selection, one potential explanation for this unique activity of posaconazole in prophylaxis is its ability to concentrate to high levels within the membranes of host cells, leading to high local drug concentrations within the lung that prevent the growth of inhaled spores (Campoli et al. 2011; Campoli et al. 2013; Sheppard et al. 2014). This pharmacokinetic property may be less relevant during established

disease in which fungal hyphae grow within areas of necrotic tissue. Finally, isavuconazole has been recently approved for the treatment of invasive aspergillosis and mucormycosis, and initial studies in small groups of patients are starting to explore its potential role in prophylaxis (Bose et al. 2020; Cornely et al. 2015). Although isavuconazole exhibits a broad antifungal spectrum of action, predictable pharmacokinetics and a good safety profile, without a randomised controlled trial there is insufficient evidence to support the use of prophylactic isavuconazole.

Multiple other agents, including echinocandins and aerosolised liposomal amphotericin B plus fluconazole, have been investigated in small trials or case series. However, as with other azoles, none of these prophylactic regimens has been shown to reduce fungal mortality in randomised controlled clinical trials.

3.4 Allogeneic Haematopoietic Stem Cell Transplantation

Allogeneic HSCT recipients can potentially develop many risk factors for IFI, often for a prolonged period of time. These risks can include prior IFI, iron overload, indwelling catheters, parenteral nutrition, prolonged neutropenia, profound cellular and humoral immunosuppression and immunosuppressive therapies, CMV infection, acute and chronic graft versus host disease (GVHD), among others. These risk factors not only vary significantly between patients, but also evolve over time during transplantation and recovery. For example, while the early neutropenic phase after HSCT has long been thought of as the conventional risk period for IFI, we now know that approximately two-thirds of IFI in this population will present after neutrophil engraftment, where CMV infection and immunosuppressive treatment for GVHD drive the risk of infection (Garcia-Vidal et al. 2008; Girmenia et al. 2014; Martino et al. 2002). Therefore, antifungal prophylaxis practice must recognise this and differentiate the risk of allogeneic HSCT recipients during the pre-engraftment period (Table 3.3), and during periods of significant

Table 3.3 Guidelines recommendations on primary antifungal prophylaxis in adult allogeneic HSCT recipients during the pre-engraftment period

Antifungal agent	ECIL-6 Low risk[a]	High risk[a]	ESCMID-ECMM-ERS[c]	NCCN	AGIHO-DGHO[d] Moulds	Candida
Fluconazole	A-I[b]	A-III against	–	1	–	A-I
Itraconazole	B-I	B-I	D-I	–	C-I	C-I
Posaconazole	B-II	B-II	B-II	2B	B-IIt	B-IIt
Voriconazole	B-I	B-I	C-I	2B	C-I	B-IIt
Micafungin	B-I	C-I	C-I	1	C-I[d]	B-IIt[e]
Liposomal AmB	C-II	C-II	–	2B (AmB products)	–	–
Aerosolised liposomal AmB	C-III	B-II	B-II	–	–	–

AGIHO-DGHO: Infectious Diseases Working Party of the German Society for Haematology and Medical Oncology; AML/MDS: acute myeloid leukaemia/myelodysplastic syndromes; AmB: amphotericin B; ECIL: European Conference on Infections in Leukaemia; ECMM: European Confederation of Medical Mycology; ERS: European Respiratory Society; ESCMID: European Society of Clinical Microbiology and Infectious Diseases
[a]Pre-engraftment risk of mould infections
[b]Only when combined with a mould-directed diagnostic approach (biomarker and/or CT scan-based) or a mould-directed therapeutic approach (empirical antifungal therapy)
[c]ESCMID-ECMM-ERS guidelines also recommend D-III for any antifungal agent after neutrophil recovery in patients without GVHD
[d]AGIHO-DGHO guidelines: day 1 to 100 without GvHD
[e]Only during neutropenia

GVHD (Table 3.4) (Maertens et al. 2018; Ullmann et al. 2016).

As in AML/MDS, across all guidelines, posaconazole is the drug of choice for antifungal prophylaxis in GVHD, as it reduces the incidence of IFI and its associated mortality (Ullmann et al. 2007). Given the high risk of invasive mould infection and their associated mortality in these patients, ECIL also strongly recommends against the use of fluconazole as prophylaxis in GVHD patients, as well as in the pre-engraftment period for patients at high-risk for mould infections. Fluconazole, however, remains the drug of choice for prevention of *Candida* infections in patients with low risk of moulds during the pre-engraftment period. If the risk of moulds is high, no drug stands out for a strong recommendation as chemoprophylaxis in the early phase after allogeneic HSCT. The posaconazole pivotal studies did not include allogeneic HSCT recipients during the early neutropenic period. Therefore, efficacy and safety data can only be inferred from the trials in AML/MDS and GVHD and from retrospective analyses (Sánchez-Ortega et al. 2011), and a strong recommendation for its use cannot be made. The pivotal prophylaxis trials of voriconazole in allogeneic HSCT did not observe a reduction in the incidence of IFI, or improved patient outcomes when compared to therapy with fluconazole or itraconazole (Marks et al. 2011; Wingard et al. 2010). Concerns about the increased toxicity of voriconazole over other azoles raise doubts about its use in this setting. In addition to the well-known voriconazole hepatic and CNS toxicities, the use of this agent in allogeneic HSCT and solid-organ transplants is associated with an increased risk of secondary squamous cell carcinoma (Wojenski et al. 2015; Tang et al. 2019). This risk can be as high as 19% at 5 years and increases with time of exposure to voriconazole, providing a strong cautionary argument against its use for prophylaxis in allogeneic HSCT recipients. Alternatives to posaconazole in GVHD and decisions on anti-mould chemoprophylaxis pre-engraftment have all limited evidence for recommendation (Table 3.4). Decisions

Table 3.4 Guidelines recommendations on primary antifungal prophylaxis in adult allogeneic HSCT recipients with significant graft-versus-host disease

Antifungal agent	ECIL-6[a]	ESCMID-ECMM-ERS[b]	NCCN	AGIHO-DGHO[c]	IDSA-ASCO
Fluconazole	A-III against	–	–	–	–
Itraconazole OS	B-I	C-II	–		Mould-active Triazole (posaconazole)[d]
Posaconazole	A-I	A-I	1	A-I (OS)	
Voriconazole	B-I	C-II	2B		
Micafungin	C-II	C-III	2B (echinocandin)	–	–
Liposomal AmB	C-II	–	2B (AmB products)	–	–

AGIHO-DGHO: Infectious Diseases Working Party of the German Society for Haematology and Medical Oncology; AML/MDS: acute myeloid leukaemia/myelodysplastic syndromes; AmB: amphotericin B; ECIL: European Conference on Infections in Leukaemia; ASCO: American Society of Clinical Oncology; ECMM: European Confederation of Medical Mycology; ERS: European Respiratory Society; ESCMID: European Society of Clinical Microbiology and Infectious Diseases; GVHD: graft-versus-host disease; IDSA: Infectious Diseases Society of America; OS: oral solution
[a]High-risk GVHD: grade III–IV acute GvHD, grade II acute GVHD of alternative donor transplants, GVHD unresponsive to standard corticosteroid therapy and acute GVHD followed by chronic GVHD
[b]Moderate to severe GVHD and/or intensified immuno-suppression
[c]To prevent Invasive aspergillosis
[d]Risk of invasive aspergillosis >6% (type: evidence-based, benefits outweigh harms; evidence quality: intermediate; strength of recommendation: moderate)

should be individualised based on specific patient characteristics and the balance of efficacy and safety for each drug.

The use of azoles in allogeneic HSCT recipients can increase the exposure to calcineurin inhibitors and their potential toxicity, warranting a recommendation for close monitoring of their blood levels and subsequent dose adjustment. However, it is less clear whether an upfront reduction of the dose of calcineurin inhibitor is required, in particular during the early phase of allogeneic HSCT when the potential occurrence of subtherapeutic levels of the immunosuppressive drug, even transiently, has a strong negative impact on the risk of GVHD and on the outcome of allogeneic HSCT (Kanda et al. 2006; Yee et al. 1988). We therefore recommend avoiding an upfront reduction of the dose of calcineurin inhibitors in favour of close monitoring of blood levels and clinical toxicity. For posaconazole in patients receiving cyclosporin A, this strategy is safe and effective in the early phase of allogeneic HSCT (Sánchez-Ortega et al. 2012).

Clinical decisions regarding the duration of antifungal prophylaxis in allogeneic HSCT are challenging. In patients treated for GVHD, antifungal prophylaxis should be maintained while GVHD is active and requires enhanced immunosuppressive therapy such as high-dose corticosteroids. In patients treated during the pre-engraftment period, antifungal prophylaxis should be maintained at least until neutrophil recovery, and probably longer, up to day +75 to +100 for patients with additional risk factors as described above.

3.5 Autologous Haematopoietic Stem Cell Transplantation

Autologous HSCT recipients have overall a low risk of IFI, and in particular a low risk of mould infections. Therefore, anti-mould chemoprophylaxis is not recommended. However, mucositis remains a risk factor for candidaemia after autologous HSCT, and fluconazole (400 mg daily) should be considered in these patients during the neutropenic phase (Table 3.5).

Table 3.5 Guidelines recommendations on primary antifungal prophylaxis for other haematological malignancies

	ECIL-6	ESCMID-ECMM-ERS	NCCN
Autologous HCT	Fluconazole B-III (Candida)	D-III for any mould active agent	Mucositis: 1 fluconazole and micafungin No mucositis: 2B no prophylaxis
ALL	No standard of care Fluconazole C-III (yeasts)	Liposomal AmB D-I	2A: Fluconazole and micafungin 2B: AmB products
MDS[a]	Not recommended		–
Lymphoma, MM, CLL	Not recommended[b]		No prophylaxis[c]

ALL: acute lymphoblastic leukaemia; AmB: amphotericin B; CLL: chronic lymphocytic leukaemia; ECIL: European Conference on Infections in Leukaemia; ECMM: European Confederation of Medical Mycology; ERS: European Respiratory Society; ESCMID: European Society of Clinical Microbiology and Infectious Diseases; HSCT: hematopoietic stem cell transplantation; MDS: myelodysplastic syndromes; MM: multiple myeloma
[a]Low-to-intermediate risk MDS (supportive care treatment, lenalidomide or hypomethylating agents)
[b]It might be considered if prolonged neutropenia (>6 months), elderly patients and advanced and unresponsive CLL disease, although it is important to consider long-term toxicity and selection pressure
[c]Treatment modality and the type of malignancy affect risk level

3.6 Novel Therapeutic Agents and Fungal Risk in Other Haematological Malignancies

Traditionally, patients with haematological malignancies beyond AML/MDS and HSCT recipients, who normally do not have neutropenia longer than 7 days, are not at increased risk of IFI and would not be considered for antifungal prophylaxis. More recently, a growing number of novel molecular-targeting agents are being approved for patients with haematological malignancies every year (available at https://www.fda. gov/drugs/resources-information-approved-drugs/hematologyoncology-cancer-approvals-safety-notifications). Many of these new agents modulate and target immune responses, and their use opens up a whole new spectrum of patients with haematological malignancies potentially at risk of IFI (Marschmeyer et al. 2019). It is worth noting that approvals of these new drugs are based on an overall evidence of improved outcomes and a beneficial balance of their antineoplastic efficacy and their safety against potential unforeseen toxicity and risks. As such, assessing the risk of fungal infections plays a minor role in the licensing path for these agents, and pivotal studies of these agents often fail to

monitor IFI rates in detail. Despite these caveats, the overall risk and incidence with the majority of these new agents appear to be very low. Therefore, while there is a need for heightened awareness and ongoing vigilance to identify changes in fungal epidemiology associated with the use of these novel agents, the available evidence does not support recommendations for antifungal prophylaxis for the majority of patients with multiple myeloma, lymphoma, chronic lymphocytic leukaemia, myeloproliferative disorders and other haematological malignancies treated with novel agents (Table 3.5).

One potential exception to this rule would be patients undergoing remission-induction therapy for acute lymphoblastic leukaemia (ALL). A recent large, double-blind, randomised study in these patients has identified an unmet need for these patients (Cornely et al. 2017b). In this trial, the rate of IFI in ALL was 11.7% in the placebo arm, clearly identifying this population as one that is at high risk of IFI, and where primary prophylaxis would be indicated. Unfortunately, 5 mg/kg liposomal amphotericin B given twice weekly was not associated with a statistically significant reduction in the rate of IFI. Although prophylaxis with azoles has become standard of care for other patient groups at similar risk (e.g. AML/MDS), the use of mould-active azoles in

ALL is not recommended because of potentially hazardous neurotoxic interactions with Vinca alkaloids that are part of ALL chemotherapy. Echinocandins hold potential as non-toxic agents without the risk of significant drug–drug interactions; however, there is a lack of data supporting their use. At this point, there is therefore no obvious best agent for use in this population, and future studies are required.

An additional development in the therapy of ALL, as well as for other B-cell malignancies, is the arrival of chimeric antigen receptor-modified T (CAR-T) cells. CAR-T cells are revolutionising the treatment of relapsed/refractory haematological malignancies but have also severe toxicities that can be life-threatening (Brudno and Kochenderfer 2019). CAR-T cell cytokine release syndrome and its treatment with tocilizumab and corticosteroids may increase the risk of opportunistic IFI, in particular moulds. However, reports on the occurrence of mould infections in CAR-T patients remain scarce, with low rates of IFI, seen predominantly in patients with other concomitant risk factors (Haidar et al. 2019). Some groups have advocated for a risk stratification approach to antifungal prophylaxis based on local rates of IFI, a prior history of mould infection, prolonged neutropenia longer than 3 weeks and treatment with corticosteroids longer than 1 week. However, validation of such strategies is required. At this time, broad use of antifungal prophylaxis in CAR-T cell recipients is not recommended.

Ibrutinib, a Bruton's tyrosine kinase inhibitor approved for the treatment of an increasing number of B-cell malignancies and for patients with chronic GVHD, has been associated with an increased risk of mould IFI. At least part of this risk stems from the use of this agent in heavily pre-treated patients, often in combination with other chemotherapy and immunomodulatory agents, rather than the drug itself (Marschmeyer et al. 2019). The incidence of invasive yeast and mould infections was overall low in the pivotal trials as well as in observational retrospective studies on this topic (Ghez et al. 2018; Varughese et al. 2018). However, the use of ibrutinib in lymphoma patients with central nervous system involvement seems to associate with an increased

risk of cerebral fungal disease (Ghez et al. 2018; Grommes and Younes 2017). As with other novel agents, these findings suggest a need for increased awareness and vigilance but do not support the use of primary antifungal prophylaxis in patients treated with ibrutinib at this time unless driven by other concomitant risk factors such as severe chronic GVHD, or elderly chronic lymphocytic leukaemia (CLL) cases with very prolonged neutropenia and advanced unresponsive disease.

Venetoclax is a BCL-2 inhibitor used in the treatment of CLL, and more recently, also in patients with AML. Use of this agent is commonly associated with severe neutropenia, a well-established risk factor for IFI (Roberts et al. 2016; Stilgenbauer et al. 2016). However, neutropenia can be managed easily withholding treatment and using GCSF and there is no evidence linking this adverse effect to an increased incidence of IFI. Use of antifungals in combination with venetoclax requires careful consideration of potential drug–drug interaction with CYP3A inducers or inhibitors, such as azoles.

Patients with low-grade MDS and chronic myeloproliferative disorders treated with novel drugs such as lenalidomide or hypomethylating agents have a low incidence of IFI, despite the presence of multiple risk factors for fungal infection (Maertens et al. 2018). A single-centre analysis of 948 courses of azacitidine in 121 consecutive AML/MDS patients reported an incidence of proven/probable IFI of only 0.21% per azacitidine treatment cycle and 1.6% per patient treated for the whole series (Pomares et al. 2016). Although IFI rates were slightly higher among patients with severe neutropenia (0.73% per azacitidine treatment cycle and 4.1% per patient treated), these rates fall well below the reasonable threshold for use of antifungal prophylaxis. Finally, there appears to be no increased risk of IFI in patients with chronic myeloid leukaemia treated with tyrosine kinase inhibitors or in patients with other chronic myeloproliferative disorders, and therefore primary antifungal prophylaxis is not recommended for these patients.

In summary, the risk of IFI with new targeted and immunomodulatory agents for patients with haematological malignancies remains small in comparison with the number of patients who benefit from new drugs. Continued awareness and post-licensure surveillance are needed to ensure the detection of special populations at risk for IFI, as has been reported with cerebral IFI in some patients treated with ibrutinib.

3.7   Aplastic Anaemia

Patients with severe aplastic anaemia (AA) undergo very prolonged periods of profound neutropenia and monocytopenia, receive intensive immunosuppressive treatment with cyclosporine A, anti-thymocyte globulin and corticosteroids, and many undergo allogeneic HSCT. Undoubtedly, these are patients with a high risk for IFI, in particular for mould infections (Bacigalupo et al. 2000; Valdez et al. 2009; Weinberger et al. 1992). In the absence of randomised controlled trials of antifungal prophylaxis in this setting, evidence can be extrapolated from studies in AML/MDS patients, for whom profound neutropenia is also the main risk factor (Cornely et al. 2007; Marks et al. 2011; Robenshtok et al. 2007; Ullmann et al. 2007; Wingard et al. 2010). Primary antifungal prophylaxis with activity against both yeasts and moulds should be used in patients with severe AA. Despite limitations in the evidence available in this indication, the recommended drug would be posaconazole, which is more effective than fluconazole and voriconazole, and has a better safety profile than the latter. Antifungal prophylaxis should be considered from diagnosis and the start of immunosuppressive therapy and continued for as long as severe neutropenia and/or lymphopenia are present. Specific recommendations for AA patients undergoing allogeneic HSCT recipients have been discussed above.

3.8   Secondary Prophylaxis

Secondary prophylaxis to prevent recurrence of prior mould infections during a subsequent period of immunosuppression is common practice, in particular in patients with AML/MDS receiving

Table 3.6 Guidelines recommendations on secondary antifungal prophylaxis for adult patients undergoing intensive chemotherapy or HSCT

Antifungal agent	AGIHO-DGHO (previous IFD)	ESCMID-ECMM-ERS (previous IA)
Posaconazole	B-III	–
Voriconazole	B-II	A-IIh
Caspofungin	B-III	–
Caspofungin → Itraconazole OS	–	B-IIh
Liposomal AmB → Voriconazole	–	C-II
Surgery[a] → secondary prophylaxis	–	B-III

AGIHO-DGHO: Infectious Diseases Working Party of the German Society for Haematology and Medical Oncology; AmB: amphotericin B; ECMM: European Confederation of Medical Mycology; ERS: European Respiratory Society; ESCMID: European Society of Clinical Microbiology and Infectious Diseases; HSCT: hematopoietic stem cell transplantation; IA: invasive aspergillosis; IFD: invasive fungal disease; OS: oral solution
[a]Timing and methods of surgery important and concomitant administration of appropriate antifungal compound justified.

further chemotherapy, and in allogeneic HSCT recipients during the early neutropenic period and later if they develop GVHD. There are no large controlled randomised trials in this setting and evidence comes from open-label, single-arm trials and retrospective studies in relatively small numbers of patients (Cordonnier et al. 2010; De Fabritiis et al. 2007; Kruger et al. 2005). Antifungal agents to be considered in this indication are listed in Table 3.6. In the absence of robust clinical trials, decisions regarding secondary prophylaxis and choice of agent should be individualised, taking into consideration patient risk factors, concomitant medications and antifungal treatment history.

3.9   Primary Prophylaxis as Part of the Antifungal Management Continuum

The high incidence of IFI, high IFI-related mortality and the reduction of these with effective primary antifungal chemoprophylaxis in randomised controlled trials have established this strategy as a standard of care in high-risk haematology patients. Unlike empirical, pre-emptive and directed treatment, primary prophylaxis is the only strategy of the antifungal management continuum with this level of evidence of improved patient outcomes. The adoption of anti-mould prophylaxis in clinical practice in the past decade took place in parallel with the development of novel IFI diagnostic tools (Lagrou et al. 2019). As the performance of diagnostic tests is sensitive to the pre-test probability of disease (Fagan 1975; Griner et al. 1981), it is important to consider the effects of effective antifungal prophylaxis on the utility of diagnostic-based antifungal use. The serum galactomannan biomarker has a sensitivity and a specificity of approximately 70% and 90%, respectively, for the diagnosis of invasive aspergillosis in haemato-oncology patients. When the test is used in a high prevalence setting of invasive aspergillosis (15%), as is observed in some high-risk haematology populations in the absence of antifungal prophylaxis, the test has a reasonable positive predictive value (PPV) of approximately 50%. However, in a clinical scenario of low pre-test prevalence of invasive aspergillosis (2%), as is observed during posaconazole prophylaxis, the PPV of serum galactomannan drops to only 12% (Donnelly and Leeflang 2010). In this situation, only approximately one out of every ten patients with a positive serum galactomannan test result would represent a true case of invasive aspergillosis, rendering the strategy ineffective (Cornely 2014). Importantly, the PPV of the galactomannan test would be predicted to rise to useful levels when used in the context of radiologically documented suspected breakthrough of antifungal prophylaxis, as a function of the increased pre-test probability of fungal disease.

These concepts are well illustrated by the results of a single-centre study of 262 consecutive high-risk episodes receiving posaconazole primary prophylaxis in combination with serum galactomannan surveillance. As with other studies, prophylaxis was associated with a low incidence of proven and probable invasive aspergillosis (1.9%). In this population, the vast majority of galactomannan tests were negative (96.7% in 83.65 risk episodes). Of the 35 positive serum galactomannan tests, 30 were found to be false positive, resulting in a low PPV of only 11.8% (Duarte et al. 2014b). Beyond validating the low PPV of the GM assay as a screening tool during antifungal prophylaxis, this study also confirmed the utility of GM testing to diagnose fungal breakthrough infections. In evaluable cases with positive serum galactomannan tests and a clinical suspicion of IFI, the performance of the serum galactomannan test improved, with a PPV of 89.6%. Thus, while effective anti-mould prophylaxis renders routine surveillance with serum galactomannan unreliable, the test remains useful to diagnose suspected breakthrough invasive aspergillosis in patients receiving effective antifungal prophylaxis (Cornely 2014; Duarte et al. 2014b).

These findings were reproduced independently in patients receiving prophylaxis with micafungin (Vena et al. 2017), and were adopted by the executive summary 2017 of the ESCMID-ECMM-ERS guidelines to help guide the combined use of effective antifungal prophylaxis to improve patient outcome, and serum GM testing to rationalise antifungal treatment. Together, these approaches have contributed to a dynamic reconfiguration of the antifungal management continuum of high-risk haematology patients in real-life practice and serve as important tools for multidisciplinary teams (Lagrou et al. 2019).

References

Bacigalupo A, Brand R, Oneto R, Bruno B, Socie G, Passweg J et al (2000) Treatment of acquired severe aplastic anemia: bone marrow transplantation compared with immunosuppressive therapy–the European Group for Blood and Marrow Transplantation experience. Semin Hematol 37:69–80

Baddley JW, Andes DR, Marr KA et al (2010) Factors associated with mortality in transplant patients with invasive aspergillosis. Clin Infect Dis 50:1559–1567

Bose P, McCue D, Wurster S et al (2020. Online ahead of print) Isavuconazole as primary anti-fungal prophylaxis in patients with acute myeloid leukemia or Myelodysplastic syndrome: an open-label, prospective, phase II study. Clin Infect Dis. https://doi.org/10.1093/cid/ciaa358

Brudno JN, Kochenderfer JN (2019) Recent advances in CAR T-cell toxicity: mechanisms, manifestations and management. Blood Rev 34:45–55

Campoli P, Al Abdallah Q, Robitaille R et al (2011) Concentration of antifungal agents within host cell membranes: a new paradigm governing the efficacy of prophylaxis. Antimicrob Agents Chemother 55:5732–5739

Campoli P, Perlin DS, Kristof AS et al (2013) Pharmacokinetics of posaconazole within epithelial cells and fungi: insights into potential mechanisms of action during treatment and prophylaxis. J Infect Dis 208:1717–1728

Chamilos G, Luna M, Lewis RE et al (2006) Invasive fungal infections in patients with hematologic malignancies in a tertiary care cancer center: an autopsy study over a 15-year period (1989-2003). Haematologica 91:986–989

Cordonnier C, Rovira M, Maertens J et al (2010) Voriconazole for secondary prophylaxis of invasive fungal infections in allogeneic stem cell transplant recipients: results of the VOSIFI study. Haematologica 95:1762–1768

Cornely OA (2014) Galactomannan testing during Mold-active prophylaxis. Clin Infect Dis 59:1703–1704

Cornely OA, Maertens J, Winston DJ et al (2007) Posaconazole vs. fluconazole or itraconazole prophylaxis in patients with neutropenia. N Engl J Med 356:348–359

Cornely OA, Bohme A, Schmitt-Hoffmann A et al (2015) Safety and pharmacokinetics of isavuconazole as antifungal prophylaxis in acute myeloid leukemia patients with neutropenia: results of a phase 2, dose escalation study. Antimicrob Agents Chemother 59:2078–2085

Cornely OA, Duarte RF, Haider S et al (2016) Phase 3 pharmacokinetics and safety study of a posaconazole tablet formulation in patients at risk for invasive fungal disease. J Antimicrob Chemother 71:718–726

Cornely OA, Robertson MN, Haider S et al (2017a) Pharmacokinetics and safety results from the phase 3 randomized, open-label, study of intravenous posaconazole in patients at risk of invasive fungal disease. J Antimicrob Chemother 72:3406–3413

Cornely OA, Leguay T, Maertens J et al (2017b) Randomized comparison of liposomal amphotericin B versus placebo to prevent invasive mycoses in acute lymphoblastic leukaemia. J Antimicrob Chemother 72:2359–2367

De Fabritiis P, Spagnoli A, Di Bartolomeo P et al (2007) Efficacy of caspofungin as secondary prophylaxis in patients undergoing allogeneic stem cell transplantation with prior pulmonary and/or systemic fungal infection. Bone Marrow Transpl 40:245–249

Donnelly JP, Leeflang MM (2010) Galactomannan detection and diagnosis of invasive aspergillosis. Clin Infect Dis 50:1070–1071

Duarte RF, López-Jiménez J, Cornely OA et al (2014a) Phase 1b study of new posaconazole tablet for prevention of invasive fungal infections in high-risk patients with neutropenia. Antimicrob Agents Chemother 58:5758–5765

Duarte RF, Sánchez-Ortega I, Cuesta I et al (2014b) Serum Galactomannan–based early detection of invasive Aspergillosis in hematology patients receiving effective Antimold prophylaxis. Clin Infect Dis 59:1696–1702

Eckmanns T, Ruden H, Gastmeier P et al (2006) The influence of high-efficiency particulate air filtration on mortality and fungal infection among highly immunosuppressed patients: a systematic review. J Infect Dis 193(10):1408–1418

Fagan TJ (1975) Nomogram for Bayes theorem. N Engl J Med 293:257

Garcia-Vidal C, Upton A, Kirby KA, Marr KA (2008) Epidemiology of invasive mold infections in allogeneic stem cell transplant recipients: biological risk factors for infection according to time after transplantation. Clin Infect Dis 47:1041–1050

Ghez D, Calleja A, Protin C et al (2018) French innovative leukemia organization (FILO) CLL group. Early-onset invasive aspergillosis and other fungal infections in patients treated with ibrutinib. Blood 131:1955–1959

Girmenia C, Raiola AM, Piciocchi A et al (2014) Incidence and outcome of invasive fungal diseases after allogeneic stem cell transplantation: a prospective study of the Gruppo Italiano Trapianto Midollo Osseo (GITMO). Biol Blood Marrow Transplant 20:872–880

Goodman JL, Winston DJ, Greenfield RA et al (1992) A controlled trial of fluconazole to prevent fungal infections in patients undergoing bone marrow transplantation. N Engl JMed 326:845–851

Griner PF, Mayewski RJ, Mushlin AI et al (1981) Selection and interpretation of diagnostic tests and procedures. Principles and applications. Ann Intern Med 94:557–592

Grommes C, Younes A (2017) Ibrutinib in PCNSL: the curios cases of clinical responses and aspergillosis. Cancer Cell 31:731–733

Haidar G, Dorritie K, Farah R et al (2019) Invasive Mold infections after chimeric antigen receptor–modified T-cell therapy: a case series, review of the literature, and implications for prophylaxis. Clin Infect Dis, Online ahead of print. https://doi.org/10.1093/cid/ciz1127

Hayes-Lattin B, Leis JF, Maziarz RT (2005) Isolation in the allogeneic transplant environment: how protective is it? Bone Marrow Transplant 36(5):373–381

Kanda Y, Hyo R, Yamasita T et al (2006) Effect of blood cyclosporine concentration on the outcome of hematopoietic stem cell transplantation from an HLA-matched sibling donor. Am J Hematol 81:838–844

Kruger WH, Zollner B, Kaulfers PM et al (2003) Effective protection of allogeneic stem cell recipients against aspergillosis by HEPA air filtration during a period of construction–a prospective survey. J Hematother Stem Cell Res 12:301–307

Kruger WH, Russmann B, de Wit M et al (2005) Haemopoietic cell transplantation of patients with a history of deep or invasive fungal infection during prophylaxis with liposomal amphotericin B. Acta Haematol 113:104–108

Lagrou K, Duarte RF, Maertens J (2019) Standards of CARE: what is considered 'best practice' for the management of invasive fungal infections? A haematologist's and a mycologist's perspective. J Antimicrob Chemother 74(Suppl 2):ii3–ii8

Lewis RE, Cahyame-Zuniga L, Leventakos K et al (2013) Epidemiology and sites of involvement of invasive fungal infections in patients with haematological malignancies: a 20-year autopsy study. Mycoses 56:638–645

Maertens J, Cornely OA, Ullmann AJ et al (2014) Phase 1B study of the pharmacokinetics and safety of posaconazole intravenous solution in patients at risk for invasive fungal disease. Antimicrob Agents Chemother 58:3610–3617

Maertens JA, Girmenia C, Brüggemann RJ et al (2018) European guidelines for primary antifungal prophylaxis in adult haematology patients: summary of the updated recommendations from the European conference on infections in leukemia. J Antimicrob Chemother 73:3221–3230

Marks DI, Pagliuca A, Kibbler CC et al (2011) Voriconazole versus itraconazole for antifungal prophylaxis following allogeneic haematopoietic stem-cell transplantation. Br J Haematol 155:318–327

Marschmeyer G, Neuburger S, Fritz L et al (2009) A prospective, randomised study on the use of well-fitting masks for prevention of invasive Aspergillosis in high-risk patients. Ann Oncol 20:1560–1564

Marschmeyer G, De Greef J, Mellinghoff SC et al (2019) Infections associated with immunotherapeutic and molecular targeted agents in hematology and oncology. A position paper by the European conference on infections in leukemia (ECIL). Leukaemia 33:844–862

Martino R, Subirá M, Roviera M et al (2002) Invasive fungal infections after allogeneic peripheral blood stem cell transplantation: incidence and risk factors in 395 patients. Br J Haematol 116:475–482

Mellinghoff SC, Panse J, Alakel N et al (2018) Primary prophylaxis of invasive fungal infections in patients with haematological malignancies: 2017 update of the recommendations of the infectious diseases working party (AGIHO) of the German Society for Haematology and Medical Oncology (DGHO). Ann Hematol 97:197–207

Nihtinen A, Anttila VJ, Richardson M et al (2007) The utility of intensified environmental surveillance for pathogenic moulds in a. stem cell transplantation ward during construction work to monitor the efficacy of HEPA filtration. Bone Marrow Transplant 40:457–460

Oren I, Haddad N, Finkelstein R, Rowe JM (2001) Invasive pulmonary aspergillosis in neutropenic patients during hospital construction: before and after chemoprophylaxis and institution of HEPA filters. Am J Hematol 66(4):257–262

Pagano L, Caira M, Candoni A et al (2010) Invasive aspergillosis in patients with acute myeloid leukemia: a SEIFEM-2008 registry study. Haematologica 95:644–650

Pomares H, Arnan M, Sánchez-Ortega I, Sureda A, Duarte RF (2016) Invasive fungal infections in AML/MDS patients treated with azacitidine: a risk worth considering antifungal prophylaxis? Mycoses 59:516–519

Raad I, Hanna H, Osting C et al (2015) Masking of neutropenic patients on transport from hospital rooms is associated with a decrease in nosocomial aspergillosis during construction. Infect Contr Hosp Epidemiol 23:41–43

Robenshtok E, Gafter-Gvili A, Goldberg E et al (2007) Antifungal prophylaxis in cancer patients after chemotherapy or hematopoietic stem-cell transplantation: systematic review and meta-analysis. J Clin Oncol 25:5471–5489

Roberts AW, Davids MS, Pagel JM et al (2016) Targeting BCL2 with venetoclax in relapsed chronic lymphocytic leukemia. N Engl J Med 374:311–322

Sánchez-Ortega I, Patiño B, Arnan M et al (2011) Clinical efficacy and safety of primary antifungal prophylaxis with posaconazole vs itraconazole in allogeneic blood and marrow transplantation. Bone Marrow Transplant 46:733–739

Sánchez-Ortega I, Vázquez L, Montes C et al (2012) Effect of posaconazole on cyclosporine blood levels and dose adjustment in allogeneic blood and marrow transplant recipients. Antimicrob Agents Chemother 56:6422–6424

Schelenz S, Hagen F, Rhodes JL et al (2016) First hospital outbreak of the globally emerging Candida Auris in a European hospital. Antimicrob Resist Infect Control 5:35

Schlesinger A, Paul M, Gafter-Gvili A et al (2009) Infection-control interventions for cancer patients after chemotherapy: a systematic review and meta-analysis. Lancet Infect Dis 9:97–107

Sheppard DC, Campoli P, Duarte RF (2014) Understanding antifungal prophylaxis with posaconazole in hematology patients: an evolving bedside to bench story. Haematologica 99:603–604

Slavin MA, Osborne B, Adams R et al (1995) Efficacy and safety of fluconazole prophylaxis for fungal infections after marrow transplantation—a prospective, randomized, double-blind study. J Infect Dis 171:1545–1552

Stilgenbauer S, Eichhorst B, Schetelig J et al (2016) Venetoclax in relapsed or refractory chronic lymphocytic leukaemia with 17p deletion: a multicentre, open-label, phase 2 study. Lancet Oncol 17:768–778

Tang H, Shi W, Song Y, Han J (2019) Voriconazole exposure and risk of cutaneous squamous cell carcinoma among lung or hematopoietic cell transplant patients: a systematic review and meta-analysis. J Am Acad Dermatol 80:500–507.e10

Taplitz RA, Kennedy EB, Bow EJ et al (2018) Antimicrobial prophylaxis for adult patients with cancer related immunosuppression: ASCO and IDSA clinical practice guideline update. J Clin Oncol 36:3043–3054

Ullmann AJ, Lipton JH, Vesole DH et al (2007) Posaconazole or fluconazole for prophylaxis in severe graft-versus-host disease. N Engl J Med 356:335–347

Ullmann AJ, Schmidt-Hieber M, Bertz H et al (2016) Infectious diseases in allogeneic haematopoietic stem cell transplantation: prevention and prophylaxis strategy guidelines 2016. Ann Hematol 95(9):1435–1455

Ullmann AJ, Aguado JM, Arikan-Akdagli S et al (2018) Diagnosis and management of Aspergillus diseases: executive summary of the 2017 ESCMID-ECMM-ERS guideline. Clin Microbiol Infect 24(Suppl 1):e1–e38

Valdez JM, Scheinberg P, Young NS, Walsh TJ (2009) Infections in patients with aplastic anemia. Semin Hematol 46:269–276

Varughese T, Taur Y, Cohen N et al (2018) Serious infections in patients receiving ibrutinib for treatment of lymphoid malignancies. Clin Infect Dis 67:687–692

Vena A, Bouza E, Alvarez-Uria A et al (2017) The misleading effect of serum galactomannan testing in high-risk haematology patients receiving prophylaxis with micafungin. Clin Microbiol Infect 23:1000.e1–4

Weinberger M, Elattar I, Marshall D et al (1992) Patterns of infection in patients with aplastic anemia and the emergence of Aspergillus as a major cause of death. Medicine (Baltimore) 71:24–43

Wingard JR, Carter SL, Walsh TJ et al (2010) Randomized, double-blind trial of fluconazole versus voriconazole for prevention of invasive fungal infection after allogeneic hematopoietic cell transplantation. Blood 116:5111–5118

Wojenski DJ, Bartoo GT, Merten JA et al (2015) Voriconazole exposure and the risk of cutaneous squamous cell carcinoma in allogeneic hematopoietic stem cell transplant patients. Transpl Infect Dis 17:250–258

Yee GC, Self SG, McGuire TR et al (1988) Serum cyclosporine concentration and risk of acute graft-versus-host disease after allogeneic marrow transplantation. N Engl J Med 319:65–70

Antiviral Prophylaxis

4

Johan A. Maertens and Zdeněk Ráčil

Viral infections account for a great majority of acute infections in humans, resulting in significant morbidity and greatly contributing to permanent disability and mortality in many immunocompromised patients, including those receiving treatments for hematological disorders, such as patients diagnosed with acute and chronic leukemia, lymphoma, and myeloma. However, within the hematology population, recipients of hematopoietic cell transplantation (HCT) appear to have the greatest risk. In this latter group, some viral infections are more phase-dependent, whereas other infections may be encountered in all transplant phases. For instance, infections with adenovirus and respiratory viruses are diagnosed in all phases after HCT, whereas manifestations of herpes simplex virus 1 and 2 are mostly seen during the pre-engraftment period, infections due to cytomegalovirus and human herpes virus-6 in the early post-engraftment phase, and

infections by Epstein–Barr virus and varicella-zoster virus often after day 100 post-transplant.

To date, pharmacological prophylaxis is only tested and approved for a small fraction of these viral pathogens. For most viruses, such as the respiratory viruses, antiviral prophylaxis is not available and/or not recommended (Table 4.1). In these latter settings, infection control measures and vaccination strategies, and adequate donor selection policies remain the first lines of prevention. However, addressing these topics is beyond the scope of this chapter, which focuses exclusively on the use of pharmacological antiviral prophylaxis in adult hematology patients.

4.1 Herpes Viruses

Seven of eight herpes viruses are well known for causing clinical syndromes in hematology patients: herpes simplex virus (HSV) type 1 and 2, varicella-zoster virus (VZV), Epstein–Barr virus (EBV), cytomegalovirus (CMV), human herpes virus (HHV)-6, and HHV-8. HHV-7 is an uncommon cause of morbidity in these patients. Primary infection (usually preceding the diagnosis of the hematological disorder) is normally resolved by the host's innate immune system, whereafter these viruses establish latency in specific host cells. However, during episodes of disrupted host immunity (resulting from disease or its treatment), these organisms can re-establish

J. A. Maertens (✉)
Department of Hematology, University Hospitals Leuven, Leuven, Belgium

Department of Microbiology, Immunology and Transplantation, University of Leuven, Leuven, Belgium
e-mail: johan.maertens@uzleuven.be

Z. Ráčil (✉)
Institute of Heamtology and Blood Transfusion, Prague, Czech Republic
e-mail: Zdenek.Racil@uhkt.cz

© Springer Nature Switzerland AG 2021

O. A. Cornely, M. Hoenigl (eds.), *Infection Management in Hematology*, Hematologic Malignancies, https://doi.org/10.1007/978-3-030-57317-1_4

Table 4.1 Antiviral prophylaxis in adult hematology patients: based on recommendations of European Conference on Infections in leukemia (ECIL) and European Blood and Marrow Transplantation (EBMT) handbook

Viral pathogen	Recommended antiviral prophylaxis	Comments
Herpes simplex virus type 1 and 2	• Oral acyclovir 3 × 200 mg to 2 × 800 mg/day. • Intravenous acyclovir 250 mg/m² or 5 mg/kg every 12 h.	Oral valacyclovir 2 × 500 mg/day or famciclovir 2 × 500 mg/day are lower recommended alternatives
Varicella-zoster virus	• Oral acyclovir 800 mg bid or valacyclovir 500 mg once or twice daily.	Post-exposure prophylaxis with acyclovir 800 mg five times daily, valacyclovir 1000 mg three times daily, or famciclovir 500 mg three times daily
Epstein–Barr virus	No prophylaxis recommended	
Cytomegalovirus	Letermovir 480 mg (or 240 mg if co-administered with cyclosporine)/day	
Human herpes virus type 6	No prophylaxis recommended/available	Foscarnet has been used with non-conclusive results
Human herpes virus type 7	No prophylaxis recommended/available	
Human herpes virus type 8	No prophylaxis recommended/available	
Influenza virus	No prophylaxis recommended	• Post-exposure prophylaxis with oseltamivir 75 mg twice daily for 10 days. • Isolation and infection control measures to prevent horizontal transmission. • Annual vaccination.
Respiratory syncytial virus	No prophylaxis recommended	Infection control measures
Parainfluenza virus	No prophylaxis recommended	Infection control measures
Human metapneumovirus	No prophylaxis recommended	Infection control measures
Rhinovirus	No prophylaxis recommended/available	Infection control measures
Human coronavirus	No prophylaxis recommended/available	Infection control measures
Enterovirus	No prophylaxis recommended/available	Infection control measures
Adenovirus	No prophylaxis recommended	Infection control measures
Human bocavirus	No prophylaxis recommended/available	
Polyoma JC virus	No prophylaxis recommended/available	
BK virus	No prophylaxis recommended/available	
Parvovirus B19	No prophylaxis recommended/available	
Human papillomavirus	No prophylaxis recommended/available	
Hepatitis A virus	No prophylaxis recommended/available	Vaccination of HAV-seronegative patients
Hepatitis B virus	Tenofovir or entecavir once daily	For at-risk patients: see chapter on vaccination
Hepatitis C virus	No prophylaxis recommended	
Hepatitis D virus	No prophylaxis recommended/available	
Hepatitis E virus	No prophylaxis available	
Norovirus	No prophylaxis recommended/available	Infection control measures
Zika virus	No prophylaxis recommended/available	Testing of blood products and grafts for the presence of Zika virus

lytic viral replication and disease, whereas HHV-8 and EBV are also able to induce malignant proliferations of latency-infected cells.

Although HHV-6, HHV-7, HHV-8, and EBV can cause life-threatening complications, including encephalitis, myelitis, and the development of malignant tumors, antiviral chemoprophylaxis is not recommended (Ljungman et al. 2008). Herein, we will review aspects of infection and reactivation of the four remaining herpes viruses and the role of chemoprophylaxis in hematology patients. Of note, antiviral drugs that rely on viral kinases for their activation (such as acyclovir and ganciclovir) are only effective during the lytic phases (primary infection or reactivation) as these kinases are not expressed during latency.

4.1.1 Herpes Simplex Virus (HSV)

Up to 80% of adult patients with hematological diseases are HSV-seropositive. Following primary infection, the virus establishes latency in the neuronal cells of sensory nerve ganglia, waiting to reactivate during periods of immunosuppression. HSV type 1, and to a lesser extent HSV type 2, are common causes of mucocutaneous lesions. They usually result from viral reactivation, whereas primary infection is unusual. Most lesions are localized in the orofacial region and less frequently in the esophageal and anogenital area. In patients with concurrent chemotherapy-induced or radiation therapy-associated mucosal damage, diagnosis can be suspected on clinical grounds but should ideally be confirmed by appropriate diagnostic techniques such as viral culture and/or detection of HSV DNA by PCR. Although more severe disease manifestations such as hepatitis, pneumonitis, meningitis, and encephalitis have all been reported, these appear to be rare (Levin et al. 2016).

Reactivation of HSV is very frequent following intensive chemotherapy for acute leukemia and in HSV-seropositive stem cell transplant recipients, both autologous and allogeneic. Rates as high as 60% and 80%, respectively, have been reported, especially during the first month after transplantation (Bustamante and Wade 1991; Meyers et al. 1980). These exceptional high rates of reactivation and their associated morbidity justify the use of prophylaxis in HSV-seropositive patients; conversely, antiviral prophylaxis is not recommended in HSV-seronegative patients.

Following a number of successful prophylaxis studies, acyclovir has become a drug of choice for many immunocompromised patients at risk of HSV reactivation (Saral et al. 1981; Gluckman et al. 1983; Hann et al. 1983; Shepp et al. 1987;

Bergmann et al. 1995). When given intravenously or orally, this nucleoside analog requires the first activation by triphosphorylation whereby the conversion to acyclovir monophosphate involves a thymidine kinase encoded by HSV (or varicella-zoster virus: see below). Newer antiviral compounds (such as valaciclovir and famciclovir) with greatly improved oral bioavailability compared to that of oral acyclovir are also commonly used, although less studied (Balfour 1999; Orlowski et al. 2004). The European Conference on Infections in Leukemia (ECIL) recommends the following dosing regimens: oral acyclovir 3×200 mg to 2×800 mg/day, oral valaciclovir 2×500 mg/day, or famciclovir 2×500 mg/ day. Obviously, in patients with severe mucositis, the intravenous route is preferred using acyclovir 250 mg/m^2 or 5 mg/kg every 12 h. Prophylaxis is continued for 3–5 weeks after the start of chemotherapy or after transplantation but may be significantly prolonged in the setting of graft-versus-host disease and/or corticosteroid treatment (Styczynski et al. 2009).

Resistance to acyclovir, although emerging (e.g., following T-cell-depleted allogeneic transplants), remains a rare event and is associated with viral thymidine kinase deficiency (Chen et al. 2000). These resistant strains remain, however, susceptible to antiviral drugs that do not require viral thymidine kinase for activation, including foscarnet or cidofovir (Styczynski et al. 2009; Chen et al. 2000; Blot et al. 2000).

4.1.2 Varicella-Zoster Virus (VZV)

Primary infection with VZV, usually during childhood and early adulthood years, causes varicella (or "chickenpox"), a highly contagious disease that is—unlike other herpes viruses—transmissible via the respiratory route. Hereafter, the virus establishes latency in the dorsal root and cranial ganglia. In VZV-seropositive immunocompromised patients, reactivation usually manifests as painful herpes zoster (or "shingles"), frequently involving multiple dermatomes. In addition, VZV-seronegative hematology patients who are exposed to individuals with VZV manifestations are at increased risk of developing varicella, especially when receiving corticosteroids at the same time. These varicella cases may present as a generalized, vesicular rash, with or without visceral dissemination (Dowell and Bresee 1993; Hill et al. 2005).

The incidence of VZV disease among hematology patients varies widely and depends largely on factors that affect the cell-mediated immune competence, such as patient's age, underlying tumor type, and antineoplastic treatment. Especially patients with underlying lymphoproliferative disorders and VZV-seropositive cell transplant recipients (autologous as well as allogeneic) carry a high risk for VZV disease and severe complications. In the absence of adequate prophylaxis, up to 25% of adult patients with acute lymphoblastic leukemia or Hodgkin's lymphoma develop VZV disease (Novelli et al. 1988). Even higher rates have been reported in seropositive transplant recipients. These infections typically occur at a median of 5–6 months post-engraftment, but may appear years later, especially in patients suffering from chronic graft-versus-host disease (Atkinson et al. 1980). More recently, the risk of VZV infection has also significantly increased in other patient populations due to the introduction of therapies that profoundly impact on cellular immunity: purine analogs (fludarabine, pentostatin, and cladribine), alemtuzumab, temozolomide, and the proteasome inhibitor bortezomib.

Specific measures for minimizing the risk of transmission (e.g., airborne and contact isolation) and vaccination guidelines are reviewed elsewhere. Epidemiological studies are needed to discern the effect of new VZV vaccines on the risk of VZV reactivation in cancer patients (Winston et al. 2018). Meanwhile, there is a firm recommendation for the use of chemoprophylaxis in VZV-seronegative patients at high-risk following exposure to varicella or herpes zoster: uncontrolled data suggest that post-exposure prophylaxis with therapeutic doses of acyclovir (800 mg five times daily), valacyclovir (1000 mg three times daily), or famciclovir (500 mg three times daily) reduces both the incidence and severity of VZV manifestations. Post-exposure prophylaxis should commence as soon as possible and be given until 21 days after exposure. In VZV-seropositive patients, post-exposure prophylaxis remains optional (Styczynski et al. 2009).

Several retrospective and three prospective randomized placebo-controlled studies have examined the role of acyclovir prophylaxis primarily in cell transplant recipients (Ljungman et al. 1986; Perren et al. 1988; Boeckh et al. 2006). While acyclovir effectively prevents herpes zoster infection during the treatment period (when given for up to 12 months), late reactivations after discontinuation of prophylaxis are frequent, especially in chronically immunosuppressed patients. Presumably, prolonged antiviral prophylaxis prevents VZV-specific immune reconstitution, resulting in a rebound phenomenon. The EBMT recommends prophylaxis with oral acyclovir (800 mg twice daily) or oral valacyclovir (500 mg twice daily) for at least one year (and longer in the presence of graft-versus-host disease and immunosuppressive therapy) in VZV-seropositive allogeneic transplant recipients (Erard et al. 2007; www.ebmt.org/education/ebmt-handbook n.d.). However, the optimal duration of chemoprophylaxis is a matter of ongoing debate and may be better guided by measuring specific T-cell immune responses. The role of prophylaxis in the autologous setting is unclear.

4.1.3 Cytomegalovirus (CMV)

Human cytomegalovirus is a common opportunistic infection after HCT but is encountered less frequently among patients undergoing cytotoxic therapy. Notable exceptions are the combined use of fludarabine and high-dose cyclophosphamide, following alemtuzumab therapy, and more recently the use of idelalisib for chronic lymphocytic leukemia. CMV is transmitted through infected body fluids such as saliva, blood, urine, semen, tears, and breast milk. Seroprevalence rates in adults range from 30–40% in most industrialized countries to almost 100% in the developing world.

An acute CMV infection in an immunocompetent host often remains unnoticed, although prolonged fever, pharyngitis, and/or mild hepatitis can occur. Primo-infections are self-limiting in most cases. The immune system effectively eliminates the virus from the infected tissues, but the viral genome remains latent within the host cells whereby reactivation can occur at any time. Uncontrolled viral replication gives rise to CMV infection and subsequent disease in patients with severely compromised T-cell immunity such as HIV-infected patients, cancer patients, and transplant recipients.

CMV infection is defined as the isolation of virions or detection of nucleic acids or viral proteins (antigens such as pp65) in any body fluid or tissue specimen. The infection is called symptomatic in case of fever and/or bone marrow suppression. CMV disease is defined by the presence of organ involvement (lung, digestive tract, liver, retina, and central nervous system) (Ljungman et al. 2017). CMV primo-infection or reactivation can result in substantial morbidity and mortality in the immunocompromised host. Moreover, CMV reactivation is associated with an increased risk of other opportunistic infections, graft failure, and possibly also graft-versus-host disease in HCT recipients because of the indirect effects on the immune system (Boeckh and Geballe 2011). The risk of CMV reactivation depends on the serological status of recipient and donor (highest risk for seropositive recipients with a seronegative donor), the degree of T-cell depletion, and the intensity of immunosuppression.

The nucleoside analog ganciclovir (GCV), its oral prodrug valganciclovir (VGCV), the nucleotide analog cidofovir (CDV), and the anion pyrophosphate analog foscarnet (PFA) are all approved for CMV treatment. Unfortunately, these drugs are myelosuppressive (GCV and VGCV), nephrotoxic (CDV and PFA), and causes of electrolyte disturbances (PFA) (Griffiths and Lumley 2014). The risk of these side effects increased with concomitant administration of other myelosuppressive or nephrotoxic drugs that are often used in at-risk patients. For these reasons, these drugs, although proven effective to prevent reactivation in clinical studies, have not gained major popularity as prophylactic agents in the vulnerable hematology population.

The nucleosides GCV and VGCV are first activated by triphosphorylation; the active product acts as a competitive substrate for CMV DNA polymerase during viral DNA synthesis. The first step of the phosphorylation process is catalyzed by the viral kinase UL97, the subsequent second step and third step are catalyzed by host cellular kinases. Mutations in UL97 are a major cause of resistance against the first-line agents GCV and VGCV. CDV also inhibits CMV DNA polymerase following phosphorylation by cellular kinases. CDV competitively inhibits the incorporation of deoxycytidine triphosphate by viral DNA polymerase during viral DNA replication, whereas PFA (does not require phosphorylation) directly inhibits polymerase function by blocking the pyrophosphate binding site. The viral DNA polymerase is encoded by UL54. Mutations of UL54 result in varying degrees of cross-resistance among GCV, CDV, and PFA (Hecke et al. 2019).

There are two accepted strategies to prevent CMV manifestations in immunocompromised patients: a preemptive and a prophylactic approach (Maertens and Lyon 2017). The main goal of the preemptive approach is to prevent CMV disease in patients with documented CMV infection, while prophylaxis focuses on the prevention of CMV reactivation/infection. Both strategies are used in concert with general measures regarding optimal donor selection and transfusion of blood products aiming to prevent CMV transmission from one person to another.

Following HSCT, preemptive management is nowadays standard practice of care in most transplant centers and is also recommended by international guidelines. Patients are monitored at least weekly for CMV reactivation using quantitative PCR for the detection of viral DNA (Ljungman et al. 2008). Treatment with antiviral drugs (usually oral valganciclovir or intravenous ganciclovir) is initiated as soon as (mostly asymptomatic) CMV reactivation is confirmed to prevent progression to clinical disease. Preemptive anti-CMV therapy has proven to be very successful; overall, the incidence of tissue-invasive CMV disease has been reduced to less than 3% in recent large clinical trials and to around 10% in daily clinical practice (Green et al. 2016).

Although a preemptive approach successfully prevents CMV end-organ disease, this surveillance-based strategy still allows for CMV reactivation (Green et al. 2016). However, a retrospective analysis of the Fred Hutchinson Cancer Research Center (Seattle) database suggests a negative effect of any degree of reactivation, especially during the first 2 months after transplant (Green et al. 2016). In addition, in a large CIBMTR analysis, CMV reactivation remains associated with increased non-relapse mortality rates, even in the current era of preemptive therapy (Teira et al. 2016). So, despite the proven effectiveness of preemptive therapy in preventing life-threatening CMV disease, allowing low-level CMV reactivation still comes with negative long-term effects, which could potentially be prevented by a prophylactic approach.

On the other hand, routine prophylaxis would expose many patients to the toxic effects of the available antiviral armamentarium, while only 40–80% of these patients may actually need preemptive therapy. Especially the prophylactic use of ganciclovir is problematic in this setting because of the high rates of neutropenia, the increased risk for bacterial and fungal infections, and the occurrence of late-onset CMV disease. Hence, the unmet need for an efficacious anti-CMV drug without dose-limiting toxicities such as bone marrow suppression and renal toxicity. Fortunately, several new antiviral drugs have been developed in recent years.

Brincidofovir is an oral, lipid-conjugated formulation of cidofovir, which is dosed twice weekly. It displays broad antiviral activity beyond CMV and is less nephrotoxic compared to cidofovir (Marty et al. 2013). Contrary to the initial positive results of a dosed-ranging phase 2 trial, the subsequent phase 3 trial failed to meet its primary endpoint of preventing clinically significant CMV infections within 24 weeks after HSCT (Marty et al. 2016). Brincidofovir causes GI toxicity, histologically characterized by epithelial apoptosis and crypt injury (Detweiler et al. 2018). These features mimic those seen in acute intestinal graft versus host disease and mycophenolate mofetil toxicity and may result in an increased

use of corticosteroids, thereby further increasing the risk of CMV reactivation.

Maribavir is an oral drug with specific activity against CMV by competitively inhibiting the CMV protein kinase UL97, thereby preventing nuclear egress of virions. The results of the dose-escalating phase 2 study were promising (Winston et al. 2008), but a placebo-controlled phase 3 study did not meet its primary endpoint of preventing CMV disease following HSC allograft. The tolerability was good with dysgeusia being the most common side effect (Marty et al. 2011).

Letermovir demonstrates potent, selective, and reversible inhibition of CMV replication by targeting the pUL56, pUL51, or both subunits of the viral terminase complex, a mechanism of action, which differs from that of currently marketed anti-CMV drugs (Razonable and Melendez 2015). This enzyme plays an important role in the cleavage of viral DNA concatemers into unit-length genome and packaging into procapsids to form mature virions. Mechanism-based side effects are unlikely due to the lack of a mammalian counterpart to the viral terminase complex. Letermovir is highly specific for human CMV and lacks inhibitory activity against other pathogenic viruses.

Letermovir can be given both orally (480 mg [240 mg when co-administered with cyclosporine] once daily) and intravenously. The drug is a weak-to-moderate inhibitor of CYP3A (resulting in increased serum levels of, e.g., sirolimus, tacrolimus), a weak–to-moderate inducer of CYP2C9/19 (decreasing levels of, e.g., voriconazole), and an inhibitor of organic anion transporting polypeptide (OATP)1B1/3. There is no significant interaction with mycophenolate or posaconazole. However, letermovir is contraindicated in patients taking pimozide or ergot alkaloids and in patients receiving simvastatin plus cyclosporine (Kim 2018).

The potential benefit of letermovir was first shown in a double-blind, placebo-controlled, dose-ranging phase 2 study in allogeneic HCT recipients. The incidence of CMV prophylaxis failure (defined as CMV viremia and/or CMV end-organ disease or study drug discontinuation prior to day 84 due to any reason) decreased across increasing letermovir dose groups (60 mg

QD, 120 mg QD, or 240 mg QD) and was highest in the placebo group (Chemaly et al. 2014a). Based on further analysis of the exposure–response curves and the favorable safety profile, the dose selected for the pivotal phase 3 registration study was 240 mg QD with concomitant cyclosporine administration and 480 mg QD without cyclosporine. Adult CMV seropositive patients undergoing allogeneic HCT were randomized 1:1 to letermovir or placebo within a median of 9 days (range, 0–28) after transplantation. At baseline, one-third of patients had engrafted. Patients who had undetectable plasma CMV DNA within 5 days of randomization received letermovir or placebo, for up to 14 weeks after transplantation. Overall, a significantly lower risk of clinically significant CMV infection (disease as well as pre-emptive therapy) among letermovir recipients than among placebo recipients by week 24 after transplantation (37.5% vs. 60.6%, P < 0,001) was noticed. Of these, 1.5% of letermovir subjects and 1.8% of placebo subjects were diagnosed with CMV end-organ disease, mainly gastrointestinal. In addition, all-cause mortality at week 24 after transplantation was significantly lower in the letermovir group compared to the placebo group (10.2% vs. 15.9%, P = 0.03), although the significance was not sustained at week 48 (p = 0.12). In general, the beneficial effect of letermovir was more pronounced in the high-risk stratum, including patients undergoing haploidentical or HLA-mismatched transplantation, cord blood recipients, and transplantations with ex-vivo T-cell-depleted grafts (Marty et al. 2017).

Letermovir is generally well tolerated, with gastrointestinal side effects being the most common ones. There was no evidence of increased myelotoxicity or nephrotoxicity (Marty et al. 2017). However, it has also become clear that extended prophylaxis (beyond week 14) may be needed, especially in patients with delayed recovery of CMV-specific T-cell immunity; many of these patients belong to the higher risk stratum including recipients of T-cell-depleted grafts, cord blood graft transplants or patients on augmented immunosuppression to treat GvHD. As for VZV, the optimal duration of prophylaxis might be better guided by functional assessments of CMV-specific cell-mediated immunity (e.g., by QuantiFERON-CMV or T-Track-CMV assays). Such approaches might even prove to be cost-effective compared to routine prophylaxis (Westall et al. 2019).

4.2   Respiratory Viruses

Community-acquired respiratory viruses are now recognized as common causes of acute respiratory illness in immunocompromised cancer patients. Contrary to immunocompetent individuals, hematology patients (in particular leukemia patients and HCT recipients) usually present with prolonged viral shedding and high rates of disease progression to the lower respiratory tract with clinico-radiological signs of pneumonia, resulting in mortality rates between 10 and 50% (Green 2017; Chemaly et al. 2014b; Hirsch et al. 2013). These viral infections often precede bacterial and fungal infections. The most common human pathogenic viruses causing respiratory infection in hematology patients include influenza viruses, respiratory syncytial virus (RSV), and parainfluenza viruses (PIV) (Wade 2006). However, all respiratory viruses can cause infections, including rhinoviruses, coronaviruses, human metapneumovirus (hMPV), adenovirus, human bocavirus, and enteroviruses. Some of these viruses show seasonality in temperate climates (e.g., influenza and RSV) whereas others remain a threat throughout the year (e.g., PIV). Although not generally considered respiratory viruses, also CMV, HSV, and VZV can present as lower respiratory tract infections.

For most of these community respiratory viruses, specific antiviral therapy is not (yet) available. Notable exceptions are influenza A and B infections, which can preferentially be treated with the oral neuraminidase inhibitor oseltamivir (75 to 150 mg bid for 10 days, mainly to prevent complications), and adenovirus infections, which may respond to cidofovir. For RSV, hMPV, and PIV, ribavirin (intravenous, aerosolized, or oral) with or without the concomitant administration of intravenous immunoglobulins has been used with variable success. No specific therapy is available for rhinovirus, coronavirus, and enterovirus infections, but most patients respond well to supportive measures.

Primary antiviral chemoprophylaxis is not recommended for any of these respiratory pathogens. Annual inactivated influenza vaccination of at-risk patients, their health care workers, and household contacts remains the mainstay of influenza prevention in immunocompromised persons (Hirsch et al. 2013). For all other respiratory viruses, no licensed vaccines are available. However, ECIL-4 experts recommend post-exposure prophylaxis for 10 days with oseltamivir for HCT recipients who are less than 1 year after transplant and for leukemia patients undergoing chemotherapy after exposure to a confirmed or probable case of influenza, regardless of their vaccination status (Hirsch et al. 2013).

These infections are transmitted from person-to-person through small-particle aerosols, large droplets, or direct or indirect contact with virus-containing secretions. Autoinoculation of mucosal surfaces following contamination of hands is a very common route of transmission. Routine infection control measures play a key role in containing the spread of the infection and preventing nosocomial outbreaks. Hand hygiene is of utmost importance. In addition, the use of surgical masks might be beneficial. Patients with documented infection should be isolated and strict protection measurements should be applied to visitors and health care workers (including wearing gloves, gowns, masks, and eye protection) (Hirsch et al. 2013). Finally, reducing the dose of corticosteroids (if applicable) should be attempted, since corticosteroids have been identified as an independent risk factor for disease progression and overall mortality for most respiratory viruses (except for influenza virus).

4.3   Hepatotropic Viruses

Increasing numbers of patients with hematological conditions and recipients (as well as donors) of HCT have evidence of resolved or active hepatitis B (HBV) or hepatitis C (HCV) viral infection. In addition, hepatitis E virus (HEV) is becoming more prevalent (von Felden et al.

2019). HBV reactivation during immunosuppressive therapy is common, not only in HBV surface antigen (HBsAg)-positive patients, but even in case of resolved infection, and may result in hepatitis flares and even liver failure. HBsAg-positive individuals are at high risk of reactivation during most immunosuppressive therapies with a clear dose/duration–risk association. HBsAg-negative/anti-HB core antibody-positive patients are at lower risk except for allogeneic HCT recipients (frequently showing delayed reactivation) and patients receiving anti-CD20 monoclonal antibodies (such as rituximab and ofatumumab). In these two particular high-risk settings, guidelines strongly recommend antiviral prophylaxis with nucleoside or nucleotide analogs from the start of immunosuppressive therapy until at least 1 year after cessation of therapy. ECIL-5 and other guidelines recommend the once daily oral administration of the third-generation agent tenofovir or entecavir as drugs of choice (Mallet et al. 2016). These drugs are preferred to lamivudine because of their higher genetic barrier to antiviral resistance.

Patients who have successfully eliminated HCV are not at risk for reactivation during immunosuppressive therapy. However, those with chronic HCV infection (presence of HCV RNA) should receive antiviral therapy as soon as feasible (if possible even postponing the transplant/therapy till completion of the antiviral course), following the advice of a hepatologist (Mallet et al. 2016). Expert advice is also needed for patients with chronic HEV, in whom therapy with ribavirin can be considered, and for patients with hepatitis D virus co-infection. Vaccination should be considered for HAV-negative hematology patients undergoing immunosuppressive therapies.

4.4   Polyomaviruses

Reactivation of the neurotropic John Cunningham polyomavirus may cause progressive multifocal leukoencephalopathy. Cases have occasionally been described following HCT and after the use of immunomodulatory drugs such as rituximab, natalizumab, and brentuximab. No prophylaxis can be given.

Reactivation of the polyomavirus BK plays a key role in the development of post-transplant hemorrhagic cystitis (HC) and renal dysfunction. The incidence of HC is clearly on the rise since the introduction of un-manipulated haplo-HCT followed by high-dose cyclophosphamide to prevent graft versus host disease. Antiviral prophylaxis is not recommended.

4.5   Other Viruses

Norovirus can cause severe and complicated gastroenteritis. Unfortunately, no antiviral prophylaxis can be given. Strict isolation and general infection control measures (hand hygiene) are mandatory.

Finally, more and more patients infected with human immunodeficiency virus (HIV) are diagnosed with hematologic cancer or undergo hematopoietic cell transplantation procedures (Kwon et al. 2019). Specific follow-up and decisions about antiviral prophylaxis should include the advice of an HIV expert.

References

Atkinson K, Meyers JD, Storb R, Prentice RL, Thomas ED (1980) Varicella-zoster virus infection after marrow transplantation for aplastic anemia or leukemia. Transplantation 29(1):47–50

Balfour HH (1999) Antiviral drugs. N Engl J Med 340:1255–1268

Bergmann OJ, Ellermann-Eriksen S, Mogensen SC, Ellegaard J (1995) Acyclovir given as prophylaxis against oral ulcers in acute myeloid leukaemia: randomised, double blind, placebo controlled trial. BMJ 310(6988):1169–1172

Blot N, Schneider P, Young P, Janvresse C, Dehesdin D, Tron P, Vannier JP (2000) Treatment of an acyclovir and foscarnet-resistant herpes simplex virus infection with cidofovir in a child after an unrelated bone marrow transplant. Bone Marrow Transplant 26(8):903–905

Boeckh M, Geballe AP (2011) Cytomegalovirus: pathogen, paradigm, and puzzle. J Clin Invest 121(5):1673–1680

Boeckh M, Kim HW, Flowers ME, Meyers JD, Bowden RA (2006) Long-term acyclovir for prevention of vari-cella zoster virus disease after allogeneic hematopoietic cell transplantation--a randomized double-blind placebo-controlled study. Blood 107(5):1800–1805

Bustamante CI, Wade JC (1991) Herpes simplex virus infection in the immunocompromised cancer patient. J Clin Oncol 9(10):1903–1915

Chemaly RF, Ullmann AJ, Stoelben S et al (2014a) Letermovir for cytomegalovirus prophylaxis in hematopoietic-cell transplantation. N Engl J Med 370(19):1781–1789

Chemaly RF, Shah DP, Boeckh MJ (2014b) Management of respiratory viral infections in hematopoietic cell transplant recipients and patients with hematologic malignancies. Clin Infect Dis 59(Suppl 5):S344–S351

Chen Y, Scieux C, Garrait V, Socié G, Rocha V, Molina JM, Thouvenot D, Morfin F, Hocqueloux L, Garderet L, Espérou H, Sélimi F, Devergie A, Leleu G, Aymard M, Morinet F, Gluckman E, Ribaud P (2000) Resistant herpes simplex virus type 1 infection: an emerging concern after allogeneic stem cell transplantation. Clin Infect Dis 31(4):927–935

Detweiler CJ, Mueller SB, Sung AD, Saullo JL, Prasad VK, Cardona DM (2018) Brincidofovir (CMX001) Toxicity Associated With Epithelial Apoptosis and Crypt Drop Out in a Hematopoietic Cell Transplant Patient: Challenges in Distinguishing Drug Toxicity From GVHD. J Pediatr Hematol Oncol 40(6):e364–e368

Dowell SF, Bresee JS (1993) Severe varicella associated with steroid use. Pediatrics 92(2):223–228

Erard V, Guthrie KA, Varley C, Heugel J, Wald A, Flowers ME, Corey L, Boeckh M (2007) One-year acyclovir prophylaxis for preventing varicella-zoster virus disease after hematopoietic cell transplantation: no evidence of rebound varicella-zoster virus disease after drug discontinuation. Blood 110(8):3071–3077

von Felden J, Alric L, Pischke S, Aitken C, Schlabe S, Spengler U, Teresa Giordani M, Schnitzler P, Bettinger D, Thimme R, Xhaard A, Binder M, Ayuk F, Lohse AW, Cornelissen JJ, de Man RA, Mallet V, von Felden J, Alric L, Pischke S, Aitken C, Schlabe S, Spengler U, Teresa Giordani M, Schnitzler P, Bettinger D, Thimme R, Xhaard A, Binder M, Ayuk F, Lohse AW, Cornelissen JJ, de Man RA, Mallet V (2019) J Hepatol. https://doi.org/10.1016/j.jhep.2019.04.022. [Epub ahead of print]

Gluckman E, Lotsberg J, Devergie A, Zhao XM, Melo R, Gomez-Morales M, Nebout T, Mazeron MC, Perol Y (1983) Prophylaxis of herpes infections after bone-marrow transplantation by oral acyclovir. Lancet 2(8352):706–708

Green ML (2017) Viral Pneumonia in Patients with Hematopoietic Cell Transplantation and Hematologic Malignancies. Clin Chest Med 38(2):295–305

Green ML, Leisenring W, Xie H, Mast TC, Cui Y, Sandmaier BM, Sorror ML, Goyal S, Özkök S, Yi J, Sahoo F, Kimball LE, Jerome KR, Marks MA, Boeckh M (2016) Cytomegalovirus viral load and mortality after haemopoietic stem cell transplantation in the era of pre-emptive therapy: a retrospective cohort study. Lancet Haematol 3(3):e119–e127

Griffiths P, Lumley S (2014) Cytomegalovirus. Curr Opin Infect Dis 27(6):554–559

Hann IM, Prentice HG, Blacklock HA, Ross MG, Brigden D, Rosling AE, Burke C, Crawford DH, Brumfitt W, Hoffbrand AV. Acyclovir prophylaxis against herpes virus infections in severely immunocompromised patients: randomised double blind trial Br Med J (Clin Res Ed) 1983;287(6389):384–8

Hecke SV, Calcoen B, Lagrou K, Maertens J (2019) Letermovir for prophylaxis of cytomegalovirus manifestations in adult allogeneic hematopoietic stem cell transplant recipients. Future Microbiol 14:175–184

Hill G, Chauvenet AR, Lovato J, McLean TW (2005) Recent steroid therapy increases severity of varicella infections in children with acute lymphoblastic leukemia. Pediatrics 116(4):e525–e529

Hirsch HH, Martino R, Ward KN, Boeckh M, Einsele H, Ljungman P (2013) Fourth European Conference on Infections in Leukaemia (ECIL-4): guidelines for diagnosis and treatment of human respiratory syncytial virus, parainfluenza virus, metapneumovirus, rhinovirus, and coronavirus. Clin Infect Dis 56(2):258–266

Kim ES (2018) Letermovir: First Global Approval. Drugs 78(1):147–152

Kwon M, Bailén R, Balsalobre P, Jurado M, Bermudez A, Badiola J, Esquirol A, Miralles P, López-Fernández E, Sanz J, Yanez L, Colorado M, Piñana JL, Dorado N, Solán L, Laperche CM, Anguita J, Serrano D, Díez-Martin JL, Grupo Español de Trasplante Hematopoyético y Terapia Celular (GETH) (2019) Allogeneic stem cell transplantation in HIV-1 infected patients with high-risk hematological disorders. AIDS. https://doi.org/10.1097/QAD.0000000000002209. [Epub ahead of print]

Levin MJ, Weinberg A, Schmid DS (2016) Herpes Simplex Virus and Varicella-Zoster virus. Microbiol Spectr 4(3). https://doi.org/10.1128/microbiolspec

Ljungman P, Wilczek H, Gahrton G, Gustavsson A, Lundgren G, Lönnqvist B, Ringdén O, Wahren B (1986) Long-term acyclovir prophylaxis in bone marrow transplant recipients and lymphocyte proliferation responses to herpes virus antigens in vitro. Bone Marrow Transplant 1(2):185–192

Ljungman P, de la Camara R, Cordonnier C, Einsele H, Engelhard D, Reusser P, Styczynski J, Ward K, European Conference on Infections in Leukemia (2008) Management of CMV, HHV-6, HHV-7 and Kaposi-sarcoma herpesvirus (HHV-8) infections in patients with hematological malignancies and after SCT. Bone Marrow Transplant 42(4):227–240. https://doi.org/10.1038/bmt.2008.162

Ljungman P, Boeckh M, Hirsch HH, Josephson F, Lundgren J, Nichols G, Pikis A, Razonable RR, Miller V, Griffiths PD, Disease Definitions Working Group of the Cytomegalovirus Drug Development Forum (2017) Definitions of Cytomegalovirus Infection and Disease in Transplant Patients for Use in Clinical Trials. Clin Infect Dis 64(1):87–91

Maertens J, Lyon S (2017) Current and future options for cytomegalovirus reactivation in hematopoietic cell transplantation patients. Future Microbiol 12:839–842

Mallet V, van Bömmel F, Doerig C, Pischke S, Hermine O, Locasciulli A, Cordonnier C, Berg T, Moradpour D, Wedemeyer H, Ljungman P, ECIL-5 (2016) Management of viral hepatitis in patients with haematological malignancy and in patients undergoing haemopoietic stem cell transplantation: recommendations of the 5th European Conference on Infections in Leukaemia (ECIL-5). Lancet Infect Dis 16(5):606–617

Marty FM, Ljungman P, Papanicolaou GA et al (2011) Maribavir prophylaxis for prevention of cytomegalovirus disease in recipients of allogeneic stem-cell transplants: A phase 3, double-blind, placebo-controlled, randomised trial. Lancet Infect Dis 11(4):284–292

Marty FM, Winston DJ, Rowley SD, Vance E, Papanicolaou GA, Mullane KM, Brundage TM, Robertson AT, Godkin S, Momméja-Marin H, Boeckh M, CMX001-201 Clinical Study Group (2013) CMX001 to prevent cytomegalovirus disease in hematopoietic-cell transplantation. N Engl J Med 369(13):1227–1236

Marty FM, Winston DJ, Chemaly RF et al (2016) Brincidofovir for prevention of cytomegalovirus (CMV) after allogeneic hematopoietic cell transplantation (HCT) in CMV-seropositive patients: A randomized, double-blind, placebo-controlled, parallel-group phase 3 trial. Biol Blood Marrow Transplant 22(3):S23

Marty FM, Ljungman P, Chemaly RF et al (2017) Letermovir prophylaxis for cytomegalovirus in hematopoietic-cell transplantation. N Engl J Med 377(25):2433–2444

Meyers JD, Flournoy N, Thomas ED (1980) Infection with herpes simplex virus and cell-mediated immunity after marrow transplant. J Infect Dis 142(3):338–346

Novelli VM, Brunell PA, Geiser CF, Narkewicz S, Frierson L (1988) Herpes zoster in children with acute lymphocytic leukemia. Am J Dis Child 142(1):71–72

Orlowski RZ, Mills SR, Hartley EE, Ye X, Piantadosi S, Ambinder RF, Gore SD, Miller CB (2004) Oral valacyclovir as prophylaxis against herpes simplex virus reactivation during high dose chemotherapy for leukemia. Leuk Lymphoma. 45(11):2215–2219

Perren TJ, Powles RL, Easton D, Stolle K, Selby PJ (1988) Prevention of herpes zoster in patients by long-term oral acyclovir after allogeneic bone marrow transplantation. Am J Med 85(2A):99–101

Razonable R, Melendez D (2015) Letermovir and inhibitors of the terminase complex: a promising new class of investigational antiviral drugs against human cytomegalovirus. Infect Drug Resist 8:269

Saral R, Burns WH, Laskin OL, Santos GW, Lietman PS (1981) Acyclovir prophylaxis of herpes-simplex-virus infections. N Engl J Med 305(2):63–67

Shepp DH, Dandliker PS, Flournoy N, Meyers JD (1987) Sequential intravenous and twice-daily oral acyclovir for extended prophylaxis of herpes simplex virus infection in marrow transplant patient. Transplantation 43(5):654–658

Styczynski J, Reusser P, Einsele H, de la Camara R, Cordonnier C, Ward KN, Ljungman P, Engelhard D, Second European Conference on Infections in Leukemia (2009) Management of HSV, VZV and EBV infections in patients with hematological malignancies and after SCT: guidelines from the Second European Conference on Infections in Leukemia. Bone Marrow Transplant 43(10):757–770

Teira P, Battiwalla M, Ramanathan M, Barrett AJ, Ahn KW, Chen M, Green JS, Saad A, Antin JH, Savani BN, Lazarus HM, Seftel M, Saber W, Marks D, Aljurf M, Norkin M, Wingard JR, Lindemans CA, Boeckh M, Riches ML, Auletta JJ (2016) Early cytomegalovirus reactivation remains associated with increased transplant-related mortality in the current era: a CIBMTR analysis. Blood 127(20):2427–2438

Wade JC (2006) Viral infections in patients with hematological malignancies. Hematology Am Soc Hematol Educ Program 2006:368–374

Westall GP, Cristiano Y, Levvey BJ, Whitford H, Paraskeva MA, Paul E, Peleg AY, Snell GI (2019) A Randomized Study of Quantiferon CMV-directed Versus Fixed-duration Valganciclovir Prophylaxis to Reduce Late CMV After Lung Transplantation. Transplantation 103(5):1005–1013

Winston DJ, Young JA, Pullarkat V, Papanicolaou GA, Vij R, Vance E, Alangaden GJ, Chemaly RF, Petersen F, Chao N, Klein J, Sprague K, Villano SA, Boeckh M (2008) Maribavir prophylaxis for prevention of cytomegalovirus infection in allogeneic stem cell transplant recipients: a multicenter, randomized, double-blind, placebo-controlled, dose-ranging study. Blood 111(11):5403–5410

Winston DJ, Mullane KM, Cornely OA, Boeckh MJ, Brown JW, Pergam SA, Trociukas I, Žák P, Craig MD, Papanicolaou GA, Velez JD, Panse J, Hurtado K, Fernsler DA, Stek JE, Pang L, Su SC, Zhao Y, ISF C, Kaplan SS, Parrino J, Lee I, Popmihajlov Z, Annunziato PW, Arvin A, V212 Protocol 001 Trial Team (2018) Inactivated varicella zoster vaccine in autologous haemopoietic stem-cell transplant recipients: an international, multicentre, randomised, double-blind, placebo-controlled trial. Lancet 391(10135):2116–2127

www.ebmt.org/education/ebmt-handbook

Immune Response to Vaccines

Sibylle C. Mellinghoff

5.1 Introduction

The first available vaccines were developed without understanding their impact on the human immune system: In 1798, Edward Jenner experimented with cowpox to stimulate smallpox immunity (Ginglen and Doyle 2018). These early endeavours intensified and have led to an armamentarium of vaccines that are available today for infection prophylaxis.

Protection by vaccines can be categorized into early and long-term protection. While early protection is mediated by the induction of antibodies, long-term protection warrants their persistence, as well as immune memory cells. The quality of such antibodies in terms of avidity, specificity, or neutralizing capacity determines the efficacy of protection. Both, B- and T-cell-subsets are important for their induction and production (Siegrist 2018).

Novel methods allow the identification of specific molecular signatures of vaccine immunogenicity and further vaccine-associated immune parameters. This offers new opportunities of efficacy-assessment; however, correlation of these new markers with vaccine-induced protection often needs to be investigated. Further insights into vaccine immunogenicity may be used to explain the heterogeneity of vaccine responses in different populations and to improve vaccination strategies in vulnerable populations (very young, elderly and immunosuppressed) in future.

Vaccines exert protection by the induction of effector mechanisms, either cells or molecules that are able of controlling pathogens or inactivating their harmful components. Antibodies are such molecules and are produced by B lymphocytes to prevent or limit infections (Cooper and Nemerow 1984). Prevention is performed by binding toxins and thus limit their diffusion, but also blocking their enzymatic active site. Antibodies may also inhibit viral replication by blockade of viral binding. In addition, they enhance opsonophagocytosis of bacteria and thus promote their clearance by macrophages and neutrophils. By activating the complement cascade, antibodies limit infections.

Effector CD4 and cytotoxic CD8 T lymphocytes are main players in the cell-mediated vaccine response. Both are important for control and clearance of pathogens rather than prevention. CD8 T cells are capable of directly killing infected cells by excretion of perforin and granzyme. They also exert indirect killing effects by secreting specific antiviral cytokines. CD4 T

S. C. Mellinghoff (✉)
University of Cologne, Cologne, Germany
e-mail: sibylle.mellinghoff@uk-koeln.de

© Springer Nature Switzerland AG 2021
O. A. Cornely, M. Hoenigl (eds.), *Infection Management in Hematology*, Hematologic
Malignancies, https://doi.org/10.1007/978-3-030-57317-1_5

cells are of great importance for protection against intra- as well as extracellular pathogens by cytokine release. Their main subsets are depicted in Table 5.1 (Geginat et al. 2014; Bentebibel et al. 2013; Spensieri et al. 2013; Mastelic Gavillet et al. 2015; Lin et al. 2010; Kumar et al. 2013). They generate and support maintenance of B and CD8+ T-cell responses (Bentebibel et al. 2013; Spensieri et al. 2013; Mastelic Gavillet et al. 2015).

Different vaccines influence different effectors of the immune system. Table 5.2 gives an overview of selected vaccines. However, most vaccines affect both humoral and cellular immunity. CD4 T cells are required for most antibody responses while antibodies significantly influence T-cell responses to intracellular pathogens.

5.2 Vaccine Immune Response

Following injection, vaccine antigens containing pathogen-associated patterns and vaccine adjuvants recruit monocytes and neutrophils, as well as dendritic cells (DC) that patrol through the body. Those are equipped with receptors (termed pattern recognition receptors—PRR) directed against extrinsic and foreign pathogen patterns. PRR allow their brisk identification as danger and activate host cells immediately after recognition (Palm and Medzhitov 2009; Trombetta and Mellman 2005). DCs mature abruptly when exposed to pathogens at injection site or elsewhere: They secrete cytokines (e.g. IFN-α), and those, in turn, activate effector cells of innate immunity such as eosinophils, macrophages and NK cells. Activation prompts DCs to migrate towards secondary lymphoid organs. These activated migrating DCs exhibit antigens by classical MHC I and II or non-classical CD1 molecules, which allow selection of antigen-specific T lymphocytes (Lanzavecchia and Sallusto 2001). Activated T cells trigger terminal maturation of DC, which consequently induces further expansion and differentiation of lymphocytes. B cells, activated by DCs and T cells, differentiate into plasma cells that produce antibodies against the vaccine. While this process leads to both humoral and cellular immunity, the vaccine itself can also wander into lymph nodes and cause particularly humoral immunity by B-cell induction. In this

Table 5.1 CD4 subsets and production of cytokines

Subset	Cytokine	Task
Tfh	IL-21	B-cell help
Th1	IFNγ, TNFα/β, IL-2	Protection against intracellular pathogens
Th2	IL-4, 5, 13	Response to extracellular pathogens
Th9	IL-9	Response to extracellular pathogens
Th17	IL-17, 22, 26	Mucosal defence

IFN, interferon; *IL*, interleukin; *Tfh*, follicular T-helper cell; *Th*, T-helper cell; *TNF*, tumour necrosis factor

Table 5.2 Vaccine-induced immunity (along (Siegrist 2018))

Vaccine	Type of vaccine	Serum IgG	Mucosal IgG	Mucosal IgA	T cells
Diphtheria toxoid	Toxoid	+	(+)		
Hepatitis A	Killed	+			
Hepatitis B (HBsAg)	Protein	+			
Hib PS	PS	+	(+)		
Influenza	Killed	+	(+)		
Measles	Live attenuated	+	+	+	+ (CD8)
Mumps	Live attenuated	+			
Pneumococcal PS	PS	+	(+)		
Pneumococcal conjugate	PS protein	+	+		+ (CD4/8)
Tetanus	Toxoid	+			
VZV	Live attenuated				+ (CD4)

PS, polysaccharide; *VZV*, Varicella zoster virus

case, it will be caught by lymph node resident DCs (Siegrist 2018; Palucka et al. 2010).

Compared to inactivated vaccines, live vaccines lead to a higher intensity of innate immune response by synergistic activation of different PRRs, but also higher antigen content following replication.

5.2.1 Live Vaccines

Live viral vaccines activate both innate and adaptive immune system. Several features lead to a high level of immunogenicity: First, viral particles are small (between 20 and 200 nm) and are therefore best suitable for drainage to lymph nodes and direct interaction with B cells. Second, their surface often is highly repetitive, leading to cross-linking and consequently activation of B-cell receptors. Also, such repetitive structures are capable of binding natural antibodies and fix complement, which further activates B cells and triggers transportation to and deposition on follicular dendritic cells. In addition, viral particles express ligands for toll-like receptor (TLR), a PRR subtype, 7/8 or 9. These trigger directly B cells' isotype switching and enable DC for T-cell priming (Zabel et al. 2013; Querec et al. 2006; Lund et al. 2003). Emerging evidence suggests that the quality of the adaptive immune response is partly determined by the particular TLR triggered (Iwasaki and Medzhitov 2004). Given the pivotal role of TLRs and DCs in initiating and enhancing the adaptive immune response, there is currently much interest in exploiting these in the development of novel vaccines.

As a result of this early diffusion pattern, route and injection site are less important in live vaccines. For example, the measles vaccine has been shown to be as immunogenic when administered intramuscularly or subcutaneously (Hong Kong Measles Vaccine, C. 1967).

5.2.2 Non-Live Vaccines

Non-live vaccines activate innate response at the injection site. The preferred route is intramuscu-

larly as DCs can be found in high amounts in the well-vascularized muscles. Vaccines can consist of glycoconjugates, proteins, PS, or inactivated pathogens and contain small amounts of pathogen-recognition patterns. However, absent microbial replication limits immune activation by vaccines.

5.2.3 Vaccine Adjuvants

Vaccine adjuvants have been an essential component of modern vaccine development. They modulate parts of the innate immune system and thus enhance vaccine response. Only few adjuvants are currently included in vaccines approved for human use despite decades of development (O'Hagan and Fox 2015).

5.2.4 Stages of Immunization

Immunization by vaccination passes several stages and always starts with an extrafollicular reaction, followed by the germinal centre reaction.

Initially, the vaccine is presented outside the lymph tissue and rapidly induces IgG antibody titres. Next, B cells proliferate in the germinal centres of lymph tissue and increase IgG titres to a peak, usually after three to four weeks after vaccination. Due to short living plasma cells, antibodies decline rapidly and may even return to baseline. In case of a second exposure to the antigen, the immune memory is activated and IgG increase within days. While short-lived plasma cells undergo the same cycle as during primary immunization, long-lived plasma cells continue to produce IgG and thus declining slower (Fig. 5.1).

5.2.4.1 The Extrafollicular Vaccine Immune Reaction

Extrafollicular immune response is responsible for the fast induction of antibody production after antigen, for example vaccine, contact. B cells are bred in the bone marrow and rest in the lymph nodes thereafter. When a B cell binds an antigen

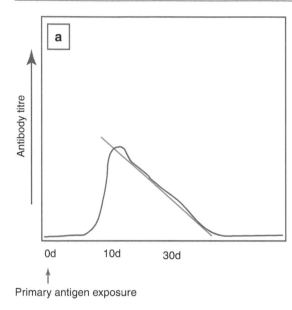

Primary antigen exposure

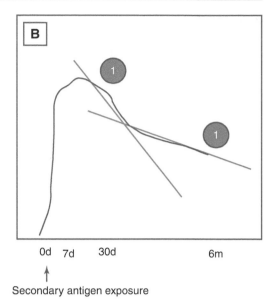

Secondary antigen exposure

Fig. 5.1 Stages of immunization: After the exposure to an antigen (**a**), a vaccine is presented to B cells outside follicles, and IgG antibody titres are produced immediately. B cells then proliferate in germinal centres and increase IgG to a peak (3–4 weeks after vaccination). Plasma cells are short-lived and thus, antibodies decline, sometimes even to baseline. When exposed to an antigen or vaccine for a second time (**b**), the immune memory is activated, and IgG increases within days to a peak. Long-lived plasma cells continue to produce IgG and thus declining slower

with its surface immunoglobulin (Ig), the cell will migrate to T cell–rich zones of secondary lymphoid organs for interaction. As soon as T cells recognize the antigen-presenting B cell, it triggers B-cell maturation into plasma cells that generate germline antibodies with low-affinity (Lee et al. 2011). Isotype switch of Ig (IgA to IgE, IgG or IgM) follows the B-cell transformation. After two cell cycles, B-cell blasts have finished the differentiation and are able to migrate to the local site of extrafollicular growth. While further contact with T cells is not required, interaction with DCs seems essential for full differentiation of plasmablasts to plasma cells (MacLennan et al. 2003).

The extrafollicular reaction is a fast immune response and Ig (IgG and IgM at low level) can be measured in blood some days after immunization (Fig. 5.1). Due to a missing selection process, Ig have germline affinity. After few days, most plasma cells are eliminated by apoptosis, and thus the role of extrafollicular immune response for efficacy of a vaccine is limited to a time span of several weeks (Siegrist 2018; MacLennan et al. 2003).

5.2.4.2 The Germinal Centre Vaccine Immune Reaction

The germinal centre (GC) immune response is essential for humoral immunity. Here, somatically mutated high-affinity memory B cells and plasma cells mediating protection against pathogens are generated (De Silva and Klein 2015).

GCs are formed transiently within peripheral lymphoid organs during T-cell dependent antibody responses (MacLennan 1994). After activation outside follicles in T cell–rich zones, B cells give rise to GC. After immunization with the antigen, formed GCs are oligoclonal: on average three B blasts colonize each follicle. After following clonal expansion, these clones of a single B cell acting against one specific antigen constitute a GC. The process is accompanied by a site-directed hypermutation mechanism that acts on the B cells' immunoglobulin-variable (Ig-v)-region genes (MacLennan 1994). The result is an isotype-switch from IgM to IgA, IgE or IgG, and the maturation of B cells concerning their affinity to a specific antigen.

GCs persist for three to four weeks. Thereafter, memory B cells proliferate in follicles in a T-cell-mediated manner for another few weeks. These cells are most probable the reservoir for plasma cells and memory cells required for long-term antibody maintenance.

5.3 Determining Factors of Vaccine Immune Response

Individuals and human populations show variation in response to vaccines. Key explanatory variables comprise host factors such as demographics, the nature of the vaccine and the vaccination schedule.

5.3.1 Host Factors

Host factors that influence the immune response to vaccination include, amongst others, age and genetic factors.

5.3.1.1 Age

It has been shown that incidence and severity of infectious diseases increase with age, which is—among other factors—due to a declining immune response of both innate and adaptive immune response (Weinberger et al. 2008). These characteristic changes of the immune system are called immunosenescence. This also entails an insufficient protection following vaccination.

Quantitative and qualitative changes within the immune system prevent local responses, impair generation of primary immune responses to neoantigens, hamper the effective induction of memory cells and decline the effect of booster vaccination. As a result, long-term protective effects of vaccination cannot be taken for granted in elderly persons. A decrease of antibody production can be seen early. In a study evaluating the impact of immunosuppression on response to influenza vaccine, a multivariate analysis showed a titre decrease of 31% with each additional 10 years after the age of 20 (Gabay et al. 2011).

Not only quantity and persistence of antibody response to vaccination are affected by age (LeMaoult et al. 1997; Frasca et al. 2005; Saurwein-Teissl et al. 2002), but also quality in

terms of specificity, isotype and affinity (Weksler 2000; Romero-Steiner et al. 1999). Lower antibody titres in elderly have so far been reported in subjects vaccinated with influenza vaccines (Gardner et al. 2001; Murasko et al. 2002), pneumococcal PS vaccines (Artz et al. 2003), as well as tetanus and tick-borne encephalitis vaccines (Hainz et al. 2005). The IgM memory B-cell pool has been shown to diminish with age and thus leading to a smaller number of antibody-producing plasma cells (Shi et al. 2005). Also, age-related differences of lymph-node structure have to be taken into account: Induction of the germinal centre is limited and leads to less antibody production (Luscieti et al. 1980), as well as reduced affinity and isotype switch (Frasca et al. 2005; Lottenbach et al. 1999). Several studies have shown diverse alterations within the antibody repertoire of the elderly (Saurwein-Teissl et al. 2002; Zheng et al. 1997; Song et al. 1997). However, reasons for changes of antibody functionality by age have not been fully understood to date. Also, T cells are affected by immunosenescence and while naïve T cells decline, large CD8 cells, possibly relicts from prior infections, increase in number (Frasca et al. 2005). CD4 cells initially increase after vaccination, but may not persist or further expand as they transfer to memory CD4 cells (Weinberger et al. 2008; Grubeck-Loebenstein et al. 2005).

Approaches to improve the efficacy of vaccines in the elderly vary and comprise the augmentation of vaccine doses (DiazGranados et al. 2014), addition of adjuvants (Deng et al. 2004) and higher frequencies of revaccination.

5.3.1.2 Genetic Factors

Different genetic factors influence the response to vaccination. The polymorphic MHC system has been investigated most in this context and was shown to affect the response to vaccination (Kimman et al. 2007). Also, the less polymorphic TLR and the cytokine immunoregulatory network differ in each individual due to the additive genetic factors (Iwasaki and Medzhitov 2004; van Duin et al. 2006). The variance due to genetic polymorphism appears to be particularly important for vaccine-induced antibody responses in young infants compared to cell-mediated and antibody response in older, immunologically mature individuals (Kimman et al. 2007; Poland and Jacobson 1998).

5.3.2 Nature of the Vaccine

Most relevantly, the nature of the vaccine influences the immune response. As discussed above, live vaccines induce a different kind and quality of immune response than inactivated vaccines. Immunogenicity also depends on the capacity of providing antigen epitopes able to bind naïve B cells, but also the ability to activate DCs and B cells (Siegrist 2018).

Also, the choice of adjuvants plays a detrimental role for the immune response. The difference in immunogenicity by simple bacterial PS and by protein-conjugated glycoconjugates underlines the important differences between extrafollicular and GC reactions in this context.

5.3.3 Schedule of Vaccination

A further determinant of vaccine antibody responses is the schedule of vaccination, which may only be investigated experimentally. Non-live antigens can be increased in dose to reach higher primary antibody responses—this is particularly useful in immunocompromised vaccinees, for example, used for hepatitis B immunization.

Few non-live vaccines (e.g. hepatitis A or human papillomavirus vaccines) induce a sustained antibody response after single vaccination, regardless age of the vaccinees. Hence, immunization schedules usually include several doses. These are to be repeated at a minimal interval of 4 weeks in order to induce consecutive waves of B cell and GC responses.

Optimal immunization schedules depend on the respective vaccine and are subject of ongoing clinical trials in order to reach most evidence for the best immune response outcome.

5.4 Specificity of Vaccine Immune Response

While low specificity means high protection to non-vaccine strains (e.g. influenza or *Streptococcus pneumoniae*), this can also potentially entail cross-reactions to allergens or self-antigens.

With regard to the B-cell axis, induction of cross-reactive antibody response is unlikely (Feikin et al. 2004; Di Genova et al. 2006). B cells identify epitopes by distant amino acids and may bind to antigenic peptides with distinct sequences. Although polyclonal stimulation has been proposed to induce memory B cells of different specificities (Bernasconi et al. 2002), this response seems not to be associated with antibody responses. Vaccination with tetanus toxoid was described to induce memory T cells, but did not modulate antibody responses to unrelated antigens (Di Genova et al. 2006). T cells, on the other hand, may have greater potential for cross-reaction due to a restricted number of amino acids presented by MHC (Oldstone 1998). Also, they are prone to be affected by cytokine changes and transient activation during infections (Di Genova et al. 2006).

References

Artz AS, Ershler WB, Longo DL (2003) Pneumococcal vaccination and revaccination of older adults. Clin Microbiol Rev 16(2):308–318

Bentebibel SE et al (2013) Induction of ICOS+CXCR3+CXCR5+ TH cells correlates with antibody responses to influenza vaccination. Sci Transl Med 5(176):176ra32

Bernasconi NL, Traggiai E, Lanzavecchia A (2002) Maintenance of serological memory by polyclonal activation of human memory B cells. Science 298(5601):2199–2202

Cooper NR, Nemerow GR (1984) The role of antibody and complement in the control of viral infections. J Invest Dermatol 83(1 Suppl):121s–127s

De Silva NS, Klein U (2015) Dynamics of B cells in germinal centres. Nat Rev Immunol 15(3):137–148

Deng Y et al (2004) Age-related impaired type 1 T cell responses to influenza: reduced activation ex vivo, decreased expansion in CTL culture in vitro, and blunted response to influenza vaccination in vivo in the elderly. J Immunol 172(6):3437–3446

Di Genova G et al (2006) Vaccination of human subjects expands both specific and bystander memory T cells but antibody production remains vaccine specific. Blood 107(7):2806–2813

DiazGranados CA et al (2014) Efficacy of high-dose versus standard-dose influenza vaccine in older adults. N Engl J Med 371(7):635–645

van Duin D, Medzhitov R, Shaw AC (2006) Triggering TLR signaling in vaccination. Trends Immunol 27(1):49–55

Feikin DR et al (2004) Specificity of the antibody response to the pneumococcal polysaccharide and conjugate vaccines in human immunodeficiency virus-infected adults. Clin Diagn Lab Immunol 11(1):137–141

Frasca D, Riley RL, Blomberg BB (2005) Humoral immune response and B-cell functions including immunoglobulin class switch are downregulated in aged mice and humans. Semin Immunol 17(5):378–384

Gabay C et al (2011) Impact of synthetic and biologic disease-modifying antirheumatic drugs on antibody responses to the AS03-adjuvanted pandemic influenza vaccine: a prospective, open-label, parallel-cohort, single-center study. Arthritis Rheum 63(6):1486–1496

Gardner EM et al (2001) Characterization of antibody responses to annual influenza vaccination over four years in a healthy elderly population. Vaccine 19(32):4610–4617

Geginat J et al (2014) Plasticity of human CD4 T cell subsets. Front Immunol 5:630

Ginglen JG, Doyle MQ (2018) Immunization. In: StatPearls. StatPearls Publishing LLC, Treasure Island (FL)

Grubeck-Loebenstein B et al (2005) Age-related differences in phenotype and function of CD4+ T cells are due to a phenotypic shift from naive to memory effector CD4+ T cells. Int Immunol 17(10):1359–1366

Hainz U et al (2005) Insufficient protection for healthy elderly adults by tetanus and TBE vaccines. Vaccine 23(25):3232–3235

Hong Kong Measles Vaccine, C (1967) Comparative trial of live attenuated measles vaccine in Hong Kong by intramuscular and intradermal injection. Bull World Health Organ 36(3):375–384

Iwasaki A, Medzhitov R (2004) Toll-like receptor control of the adaptive immune responses. Nat Immunol 5(10):987–995

Kimman TG, Vandebriel RJ, Hoebee B (2007) Genetic variation in the response to vaccination. Community Genet 10(4):201–217

Kumar P, Chen K, Kolls JK (2013) Th17 cell based vaccines in mucosal immunity. Curr Opin Immunol 25(3):373–380

Lanzavecchia A, Sallusto F (2001) Regulation of T cell immunity by dendritic cells. Cell 106(3):263–266

Lee SK et al (2011) B cell priming for extrafollicular antibody responses requires Bcl-6 expression by T cells. J Exp Med 208(7):1377

LeMaoult J et al (1997) Clonal expansions of B lymphocytes in old mice. J Immunol 159(8):3866

Lin Y, Slight SR, Khader SA (2010) Th17 cytokines and vaccine-induced immunity. Semin Immunopathol 32(1):79–90

Lottenbach KR et al (1999) Age-associated differences in immunoglobulin G1 (IgG1) and IgG2 subclass antibodies to pneumococcal polysaccharides following vaccination. Infect Immun 67(9):4935–4938

Lund J et al (2003) Toll-like receptor 9-mediated recognition of herpes simplex virus-2 by plasmacytoid dendritic cells. J Exp Med 198(3):513–520

Luscieti P et al (1980) Human lymph node morphology as a function of age and site. J Clin Pathol 33(5):454–461

MacLennan IC (1994) Germinal centers. Annu Rev Immunol 12:117–139

MacLennan IC et al (2003) Extrafollicular antibody responses. Immunol Rev 194:8–18

Mastelic Gavillet B et al (2015) MF59 mediates its B cell Adjuvanticity by promoting T follicular helper cells and thus germinal center responses in adult and early life. J Immunol 194(10):4836–4845

Murasko DM et al (2002) Role of humoral and cell-mediated immunity in protection from influenza disease after immunization of healthy elderly. Exp Gerontol 37(2-3):427–439

O'Hagan DT, Fox CB (2015) New generation adjuvants-from empiricism to rational design. Vaccine 33(Suppl 2):B14–B20

Oldstone MB (1998) Molecular mimicry and immune-mediated diseases. FASEB J 12(13):1255–1265

Palm NW, Medzhitov R (2009) Pattern recognition receptors and control of adaptive immunity. Immunol Rev 227(1):221–233

Palucka K, Banchereau J, Mellman I (2010) Designing vaccines based on biology of human dendritic cell subsets. Immunity 33(4):464–478

Poland GA, Jacobson RM (1998) The genetic basis for variation in antibody response to vaccines. Curr Opin Pediatr 10(2):208–215

Querec T et al (2006) Yellow fever vaccine YF-17D activates multiple dendritic cell subsets via TLR2, 7, 8, and 9 to stimulate polyvalent immunity. J Exp Med 203(2):413–424

Romero-Steiner S et al (1999) Reduction in functional antibody activity against Streptococcus pneumoniae in vaccinated elderly individuals highly correlates with decreased IgG antibody avidity. Clin Infect Dis 29(2):281–288

Saurwein-Teissl M et al (2002) Lack of antibody production following immunization in old age: association with CD8(+)CD28(−) T cell clonal expansions and an imbalance in the production of Th1 and Th2 cytokines. J Immunol 168(11):5893–5899

Shi Y et al (2005) Regulation of aged humoral immune defense against pneumococcal bacteria by IgM memory B cell. J Immunol 175(5):3262–3267

Siegrist C-A (2018) 2 - Vaccine Immunology. In: Plotkin SA et al (eds) Plotkin's vaccines (seventh edition). Elsevier, pp 16–34.e7

Song H, Price PW, Cerny J (1997) Age-related changes in antibody repertoire: contribution from T cells. Immunol Rev 160:55–62

Spensieri F et al (2013) Human circulating influenza-CD4+ICOS1+IL-21+ T cells expand after vaccination, exert helper function, and predict antibody responses. Proc Natl Acad Sci U S A 110(35):14330–14335

Trombetta ES, Mellman I (2005) Cell biology of antigen processing in vitro and in vivo. Annu Rev Immunol 23:975–1028

Weinberger B et al (2008) Biology of immune responses to vaccines in elderly persons. Clin Infect Dis 46(7):1078–1084

Weksler ME (2000) Changes in the B-cell repertoire with age. Vaccine 18(16):1624–1628

Zabel F, Kundig TM, Bachmann MF (2013) Virus-induced humoral immunity: on how B cell responses are initiated. Curr Opin Virol 3(3):357–362

Zheng B et al (1997) Immunosenescence and germinal center reaction. Immunol Rev 160:63–77

Vaccine-Preventable Diseases

6

Hamdi Akan, Tony Bruns, and Mathias W. Pletz

Vaccination can be accepted as the main strategy in preventing infections, but vaccination of cancer patients is a complex approach. The diversity of immunodeficiencies in different hematological disorders, and the change of immunosuppression during the course of the illness, lower vaccine responses, difficulty in conducting clinical trials with adequate patient numbers, contraindication of live attenuated vaccines in most cases, and few data on several vaccines make this a problematic area. This chapter summarizes the situation in four important vaccine-preventable diseases (influenza, herpes, zoster, HBV, and pneumococcal infection).

6.1 Influenza

Influenza is a disease caused by A, B, C, and D influenza viruses. A & B viruses are responsible for the disease. The virus carries hemagglutinin,

a surface glycoprotein and this binds to the sialic acid residues on respiratory epithelial cell surface glycoproteins. This interaction with the host cells is important for the pathogenicity of the virus. The epidemiology of the influenza infection changes rapidly over time and this is due to a change in the virus. Two major antigenic changes affecting the epidemiology such as antigenic drifts and shifts can be seen. Antigenic drift is a slow and small genetic change that occurs during time as the virus replicates. These changes accumulate and may produce a new distinct virus. Antigenic shift is a major change in the hemagglutinin and neuroaminidase proteins (hemagglutinins (H1, H2, and H3) and neuraminidases (N1 and N2) on Type A virus) and maybe the cause of a pandemic such as the H1N1 pandemic in 2009. Antigenic shifts can occur between the genomic cells of different animal and human viruses (Webster et al. 1993). While the antigenic drift is confined to Type B influenza virus, Type A virus can both have a drift and shift.

These changes have a great impact on the epidemiology and mortality of the influenza virus.

The 1918 Spanish Influenza was the result of a shift and caused the death of 50–100 million people (Johnson and Mueller 2002). Seasonal influenza vaccine is recommended for all persons aged ≥6 months (Grohskopf et al. 2017). Despite seasonal variations in effectiveness (36% in 2017–2018 and 20% in 2014–2015), vaccination was estimated to prevent 11,000–144,000

H. Akan (✉)
Department of Hematology Clinical Research Unit,
Ankara University Faculty of Medicine,
Ankara, Turkey

T. Bruns (✉)
Department of Internal Medicine IV, Jena University
Hospital, Jena, Germany
e-mail: TONY.BRUNS@med.uni-jena.de

M. W. Pletz (✉)
Institute for Infectious Diseases and Infection
Control, Jena University Hospital, Jena, Germany
e-mail: mathias.pletz@med.uni-jena.de

© Springer Nature Switzerland AG 2021
O. A. Cornely, M. Hoenigl (eds.), *Infection Management in Hematology*, Hematologic
Malignancies, https://doi.org/10.1007/978-3-030-57317-1_6

influenza-associated hospitalizations and 300–4000 influenza-associated deaths in the 2014–2015 season (Flannery et al. 2018).

In hematological malignancies, there is an increased risk of influenza-associated aspergillosis. This is an underdiagnosed situation with high mortality rates. Two papers published in 2017 showed the importance of this problem. Patients admitted to the ICUs with a diagnosis of influenza have an increased rate of aspergillosis (16%) and high mortality rates (van de Veerdonk et al. 2017; Martin-Loeches et al. 2017). The incidence and mortality are higher in patients with EORTC host criteria.

Annual influenza vaccination is the main measure to prevent influenza in several guidelines and recommendations (Grohskopf et al. 2017; Paules and Subbarao 2017). Influenza vaccination reduces the risk of death and the severity of illness, especially in high-risk patients such as elderly (Castilla et al. 2013). Influenza vaccination is also important in reducing the risk of influenza pneumonia (Grijalva et al. 2015). Influenza vaccines can be trivalent (two influenza A virus antigens plus one influenza B virus antigen), or quadrivalent (two influenza A antigens and two influenza B antigens), can be inactive or live attenuated, can be standard dose or high dose, or can be a standard trivalent vaccine containing an immune-augmenting adjuvant. The vaccine is usually administered intramuscularly, but intradermal or nasal preparations are also available (Lambkin-Williams et al. 2016; Belshe RB et al. 2004). The live attenuated vaccine is contraindicated in immunosuppressed patients.

6.1.1 Hematological Malignancies and Influenza

Hematological malignancies with immunosuppression face several problems related to influenza. Influenza-related complications and mortality might be higher in such patients (Kunisaki and Janoff 2009; Cooksley et al. 2005), influenza vaccination may yield suboptimal response (Bitterman et al. 2018; Stiver and Weinerman 1978), and influenza might delay the scheduled treatments. These are the main reasons necessitating influenza vaccine in hematological malignancies albeit the risk of suboptimal immune response.

Influenza mortality is high among patients with hematological malignancies (D) with case-fatality range between 11% and 33% (Kunisaki and Janoff 2009; Bitterman et al. 2018). A Cochrane review analyzed 6 studies with 2275 participants consisting of hematological malignancies, solid tumors, and stem cell transplant patients with influenza vaccine. The data suggest a lower mortality and infection associated outcomes in both cohorts (Bitterman et al. 2018). Several studies comparing influenza vaccination with no vaccination show a limited benefit of influenza vaccine in terms of influenza incidence and all-cause mortality, but there is a reduction in influenza-associated pneumonia (Grijalva et al. 2015). There are also several clinical studies to show the efficacy of the influenza vaccine, but the main problems in these studies are that they include different hematological malignancies; the measure of efficacy and time of vaccination are different and sample sizes are small. (Stiver and Weinerman 1978; Hodges et al. 1979; Brydak et al. 2006; Gribabis et al. 1994; Lo et al. 1993; Mazza et al. 2005; Robertson et al. 2000; Ljungman et al. 2005; Rapezzi et al. 2003) The response to influenza vaccination remains between 3% and 76% and recommendation for an influenza vaccine remains obscure. Multiple myeloma and chronic lymphocytic leukemia are typical examples of hematological malignancies with diminished responses to influenza vaccines (Gribabis et al. 1994; Robertson et al. 2000). Patients with lymphoma, in particular, seem to have some of the poorest humoral responses (Brydak et al. 2006; Lo et al. 1993; Mazza et al. 2005; Rapezzi et al. 2003).

Another concern about influenza vaccination among cancer patients is that the perception and coverage are low and information given by the physician during a consultation is important to improve the rates of vaccination (Poeppl et al. 2015).

Several attempts are being made to improve the efficacy of the influenza vaccination in immunosuppressed patients. The use of adjuvanted vaccine resulted in no difference for the outcomes (Natori et al. 2017a); high-dose influenza vaccine demonstrated significantly better immunogenicity than SD vaccine in adult transplant recipients (Natori et al. 2017b).

ECIL 7 Guidelines list shorter time between transplant and vaccination, low lymphocyte counts at vaccination, low IgG and IgM at vaccination, chronic GVHD, use of immunosuppressive drugs, and rituximab in the last 12 months as the predictors of poor immune response to influenza vaccination after HSCT (ECIL-7 2017).

Current IDSA guidelines recommend one dose of inactive influenza vaccine (IIV) annually (strong, moderate) to persons aged ≥6 months starting 6 months after HSCT (strong, moderate) and starting 4 months after if there is a community outbreak of influenza (strong, very low). For children aged 6 months–8 years who are receiving influenza vaccine for the first time, 2 doses should be administered (strong, low) (Rubin et al. 2014). ECIL-7 Guidelines recommend annual seasonal IIV, 1 dose, at the beginning of flu season in all patients >6 months after transplant and pursued during the first years following transplant, at least until 6 months after stopping any IS and as long as the patient is judged to be immunosuppressed in allogeneic transplants (AII) and annual seasonal inactivated influenza vaccination, 1 dose, at the beginning of flu season in all patients >6 months after transplant, at least as long as the patient is judged to be immunosuppressed in autologous transplants (BII). In the setting of a community outbreak, IIV can be given to both allo- and auto-HSCT recipients, from 3 months after transplant. In that case, a second dose is likely to be beneficial (BII) (ECIL-7 2017).

6.1.2 Hematopoietic Stem Cell Transplantation (HSCT) and Influenza

Hematopoietic stem cell transplant patients are different from other hematological malignancies in terms of immunosuppression, influenza immunity, and response to vaccination. Although autologous stem cell transplant patients have similar risks compared to patients receiving conventional chemotherapies, allogeneic HSCT patients differ considerably due to the prolonged use of immunosuppressive drugs and graft-versus-host-disease (GVHD). Also, the immunization of the allogeneic transplant donor may have an impact on the immune state of the transplant recipients. It is not clear whether there is an increase in the incidence of Influenza infection in such patients (Hassan et al. 2003; Ljungman 2001), but hospitalization rates and mortality due to influenza disease is considerably higher in allogeneic HSCT recipients (Ljungman 2001; Nichols et al. 2004), especially in patients developing pneumonia (Whimbey et al. 1996). All HSCT patients >6 years old are recommended to have yearly influenza vaccine, but the timing of the vaccination is crucial to achieve an immune protection.

The incidence of influenza rates among patients with HSCT varies in several studies, but the largest analysis showed that there was no difference between the influenza rate according to the donor type, and there was no association between the presence of GVHD and influenza risk (Nichols et al. 2004). The impact of influenza vaccination on mortality rates is not clear; while some studies show no difference between the vaccinated and non-vaccinated patients (Ambati et al. 2015), one study showed a slight decrease in the vaccinated group (Machado et al. 2005). The efficacy of the adjuvanted influenza vaccine was compared to non-adjuvanted vaccine and no difference was found (Natori et al. 2017a).

6.1.2.1 Timing of the Vaccination

Influenza vaccine elicits substandard serological responses due to impaired B- and T-cell reconstitution, especially in patients with graft-versus-host disease. Pretransplant vaccination of the donor and the recipient may yield seroprotective levels (Storek et al. 2003). Influenza vaccination timing during the influenza session is also important, as cases vaccinated late in the influenza season have low seroconversion rates compared to the cases vaccinated in the early influenza session (Yalçin et al. 2010). Protective effect of the vaccine is low in patients vaccinated early after stem cell transplantation (Avetisyan et al. 2008) and although this effect can be boosted by a second dose of vaccine post-transplant, the serological response is limited (Engelhard et al. 2011), but comparable to natural infection in these patients (Dhédin et al. 2014). There are reports showing a favorable response to two doses of influenza vaccine in hematological malignancies (Lo et al. 1993; Ljungman et al. 2005; van der Velden et al. 2001). Vaccination response is diminished during active chemotherapy (Ljungman et al. 2005) and a period of 6 months after HSCT (Machado et al. 2005) and 12 months after chemotherapy yield better vaccine responses unless they are not receiving rituximab maintanance (Yri et al. 2011).

6.1.2.2 Vaccination of the Household

According to IDSA Guidelines, "individuals who live in a household with immunocompromised patients age ≥6 months should receive influenza vaccine annually (strong, high). They should receive either inactivated influenza vaccine (IIV; strong, high) or live attenuated influenza vaccine (LAIV) provided they are healthy, not pregnant, and aged 2–49 years (strong, low). Exceptions include individuals who live in a household with an immunocompromised patient who was a hematopoietic stem cell transplant (HSCT) recipient within 2 months after transplant or with graft vs. host disease (GVHD) or is a patient with severe combined immune deficiency (SCID)." (Rubin et al. 2014)

6.1.2.3 Vaccination of the Donor

HSCT donors should receive their routine vaccinations, but live influenza vaccine should not be administered starting from 4 weeks before stem cell collection (Rubin et al. 2014).

6.2 Fungal Infections and Vaccination

Fungal infections, esp. Aspergillus and Candida, remain an important problem in patients with hematological malignancies. Patients with acute leukemia, allogeneic stem cell transplantation, and long-term immunosuppression are prone to fungal infections (Koehler et al. 2017; Bowden et al. 2002). The use of targeted therapies and biological drugs may be a factor in increasing the risk of fungal infections, especially with drugs causing long-term immunodeficiency (Aguilar-Company et al. 2018; Fernández-Ruiz et al. 2018).

Vaccine development against fungal infections is an area of research and several targets have been identified for vaccine development (Hamad 2012; Cassone and Casadevall 2012; Shibasaki et al. 2014). In animal studies, several vaccines proved out to be efficient (Torosantucci et al. 2005; Xin and Cutler 2011). Dendritic cell vaccines are also promising in this area (Bacci et al. 2002; Bozza et al. 2003; Fidan et al. 2014). The clinical use of antifungal vaccines is limited. There are several clinical trials assessing the efficacy of NDV-3A vaccine in vulvovaginal candidiasis, NDV-3 in *S. aureus* and Candida. The problems in developing antifungal vaccines are several; the structure of the inactive fungi is complex and less immunogenic than the live fungi. The use of fungi with diminished virulence is more immunogenic, but may pose risks in immunosuppressed patients; vaccines developed against the subunits of a fungus should be standardized and adjuvants are needed because of diminished immunogenicity, and the targets are usually protein-based and this may be a problem because of the homology between the vaccine target and human receptors.

6.3 Herpes Zoster

Herpes Zoster is an infection caused by varicella-zoster virus (VZV). VZV is a herpesvirus and among the eight herpesviruses that can cause infection in human. Varicella-zoster virus can cause two clinically distinct diseases: varicella (chickenpox) and herpes zoster (shingles) mainly characterized by skin lesions and associated different clinical patterns (Schmid and Jumaan 2010). VZV is highly contagious and transmitted by contact either with aerosolized droplets from nasopharyngeal secretions of an infected individual or by direct contact with vesicle fluid from skin lesions. After the transmission, the children develop a mild varicella disease, characterized by vesicular skin lesions. After the clinical resolution, the virus resides in sensory dorsal root ganglia and causes a latent infection, but does not produce any symptoms until reactivation. The virus mainly enters the root ganglia by retrograde axonal transport from the epidermal nerve endings and also varicella-associated viremia can be a way of transportation (Gershon et al. 2012). After the reactivation of the virus, a clinically significant infection, herpes zoster (shingles) occurs and this time, the disease is characterized not only by unilateral vesicular skin lesions but also by severe neurological pain in the affected dermatome. The virus replicates in the ganglionic neurons and causes inflammation and death of the neurons and causes postherpetic neuralgia. The incidence of postherpetic neuralgia is around 10% and increases with age (Gauthier et al. 2009; Gialloreti et al. 2010). The VZV skin lesion tends to disappear without treatment but the postherpetic pain (neuralgia) is difficult to treat. The neurological complications besides neuralgia are paresis of the arm, leg, diaphragm and urinary retention, meningoencephalitis, vasculopathy, giant cell arteritis, and eye involvement. (Gershon et al. 2015) VZV may cause Ramsay Hunt syndrome that is an acute peripheral facial neuropathy associated with erythematous vesicular rash of the skin of the ear canal, auricle, or mucous membrane of the oropharynx (Sweeney and Gilden 2001). Also, other zoster complications may be seen including pancreatitis and hepatitis (Chhabra et al. 2017). Unlike herpes simplex, asymptomatic individuals do not transmit VZV infection (Gershon and Steinberg 1990). As varicella infection or vaccination does not protect against reactivation, two separate vaccines against varicella and HZV are developed.

The incidence of Herpes Zoster in the general population was found to be 4.47 per 1000 person-years (Johnson et al. 2015). Although varicella occurs in children, herpes zoster is a disease of the adults and usually increasing age (>50), physical trauma, immunosuppression, malignancy, depression, disrupted cellular mediated immunity, HIV, and chronic lung or kidney disease are the main risk factors for the reactivation of the virus. According to a recent meta-analysis of 62 studies, female sex, race/ethnicity (white people), family history, autoimmune diseases, asthma, diabetes mellitus, and chronic obstructive pulmonary disease are risk factors for VZV (Kawai and Yawn 2017), although there are other studies showing that gender has no impact on developing VZV. (Di Legami et al. 2007; Chidiac et al. 2001) Age is a main risk factor and the incidence increases to >10/1.000 patient-years after the age of 60 while the population incidence of VZV is 3–4/1.000 patient-year. (Gershon et al. 2015) The peak incidence is in the 60–69 age group and after 80 years, there is a lower incidence, but increased hospitalization (Di Legami et al. 2007; Kim et al. 2014). The incidence in the high-risk group was 12.78 per 1000 in the United States (Johnson et al. 2015).

It is very rare to develop a second herpes zoster virus infection (1–4%). The mortality of HZV is closely related to age and the overall mortality ranged from 0 to >0.07/100,000 in the WHO European database (Bricout et al. 2015).

Diagnosis of zoster is often made clinically, and laboratory tests are limited to atypical presentations, or cases occurring after a HZV vaccination to discriminate between VZV wild-type and vaccine strains. PCR and direct immunofluorescence from vesicles can be done, and also detection of VZV DNA from saliva can be helpful (Sauerbrei et al. 2003; Sauerbrei et al. 2004).

Antiviral treatment with acyclovir, famciclovir, and valacyclovir is effective in controlling VZV infection, but 22% of patients develop postherpetic neuralgia despite treatment (Pentikis et al. 2011). The treatment should be given within 72 hours of rash observation and care must be taken in patients with renal failure; IV acyclovir is contraindicated in patients with acute renal failure. Although corticosteroid are used to treat Ramsay-Hunt syndrome, ocular zona zoster, and zoster pain, the efficacy of corticosteroids is still not clear (Clemmensen and Andersen 1984).

6.3.1 Hematological Malignancies and Herpes Zoster

The immunosuppressed patients (transplant recipients, patients receiving immunomodulatory drugs, and HIV patients) are at increased risk of herpes zoster infection and solid organ transplant recipients have 10–100-fold increase in the incidence of HZV compared to general population. The incidence among hematologic cancers (31.0/1000-person year) was greater than solid organ cancers (14.9/1000-person year) (Yenikomshian et al. 2015). While the degree of cellular immunosuppression in solid tumors is limited and the therapies do not lead to major T-cell disruptions, this is not the case for hematological malignancies. The main reason for increased HZV infections in hematological malignancies is mainly related to the underlying cellular immunity disorder such as in Hodgkin's disease and the treatment used for the malignancy. A study carried out in cancer patients showed that the incidence of herpes zoster was low for individuals affected with prostate cancer (12.3/1000-person year) and high for those with Hodgkin's lymphoma (47.8/1000-person year) (Yenikomshian et al. 2015). Another study demonstrated that 8% of the Hodgkin's lymphoma patients develop VZV infection (Je and Firat 1965). There is also a relationship between the occurrence of Herpes Zoster and subsequent development of cancer in a matched retrospective cohort study analyzing 542.575 individuals with Herpes Zoster (Iglar et al. 2013). The incidence of cancer after the development of Herpes Zoster was greater, especially after 180 days and the greatest risk was for lymphoma and leukemia.

There are several reports showing an increased risk of herpes zoster with different drugs used in the treatment of hematologic diseases such as ruxolitinib (Lussana et al. 2018), bortezomib, and lenalidomide (Chanan-Khan et al. 2008; König et al. 2014) and disseminated cases with Ibrutinib and idelalisib (Giridhar et al. 2017), and also there are other studies showing a low risk with Imatinib (Mattiuzzi et al. 2003) and TNF-alfa blockers (Winthrop et al. 2013). As the use of corticosteroids during treatment of various diseases has been shown to increase the risk of HZV infection, the increase in the herpes zoster incidence in hematological malignancies can be attributed to the use of corticosteroids. (Winthrop et al. 2013) Prophylaxis against most of the new drugs used in the treatment of hematological malignancies is not warranted and there is little evidence to support this (Sandherr et al. 2015).

6.3.2 Hematopoietic Stem Cell Transplantation and Herpes Zoster

Herpes zoster is a late-occurring complication of stem cell transplantation (SCT) and before the use of acyclovir prophylaxis, nearly half of the patients who underwent stem cell transplantation developed herpes zoster. After the introduction of effective antiviral prophylaxis, this incidence is getting very low. In a multicenter study done in USA in stem cell transplantation centers, the frequency was 4% and there were 2 disseminated cases out of 13 patients with herpes zoster (Schuster et al. 2017). The occurrence of herpes zoster is usually around 3–12 months (median 5 months) after allogeneic or autologous transplantation, but can be seen beyond this time period, especially in patients with chronic GVHD (Styczynski et al. 2009). Chronic GVHD, leukemia diagnosis, age > 50 years, cord blood transplantation, and T-cell immunodeficiency increase the risk of herpes zoster infection (Styczynski et al. 2009; Tomonari et al. 2003). There is a higher incidence of herpes zoster among bone marrow or stem cell transplant recipients (43.03/1000-person year) than among solid organ transplant recipients (17.04/1000-person year) (Chen et al. 2014). The incidence of herpes zoster varies between 8% and 30% one year following autologous stem cell transplantation. In a study analyzing multiple myeloma patients undergoing autologous stem cell transplantation, 30% of the patients showed herpes zoster reactivation despite 3 weeks of antiviral prophylaxis, but there was no negative impact on survival (Kamber et al. 2015).

6.3.2.1 Prophylaxis and Protection Measures

For autologous transplant patients and chemotherapeutic agents, the risk of HZV reactivation is low and antiviral prophylaxis is not recommended (Styczynski et al. 2009; Inazawa et al. 2017; Kim et al. 2012). In allogeneic stem cell transplantation, acyclovir or valacyclovir is effective for prophylaxis (Sandherr et al. 2015). Acyclovir 400 mg tid or qid or valacyclovir 500 mg bid or tid is a common practice, but lower doses are recommended in patients receiving proteasome inhibitors (Chanan-Khan et al. 2008). The recommended duration for VZV prophylaxis in seropositive Allogeneic SCT patients is 1 year or longer in presence of AGVHD. The risk of VZV transmission and how to avoid exposure should be explained to leukemic patients and SCT candidates and recipients. VZV-seronegative leukemic patients and SCT recipients should not have contact with people with chickenpox or zoster. Leukemic patients, who are candidates for SCT, should also avoid contact with vaccine recipients experiencing a rash after varicella vaccine before and after SCT. As there is an increased risk of VZV infection after contact with varicella in hospital setting (Gustafson et al. 1982), all patients with varicella or disseminated zoster should be placed under airborne and contact isolation. The isolation should continue as long as the rash remains vesicular and until all lesions are crusted (Styczynski et al. 2009).

Varicella zoster immunoglobulin is indicated for use in post-exposure prophylaxis of varicella for persons at high risk for severe disease who lack evidence of immunity to varicella and for whom varicella vaccine is contraindicated ((CDC) CfDCaP 2013). CDC recommends that varicella zoster immunoglobulin be administered as soon as possible after exposure and within 10 days and only recommended in immunocompromised adult patients without evidence of immunity. Due to low availability and decreasing demand, it is not a common practice to use Varicella zoster immunoglobulin in hematological malignancies and SCT patients (Food and Drug Administration 2012).

6.4 Hepatitis B Virus

The Hepatitis B virus (HBV) is a small, enveloped, hepatotropic, partially double-stranded DNA virus belonging to the *Hepadnaviridae* family. HBV can be classified into at least ten genotypes (A to J) and several subtypes, differing in their geographic distribution, carcinogenic potential, and the response to interferon treatment (Lin and Kao 2017). Its compact genome consists of 4 open reading frames encoding for 7 proteins: the secreted dimeric HBV e antigen (HBeAg), the viral capsid protein HCV core antigen (HBcAg), a polymerase with reverse transcriptase activity (HBV Pol/RT), the different-sized envelope glycoproteins (PreS1, PreS2, and HBsAg), and the transcription regulator HBV x antigen (HBx) (Tong and Revill 2016). Upon infection of hepatocytes, the compact relaxed circular (RC) DNA is released and converted to covalently closed circular (ccc) DNA form, which serves as episomal DNA for the stable transcription of viral mRNAs utilizing DNA-dependent RNA polymerases of the host (Tong and Revill 2016).

6.4.1 The Natural History of HBV Infection

HBV infection continues to represent a major global health burden despite the availability of a vaccine and effective antiviral treatment. It is currently responsible for more than 600,000 deaths per year owing to hepatic failure, cirrhosis, and liver cancer. On a global level, 257 million people live with hepatitis B infection and the serological marker of active HBV replication, the hepatitis B surface antigen (HBsAg), is found in 3.61% of individuals ranging from 5% to 9% in Africa and the Western Pacific Region to less than 1% in North America and Central Europe (Schweitzer et al. 2015).

In contrast to other hepatotropic viruses, acute HBV infection is characterized by a rather delayed viral amplification and hepatic spread (Bertoletti and Ferrari 2012). In individuals, who clear HBV, robust multi-epitope-specific T-cell responses mediate direct hepatolytic and indirect antiviral effects. In addition, neutralizing anti-HBs antibodies prevent viral spread and reinfection. Patients who develop chronic HBV infection show functional alterations of virus-specific T cells and B cells consistent with immune exhaustion and limit viral clearance by the host (Maini and Pallett 2018; Burton et al. 2018). The chronicity rate is around 90% when transmitted at birth from an HBe-Ag-positive mother and transmission prophylaxis is not administered, and it is still up to 70% when transmitted during childhood as compared to 5–10% in adult life (Vegnente et al. 1992).

In chronic HBV infection, there is a distinct association of viral replication and immune-mediated liver damage, which is reflected by the four phases of chronic HBV infection according to a revised nomenclature (European Association for the Study of the Liver 2017). This nomenclature is considering the presence or absence of hepatic inflammation (chronic HBV infection vs. chronic hepatitis B) and the presence or absence of the HBe antigen (Fig. 6.1a). Patients who clear HBsAg still harbor a pool of episomal cccDNA in hepatocytes and are susceptible to HBV reactivation, especially in the context of immunosuppressive therapies. Therefore, the term "resolved HBV infection" should not be used, as immune control over HBV does not suggest viral clearance (Werle-Lapostolle et al. 2004).

According to European guidelines (European Association for the Study of the Liver 2017), all candidates for chemotherapy or immunosuppressive therapy should therefore be screened for HBsAg, anti-HBs, and anti-HBc prior to treatment. In anti-HBc-negative patients, vaccination is recommended (European Association for the Study of the Liver 2017). This is particularly important, as the majority of patients with chronic HBV infection in the Western world are not aware of their infection. In contrast, American guidelines (Hwang et al. 2015; Reddy et al. 2015) recommend an risk-adapted screening approach and restrict screening to patients at risk of HBV infection and patients at high risk of HBV reactivation. Anti HBc should always be tested before treatment with B-cell-depleting antibodies. However, anti-HBc tests done shortly after intravenous immunoglobulin infusion must be interpreted with caution because they might indicate passive transfer (Lu et al. 2018).

6.4.2 Hepatitis B Reactivation

Reactivation of HBV replication is currently defined as a significant increase of serum HBV DNA levels, that is, ≥ 100 IU/mL in a person with previously undetectable HBV DNA or an increase of ≥ 2 $\log_{10}$ in a person with a previously stable HBV DNA (Hwang and Lok 2014). As serum aminotransferase levels are within the normal range in the early phase of reactivation, they are no longer required for diagnosis (Hoofnagle 2009). The term reactivation comprises two major scenarios: First, the reappearance of HBsAg (reverse seroconversion) or HBV DNA in a patient with previous HBV infection (anti-HBc+/HBsAg-patient) and second, an increase in viral replication in a patient with preexisting chronic hepatitis B infection (anti-HBc+/HBsAg+ patient).

Usually, HBV reactivation occurs in three phases (Fig. 6.1b) (Hwang and Lok 2014; Hoofnagle 2009). In the early phase, HBV replication abruptly increases, and reverse HBsAg seroconversion may occur. In HBeAg-negative patients, this marker may reappear. This phase is clinically asymptomatic and aminotransferase concentrations are normal or only mildly elevated. The second phase typically occurs after two to three cycles of chemotherapy (Lok et al. 1991) and is a result of the immune reconstitution within weeks and months after the onset of chemotherapy and is characterized by hepatic injury as indicated by biochemical hepatitis, symptoms, and jaundice in severe cases. During this phase, HBV DNA levels may already start to fall. The third phase is the phase of resolution and recovery, where transaminase levels and HBV DNA return to baseline (Hoofnagle 2009).

HBV reactivation has been shown to occur with systemic chemotherapy for solid cancers and leukemia, corticosteroids, B-cell depleting monoclonal antibodies, anti-TNF agents, with progression of HIV infection, after solid organ transplantation, bone marrow and hematopoietic stem cell transplantation, and after transarterial chemoembolization for hepatocellular carcinoma

Fig. 6.1 Phases of chronic HBV infection and reactivation. Representative courses of alanine aminotransferase (ALT) and HBV DNA levels (**a**) in the four phases of chronic hepatitis B virus infection and (**b**) during HBV reactivation are shown. Nomenclature according to (European Association for the Study of the Liver 2017; Hoofnagle 2009)

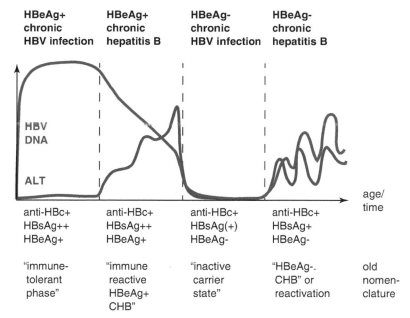

a Phases of chronic hepatitis B virus infection

HBeAg+ chronic HBV infection	HBeAg+ chronic hepatitis B	HBeAg- chronic HBV infection	HBeAg- chronic hepatitis B	
anti-HBc+ HBsAg++ HBeAg+	anti-HBc+ HBsAg++ HBeAg+	anti-HBc+ HBsAg(+) HBeAg-	anti-HBc+ HBsAg+ HBeAg-	age/ time
"immune-tolerant phase"	"immune reactive HBeAg+ CHB"	"inactive carrier state"	"HBeAg-. CHB" or reactivation	old nomen-clature

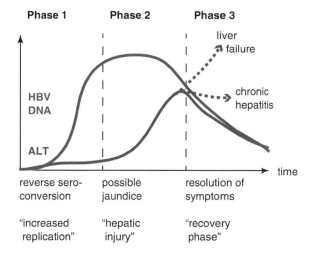

b Phases of hepatitis B virus reactivation

Phase 1	Phase 2	Phase 3	
reverse sero-conversion	possible jaundice	resolution of symptoms	time
"increased replication"	"hepatic injury"	"recovery phase"	

(Hwang and Lok 2014; Hoofnagle 2009). Although symptomatic HBV reactivation usually develops within the first 3 months after the start of systemic cancer chemotherapy, HBV reactivation can occur up to 12 months after the last administration of the B-cell-depleting antibody rituximab (Evens et al. 2011) and even later in patients undergoing allogeneic hematopoietic stem cell transplantation or lifelong immunosuppression (Hammond et al. 2009).

6.4.3 Prevention of HBV Reactivation

HBV reactivation frequently leads to the premature termination of chemotherapy or a delay in treatment schedules (Yeo et al. 2003) and carry the risk of fulminant hepatitis, liver failure, and death if not recognized early (Evens et al. 2011). The reported incidence of HBV reactivation in HBsAg+ patients is 15–50% after chemotherapy and more than 75% after bone marrow transplantation (Cornberg 2018).

Risk factors for HBV reactivation are host-related, for example, being male as opposed to being female and being at a younger age, HBV infection-related, for example, being positive for HBsAg or having higher levels of HBV DNA before treatment start as opposed to undetectable or low levels, and treatment-related, for example, treated for hematological malignancies as opposed to solid tumors (Hwang and Lok 2014). Among the solid tumors, patients undergoing treatment for breast cancer have the highest risk of reactivation, most likely due to the frequent use of corticosteroids and anthracyclin derivates, such as doxorubicin and epirubicin, in these patients. (Reddy et al. 2015) The highest risks have been observed in HBsAg+ and HBsAg-patients undergoing stem cell transplantation or receiving B-cell-depleting therapies with rituximab (Evens et al. 2011) and in HBsAg+ patients receiving anthracyclines and/or corticosteroids (Cheng et al. 2003). Although many immunosuppressive drugs have been associated with HBV reactivation, systemically collected data are missing. However, many guidelines (European Association for the Study of the Liver 2017; Reddy et al. 2015; Cornberg 2018; Perrillo et al. 2015) refer to an estimated HBV reactivation risk, which can be stratified as high (>10% probability), moderate (1–10%), or low (<1%) by the stratification by HBsAg status and therapeutic regimen (Fig. 6.2).

Similarly to immunocompetent patients, HBsAg-positive patients with evidence of chronic hepatitis B should receive a potent nucleoside (entecavir) or nucleotide analogue (tenofovir disoproxil fumarate or tenofovir alafenamid) (European Association for the Study of the Liver 2017). In patients without biochemical hepatitis who are at risk of HBV reactivation, preventive strategies are recommended. They can either be performed as antiviral prophylaxis or as preemptive therapy when an increase in viral replication is monitored. Preemptive therapy is based upon monitoring HBsAg and/or HBV DNA every 1–3 months during and after immunosuppression, and starting a potent nucleos(t)ide analogue

in case of detectable HBV DNA or reverse seroconversion independently of serum aminotransferases (European Association for the Study of the Liver 2017). The introduction of antiviral therapy should not delay the onset of chemotherapy but ideally be started before or concomitantly with cancer treatment (Hwang et al. 2015).

In patients at high risk of HBV reactivation, antiviral prophylaxis is recommended over preemptive therapy. (European Association for the Study of the Liver 2017; Reddy et al. 2015) Some (European Association for the Study of the Liver 2017; Hwang et al. 2015; Terrault et al. 2018) guidelines recommend antiviral prophylaxis in *all HBsAg+ or HBV DNA+ patients* undergoing immunosuppressive therapy, while others (Reddy et al. 2015; Cornberg 2018) only restrict this to HBsAg+ patients receiving drugs associated with a moderate or high risk of HBV reactivation.

Patients at moderate risk of HBV reactivation can receive prophylactic antiviral therapy, or they can be closely monitored and treated preemptively if there is evidence of HBV reactivation. The American Gastroenterological Association (Reddy et al. 2015) recommends antiviral prophylaxis over monitoring for patients at moderate risk of HBV reactivation, whereas the European and American Associations for the Study of the Liver (European Association for the Study of the Liver 2017; Terrault et al. 2018) recommend monitoring over prophylaxis in HBsAg-negative patients at moderate risk of reactivation.

Patients at low risk of HBV reactivation should not receive routine antiviral prophylaxis (Reddy et al. 2015), although there is controversy whether this may be appropriate in HBsAg+ patients and in conditions requiring long durations of immunosuppression (European Association for the Study of the Liver 2017). In clinical settings characterized by limited adherence to monitoring or unknown risk of viral reactivation associated with new therapies, universal prophylaxis is recommended over preemptive therapy (European Association for the Study of the Liver 2017; Reddy et al. 2015).

Given the high rates of drug resistance with first- or second-generation nucleos(t)ide analogues, antiviral prophylaxis and preemptive

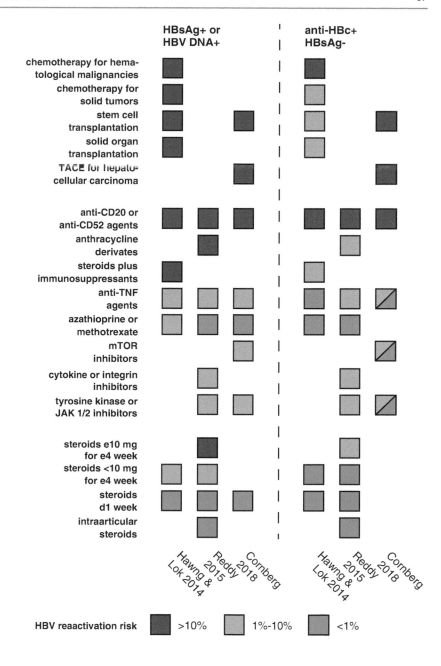

Fig. 6.2 Risk stratification for HBV reactivation. HBV reactivation risk stratified by and as assessed by systematic reviews (Reddy et al. 2015; Perrillo et al. 2015) and expert consensus (Hwang and Lok 2014; Cornberg 2018)

therapy should be performed using antiviral drugs with a high barrier to resistance, such as entecavir, tenofovir disoproxil fumarate, or tenofovir alafenamid (European Association for the Study of the Liver 2017; Reddy et al. 2015; Terrault et al. 2018). A recent network meta-analysis confirmed the superiority of entecavir and tenofovir disoproxil fumarate over lamivudine, telbivudine, and adefovir in preventing HBV reactivation in HBsAg+ patients with hematological malignancies receiving chemotherapy or hematopoietic stem cell transplantation (Zhang et al. 2017). HBV prophylaxis should continue for at least 6 (better 12) months after discontinuation of chemotherapy and for at least 12 (better 18) months after discontinuation of B-cell-depleting agents (European Association for the Study of the Liver 2017). Patients with higher baseline levels of HBV DNA are at a higher risk of hepatic flares after drug withdrawal and might benefit from prolonged or indefinite therapy (Hui et al. 2005).

6.5 Pneumococcal Disease

6.5.1 The Pathogen

A recent literature review on vaccine guidelines published between 2005 and 2016 found that pneumococcal and injectable influenza are the only two vaccines universally recommended in all cases of immunosuppression (Lopez et al. 2017).

Streptococcus pneumoniae is a Gram-positive, encapsulated diplococci. The bacterial polysaccharide capsule contributes to the overall virulence of the pathogen and protects the bacterium from phagocytosis. Uncapsulated pneumococci such as the laboratory reference strain R6 are considered to be nonpathogenic. More than 90 different capsular types (i.e., serotypes) have been described so far. Serotype distribution is constantly changing and differs by region and observation period and has been tremendously influenced by herd protection effects after the introduction of the pneumococcal conjugate vaccine for infants (Pletz et al. 2008). Currently, serotype 3, which seems not to be affected by herd protection, is in many regions the most prevalent serotype.

S*treptococcus* pneumoniae is a common colonizer in the respiratory tract, often symptomless; however, it can progress to respiratory or even systemic disease. An important feature is that pneumococcal disease will not occur without preceding nasopharyngeal colonization with the homologous strain, so pneumococcal carriage is believed to be an important source of horizontal spread of this pathogen within the community (Bogaert et al. 2004a). The main reservoir of pneumococci is the nasopharyngeal zone of healthy carriers, especially of infants. Up to 70% of infants attending children day-care centers and more than 90% of infants in some native communities but less than 5% of adults are colonized. (Bogaert et al. 2004b; Kwetkat et al. 2018)

6.5.2 Spectrum and Categorization of Pneumococcal Disease

Pneumococci are a leading cause of community-acquired respiratory tract infection, ranging from otitis media, sinusitis, acute exacerbation of COPD to community-acquired pneumonia and primary bacteremia. They can also cause a substantial proportion of early-onset (i.e., up to day 5 of hospitalization) hospital-acquired pneumonia. The longer the hospitalization before onset of pneumonia, the less likely are pneumococci as underlying pathogen (Gastmeier et al. 2009). Pneumococcal disease can be distinguished into invasive and noninvasive (Fig. 6.3). Invasive pneumococcal disease (IPD) is defined as the isolation of S. pneumoniae from a normally sterile site, for example, blood, cerebrospinal fluid, or pleural fluid. Noninvasive disease (i.e., sinusitis, otitis media) is frequent but not severe; invasive diseases are associated with a high case fatality rate but a lower incidence. Pneumococcal pneumonia can be invasive (i.e., positive blood or pleural culture, 10–15%) or noninvasive (detection from respiratory specimen only). In contrast to other noninvasive diseases (sinusitis, otitis media), the mortality rate for nonbacteremic pneumococcal pneumonia is still considerable and does not always differ from invasive pneumococcal disease (Pletz et al. 2012; Pletz et al. 2010). There is uncertainty how to classify pneumococcal pneumonias detected by urine antigen test only. However, pneumonia represents the main burden of pneumococcal disease since it has a high case fatality rate (ca. 15% of hospitalized patients) and a high incidence (Ewig et al. 2009).

Recently, a timely association between pneumonia and cardiovascular events has been detected by numerous observational studies. Besides generating enlargement and instability of atherosclerotic plaques, pneumococci have been shown to invade the myocardium and induce microlesions and heart scarring (Welte and Pletz 2017; Restrepo and Reyes 2018; Brown et al. 2014).

Besides *Staphylococcus aureus* and *Haemophilus influenzae*, pneumococci are a frequent cause of bacterial co-infections associated

Fig. 6.3 The spectrum of pneumococcal diseases. Pneumonia represents the main burden, it is frequent and severe (Pletz and Welte 2014)

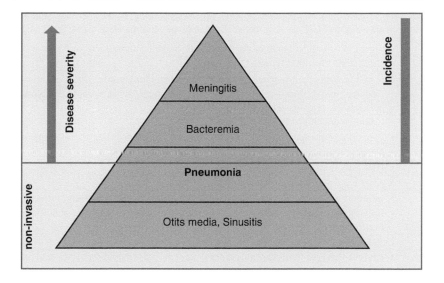

with influenza. Observational studies have shown that these co-infections can increase mortality dramatically (von Baum et al. 2011). In line with these observations, it has also been shown that pneumoccccal and influenza vaccine can act synergistically (Hedlund et al. 2003).

6.5.3 Risk Factors for Pneumococcal Disease

Besides an immature immune system (infants) or immunosenescence (elderly), immunosuppression and certain comorbidities increase the risk for pneumococcal disease.

In a recent Danish cohort study, pneumococci were the leading cause of blood stream infections in CLL patients accounting for 22% of the cases (Andersen et al. 2018). A 2018 meta-analysis on invasive pneumococcal disease showed that autologous or allogenic stem cell transplant recipients have the highest incidence of 696 and 812/100,000, respectively, compared to 10/100.000 in a healthy control cohort. The case fatality rate was 10.3–20% compared to 1,5–14% in the healthy control cohort (van Aalst et al. 2018).

Since the spleen plays a major role within the immune response to pneumococci, anatomic or functional asplenia confers the highest risk, particularly for invasive pneumococcal disease.

These "overwhelming postsplenectomy infections (OPSI)" present frequently as sepsis, often accompanied by exanthema (*Purpura fulminans*), can start within hours and are associated with a very high mortality (Theilacker et al. 2016). OPSI survivors are frequently disabled by the loss of fingers or toes due to fulminant disseminate intravascular coagulation.

In addition to vaccination, prevention of OPSI may require antibiotic prophylaxis as stand-by application or even long-term intake of penicillin after survived OPSI.

The numerous risk factors for pneumococcal disease have been recently summarized and categorized into three groups by the German Standing Committee on Vaccination (Table 6.1). Group 1 (congenital and acquired immunosuppression) is associated with a high risk for pneumococcal disease, group 2 (comorbidities other than immunosuppression) with a moderate risk, and group 3 with a risk for pneumococcal meningitis. Noteworthy, chronic kidney failure, nephrotic syndrome, and liver cirrhosis (e.g., spontaneous bacterial peritonitis due to pneumococci) are associated with immunosuppression and therefore included in group 1. However, this categorization does not consider that individual risk factors (e.g., diabetes mellitus and COPD) may occur simultaneously resulting in "risk stacking." (Morton et al. 2017)

Table 6.1 Risk factors for pneumococcal disease according to the German Standing Committee on Vaccination (https://www.rki.de/EN/Content/infections/Vaccination/recommandations/34_2017_engl.pdf?__blob=publicationFile)

1. Congenital or acquired immunodeficiencies or immunosuppression, such as the following:
• T-cell deficiency or defective T-cell function
• B-cell or antibody deficiency (e.g., hypogammaglobulinemia)
• Deficiency or dysfunction of myeloid cells (e.g., neutropenia, chronic granulomatosis, leukocyte adhesion deficiencies, and signal transduction defects)
• Complement and properdin deficiencies
• Functional hyposplenism (e.g., sickle cell anemia), splenectomy[a], or anatomical asplenia
• Neoplastic diseases
• HIV infection
• After bone marrow transplantation
• Immunosuppressive therapy[a] (e.g., due to organ transplantation or autoimmune disease)
• Immunodeficiency in the context of chronic kidney failure, nephrotic syndrome, or chronic liver insufficiency
2. Other chronic diseases, such as the following:
• Chronic diseases of the cardiovascular system or of the respiratory tract (e.g., asthma, emphysema, or COPD)
• Metabolic diseases, for example, diabetes mellitus treated with oral medication or insulin
• Neurological diseases, for example, cerebral palsy or seizure disorders
3. Anatomical and foreign-material associated risks for pneumococcal meningitis, such as
• Cerebral spine fluid fistula
• Cochlea implant[a]

[a]vaccination preferably before intervention

References

(CDC) CfDCaP (2013) Updated recommendations for use of VariZIG--United States, 2013. MMWR Morb Mortal Wkly Rep 62(28):574–576

van Aalst M, Lotsch F, Spijker R, van der Meer JTM, Langendam MW, Goorhuis A et al (2018) Incidence of invasive pneumococcal disease in immunocompromised patients: a systematic review and meta-analysis. Travel Med Infect Dis 24:89–100. https://doi.org/10.1016/j.tmaid.2018.05.016

Aguilar-Company J, Fernández-Ruiz M, García-Campelo R, Garrido-Castro AC, Ruiz-Camps I (2018) ESCMID study Group for Infections in compromised hosts (ESGICH) consensus document on the safety of targeted and biologic therapies: an infectious diseases perspective-cell surface receptors and associated signaling pathways. Clin Microbiol Infect 24:S41

Ambati A, Boas LS, Ljungman P et al (2015) Evaluation of pretransplant influenza vaccination in hematopoietic SCT: a randomized prospective study. Bone Marrow Transplant 50(6):858–864

Andersen MA, Moser CE, Lundgren J, Niemann CU (2018) Epidemiology of bloodstream infections in patients with chronic lymphocytic leukemia: a longitudinal nation-wide cohort study. Leukemia 33:662. https://doi.org/10.1038/s41375-018-0316-5

Avetisyan G, Aschan J, Hassan M, Ljungman P (2008) Evaluation of immune responses to seasonal influenza vaccination in healthy volunteers and in patients after stem cell transplantation. Transplantation 86(2):257–263

Bacci A, Montagnoli C, Perruccio K et al (2002) Dendritic cells pulsed with fungal RNA induce protective immunity to Candida albicans in hematopoietic transplantation. J Immunol 168(6):2904–2913

von Baum H, Schweiger B, Welte T, Marre R, Suttorp N, Pletz MW et al (2011) How deadly is seasonal influenza-associated pneumonia? The German competence network for community-acquired pneumonia. Eur Respir J 37(5):1151–1157. https://doi.org/10.1183/09031936.00037410

Belshe RB, Newman FK, Cannon J et al (2004) Serum antibody responses after intradermal vaccination against influenza. N Engl J Med 351(22):2286–2294

Bertoletti A, Ferrari C (2012) Innate and adaptive immune responses in chronic hepatitis B virus infections: towards restoration of immune control of viral infection. Gut 61:1754–1764. https://doi.org/10.1136/gutjnl-2011-301073

Bitterman R, Eliakim-Raz N, Vinograd I, Zalmanovici Trestioreanu A, Leibovici L, Paul M (2018) Influenza vaccines in immunosuppressed adults with cancer. Cochrane Database Syst Rev 2:CD008983

Bogaert D, De Groot R, Hermans PW (2004a) Streptococcus pneumoniae colonisation: the key to pneumococcal disease. Lancet Infect Dis 4(3):144–154. https://doi.org/10.1016/S1473-3099(04)00938-7

Bogaert D, van Belkum A, Sluijter M, Luijendijk A, de Groot R, Rumke HC et al (2004b) Colonisation by

Streptococcus pneumoniae and Staphylococcus aureus in healthy children. Lancet 363(9424):1871–1872. https://doi.org/10.1016/S0140-6736(04)16357-5

Bowden R, Chandrasekar P, White MH et al (2002) A double-blind, randomized, controlled trial of amphotericin B colloidal dispersion versus amphotericin B for treatment of invasive aspergillosis in immunocompromised patients. Clin Infect Dis 35(4):359–366

Bozza S, Perruccio K, Montagnoli C et al (2003) A dendritic cell vaccine against invasive aspergillosis in allogeneic hematopoietic transplantation. Blood 102(10):3807–3814

Bricout H, Haugh M, Olatunde O, Prieto RG (2015) Herpes zoster-associated mortality in Europe: a systematic review. BMC Public Health 15:466

Brown AO, Mann B, Gao G, Hankins JS, Humann J, Giardina J et al (2014) Streptococcus pneumoniae translocates into the myocardium and forms unique microlesions that disrupt cardiac function. PLoS Pathog 10(9):e1004383. https://doi.org/10.1371/journal.ppat.1004383

Brydak LB, Machała M, Centkowski P, Warzocha K, Biliński P (2006) Humoral response to hemagglutinin components of influenza vaccine in patients with non-Hodgkin malignant lymphoma. Vaccine 24(44–46):6620–6623

Burton AR, Pallett LJ, McCoy LE et al (2018) Circulating and intrahepatic antiviral B cells are defective in hepatitis B. J Clin Invest 128:4588–4603. https://doi.org/10.1172/JCI121960

Cassone A, Casadevall A (2012) Recent progress in vaccines against fungal diseases. Curr Opin Microbiol 15(4):427–433

Castilla J, Godoy P, Domínguez A et al (2013) Influenza vaccine effectiveness in preventing outpatient, inpatient, and severe cases of laboratory-confirmed influenza. Clin Infect Dis 57(2):167–175

Chanan-Khan A, Sonneveld P, Schuster MW et al (2008) Analysis of herpes zoster events among bortezomib-treated patients in the phase III APEX study. J Clin Oncol 26(29):4784–4790

Chen SY, Suaya JA, Li Q et al (2014) Incidence of herpes zoster in patients with altered immune function. Infection 42(2):325–334

Cheng A-L, Hsiung CA, Su I-J et al (2003) Steroid-free chemotherapy decreases risk of hepatitis B virus (HBV) reactivation in HBV-carriers with lymphoma. Hepatology 37:1320–1328. https://doi.org/10.1053/jhep.2003.50220

Chhabra P, Ranjan P, Bhasin DK (2017) Simultaneous occurrence of Varicella Zoster virus-induced pancreatitis and hepatitis in a renal transplant recipient: a case report and review of literature. Perm J 21

Chidiac C, Bruxelle J, Daures JP et al (2001) Characteristics of patients with herpes zoster on presentation to practitioners in France. Clin Infect Dis 33(1):62–69

Clemmensen OJ, Andersen KE (1984) ACTH versus prednisone and placebo in herpes zoster treatment. Clin Exp Dermatol 9(6):557–563

Cooksley CD, Avritscher EB, Bekele BN, Rolston KV, Geraci JM, Elting LS (2005) Epidemiology and outcomes of serious influenza-related infections in the cancer population. Cancer 104(3):618–628

Cornberg M (2018) Hepatitis B – Ein Ausblick auf aktualisierte Leitlinien. Dtsch Med Wochenschr 143:183–188. https://doi.org/10.1055/s-0043-114048

Dhédin N, Krivine A, Le Corre N et al (2014) Comparable humoral response after two doses of adjuvanted influenza a/H1N1pdm2009 vaccine or natural infection in allogeneic stem cell transplant recipients. Vaccine 32(5):585–591

Di Legami V, Gianino MM, Ciofi Degli Atti M et al (2007) Epidemiology and costs of herpes zoster: background data to estimate the impact of vaccination. Vaccine 25(43):7598–7604

ECIL-7 (2017. http://www.ecil-leukaemia.com/telechargements/ECIL%207%20Vaccine%20Part%20I%20and%20II%20Final.pdf. Accessed Feb 2018) Guidelines for vaccination of patients with hematological malignancies and HSCT recipients, p 2018

Engelhard D, Zakay-Rones Z, Shapira MY et al (2011) The humoral immune response of hematopoietic stem cell transplantation recipients to AS03-adjuvanted a/California/7/2009 (H1N1)v-like virus vaccine during the 2009 pandemic. Vaccine 29(9):1777–1782

European Association for the Study of the Liver (2017) Electronic address: easloffice@easloffice.eu, European Association for the Study of the Liver. EASL 2017 Clinical Practice Guidelines on the management of hepatitis B virus infection. J Hepatol 67:370–398. https://doi.org/10.1016/j.jhep.2017.03.021

Evens AM, Jovanovic BD, Su Y-C et al (2011) Rituximab-associated hepatitis B virus (HBV) reactivation in lymphoproliferative diseases: meta-analysis and examination of FDA safety reports. Ann Oncol 22:1170–1180. https://doi.org/10.1093/annonc/mdq583

Ewig S, Birkner N, Strauss R, Schaefer E, Pauletzki J, Bischoff H et al (2009) New perspectives on community-acquired pneumonia in 388 406 patients. Results from a nationwide mandatory performance measurement programme in healthcare quality. Thorax 64(12):1062–1069. https://doi.org/10.1136/thx.2008.109785

Fernández-Ruiz M, Meije Y, Manuel O et al (2018) ESCMID study Group for Infections in compromised hosts (ESGICH) consensus document on the safety of targeted and biological therapies: an infectious diseases perspective (introduction). Clin Microbiol Infect 24:S2

Fidan I, Kalkanci A, Yesilyurt E, Erdal B (2014) In vitro effects of Candida albicans and Aspergillus fumigatus on dendritic cells and the role of beta glucan in this effect. Adv Clin Exp Med 23(1):17–24

Flannery B, Chung JR, Belongia EA et al (2018) Interim estimates of 2017-18 seasonal influenza vaccine effectiveness - United States, February 2018. MMWR Morb Mortal Wkly Rep 67(6):180–185

Food and Drug Administration (2012) FDA approves VariZIG for reducing chickenpox symptoms. Food and Drug Administration, Silver Spring, MD. http://www.fda.gov/newsevents/newsroom/pressannouncements/ucm333233.htm

Gastmeier P, Sohr D, Geffers C, Ruden H, Vonberg RP, Welte T (2009) Early- and late-onset pneumonia: is this still a useful classification? Antimicrob Agents Chemother 53(7):2714–2718. https://doi.org/10.1128/AAC.01070-08

Gauthier A, Breuer J, Carrington D, Martin M, Rémy V (2009) Epidemiology and cost of herpes zoster and post-herpetic neuralgia in the United Kingdom. Epidemiol Infect 137(1):38–47

Gershon AA, Steinberg SP (1990) Live attenuated varicella vaccine: protection in healthy adults compared with leukemic children. National Institute of Allergy and Infectious Diseases Varicella vaccine collaborative study group. J Infect Dis 161(4):661–666

Gershon AA, Chen J, Davis L et al (2012) Latency of varicella zoster virus in dorsal root, cranial, and enteric ganglia in vaccinated children. Trans Am Clin Climatol Assoc 123:17–33. discussion 33-15

Gershon AA, Breuer J, Cohen JI et al (2015) Varicella zoster virus infection. Nat Rev Dis Primers 1:15016

Gialloreti LE, Merito M, Pezzotti P et al (2010) Epidemiology and economic burden of herpes zoster and post-herpetic neuralgia in Italy: a retrospective, population-based study. BMC Infect Dis 10:230

Giridhar KV, Shanafelt T, Tosh PK, Parikh SA, Call TG (2017) Disseminated herpes zoster in chronic lymphocytic leukemia (CLL) patients treated with B-cell receptor pathway inhibitors. Leuk Lymphoma 58(8):1973–1976

Gribabis DA, Panayiotidis P, Boussiotis VA, Hannoun C, Pangalis GA (1994) Influenza virus vaccine in B-cell chronic lymphocytic leukaemia patients. Acta Haematol 91(3):115–118

Grijalva CG, Zhu Y, Williams DJ et al (2015) Association between hospitalization with community-acquired laboratory-confirmed influenza pneumonia and prior receipt of influenza vaccination. JAMA 314(14):1488–1497

Grohskopf LA, Sokolow LZ, Broder KR et al (2017) Prevention and control of seasonal influenza with vaccines: recommendations of the advisory committee on immunization practices - United States, 2017-18 influenza season. MMWR Recomm Rep 66(2):1–20

Gustafson TL, Lavely GB, Brawner ER, Hutcheson RH, Wright PF, Schaffner W (1982) An outbreak of airborne nosocomial varicella. Pediatrics 70(4):550–556

Hamad M (2012) Universal fungal vaccines: could there be light at the end of the tunnel? Hum Vaccin Immunother 8(12):1758–1763

Hammond SP, Borchelt AM, Ukomadu C et al (2009) Hepatitis B virus reactivation following allogeneic hematopoietic stem cell transplantation. Biol Blood Marrow Transplant 15:1049–1059. https://doi.org/10.1016/j.bbmt.2009.05.001

Hassan IA, Chopra R, Swindell R, Mutton KJ (2003) Respiratory viral infections after bone marrow/peripheral stem-cell transplantation: the Christie hospital experience. Bone Marrow Transplant 32(1):73–77

Hedlund J, Christenson B, Lundbergh P, Ortqvist A (2003) Effects of a large-scale intervention with influenza and 23-valent pneumococcal vaccines in elderly people: a 1-year follow-up. Vaccine 21(25–26):3906–3911

Hodges GR, Davis JW, Lewis HD et al (1979) Response to influenza a vaccine among high-risk patients. South Med J 72(1):29–32

Hoofnagle JH (2009) Reactivation of hepatitis B. Hepatology 49:S156–S165. https://doi.org/10.1002/hep.22945

Hui C-K, Cheung WWW, Au W-Y et al (2005) Hepatitis B reactivation after withdrawal of pre-emptive lamivudine in patients with haematological malignancy on completion of cytotoxic chemotherapy. Gut 54:1597–1603. https://doi.org/10.1136/gut.2005.070763

Hwang JP, Lok AS-F (2014) Management of patients with hepatitis B who require immunosuppressive therapy. Nat Rev Gastroenterol Hepatol 11:209–219. https://doi.org/10.1038/nrgastro.2013.216

Hwang JP, Somerfield MR, Alston-Johnson DE et al (2015) Hepatitis B virus screening for patients with Cancer before therapy: American Society of Clinical Oncology provisional clinical opinion update. J Clin Oncol 33:2212–2220. https://doi.org/10.1200/JCO.2015.61.3745

Iglar K, Kopp A, Glazier RH (2013) Herpes zoster as a marker of underlying malignancy. Open Med 7(2):e68–e73

Inazawa N, Hori T, Nojima M et al (2017) Virus reactivations after autologous hematopoietic stem cell transplantation detected by multiplex PCR assay. J Med Virol 89(2):358–362

Je S, Firat D (1965) Varicella-Zoster Infection In Hodgkin's Disease: Clinical And Epidemiological Aspects. Am J Med 39:452–463

Johnson NP, Mueller J (2002) Updating the accounts: global mortality of the 1918-1920 "Spanish" influenza pandemic. Bull Hist Med 76(1):105–115

Johnson BH, Palmer L, Gatwood J, Lenhart G, Kawai K, Acosta CJ (2015) Annual incidence rates of herpes zoster among an immunocompetent population in the United States. BMC Infect Dis 15:502

Kamber C, Zimmerli S, Suter-Riniker F et al (2015) Varicella zoster virus reactivation after autologous SCT is a frequent event and associated with favorable outcome in myeloma patients. Bone Marrow Transplant 50(4):573–578

Kawai K, Yawn BP (2017) Risk factors for herpes zoster: a systematic review and meta-analysis. Mayo Clin Proc 92(12):1806–1821

Kim ST, Park KH, Oh SC et al (2012) Varicella zoster virus infection during chemotherapy in solid cancer patients. Oncology 82(2):126–130

Kim YJ, Lee CN, Lim CY, Jeon WS, Park YM (2014) Population-based study of the epidemiology of herpes zoster in Korea. J Korean Med Sci 29(12):1706–1710

Koehler P, Hamprecht A, Bader O et al (2017) Epidemiology of invasive aspergillosis and azole resistance in patients with acute leukaemia: the SEPIA study. Int J Antimicrob Agents 49(2):218–223

König C, Kleber M, Reinhardt H, Knop S, Wäsch R, Engelhardt M (2014) Incidence, risk factors, and implemented prophylaxis of varicella zoster virus infection, including complicated varicella zoster virus and herpes simplex virus infections, in lenalidomide-treated multiple myeloma patients. Ann Hematol 93(3):479–484

Kunisaki KM, Janoff EN (2009) Influenza in immunosuppressed populations: a review of infection frequency, morbidity, mortality, and vaccine responses. Lancet Infect Dis 9(8):493–504

Kwetkat A, Pfister W, Pansow D, Pletz MW, Sieber CC, Hoyer H (2018) Naso- and oropharyngeal bacterial carriage in nursing home residents: impact of multimorbidity and functional impairment. PLoS One 13(1):e0190716. https://doi.org/10.1371/journal.pone.0190716

Lambkin-Williams R, Gelder C, Broughton R et al (2016) An Intranasal Proteosome-Adjuvanted Trivalent Influenza Vaccine Is Safe, Immunogenic & Efficacious in the Human Viral Influenza Challenge Model. Serum IgG & Mucosal IgA Are Important Correlates of Protection against Illness Associated with Infection. *PLoS One* 11(12):e0163089

Lin C-L, Kao J-H (2017) Natural history of acute and chronic hepatitis B: the role of HBV genotypes and mutants. Best Pract Res Clin Gastroenterol 31:249–255. https://doi.org/10.1016/j.bpg.2017.04.010

Ljungman P (2001) Respiratory virus infections in stem cell transplant patients: the European experience. Biol Blood Marrow Transplant 7(Suppl):5S–7S

Ljungman P, Nahi H, Linde A (2005) Vaccination of patients with haematological malignancies with one or two doses of influenza vaccine: a randomised study. Br J Haematol 130(1):96–98

Lo W, Whimbey E, Elting L, Couch R, Cabanillas F, Bodey G (1993) Antibody response to a two-dose influenza vaccine regimen in adult lymphoma patients on chemotherapy. Eur J Clin Microbiol Infect Dis 12(10):778–782

Lok ASF, Liang RHS, Chiu EKW et al (1991) Reactivation of hepatitis B virus replication in patients receiving cytotoxic therapy: report of a prospective study. Gastroenterology 100:182–188. https://doi.org/10.1016/0016-5085(91)90599-G

Lopez A, Mariette X, Bachelez H, Belot A, Bonnotte B, Hachulla E et al (2017) Vaccination recommendations for the adult immunosuppressed patient: a systematic review and comprehensive field synopsis. J Autoimmun 80:10–27. https://doi.org/10.1016/j.jaut.2017.03.011

Lu H, Lok AS, Warneke CL et al (2018) Passive transfer of anti-HBc after intravenous immunoglobulin administration in patients with cancer: a retrospective chart review. Lancet Haematol 5:e474–e478. https://doi.org/10.1016/S2352-3026(18)30152-2

Lussana F, Cattaneo M, Rambaldi A, Squizzato A (2018) Ruxolitinib-associated infections: a systematic review and meta-analysis. Am J Hematol 93(3):339–347

Machado CM, Cardoso MR, da Rocha IF, Boas LS, Dulley FL, Pannuti CS (2005) The benefit of influenza vaccination after bone marrow transplantation. Bone Marrow Transplant 36(10):897–900

Maini MK, Pallett LJ (2018) Defective T-cell immunity in hepatitis B virus infection: why therapeutic vaccination needs a helping hand. Lancet Gastroenterol Hepatol 3:192–202. https://doi.org/10.1016/S2468-1253(18)30007-4

Martin-Loeches I, Schultz M, Vincent JL et al (2017) Increased incidence of co-infection in critically ill patients with influenza. Intensive Care Med 43(1):48–58

Mattiuzzi GN, Cortes JE, Talpaz M et al (2003) Development of Varicella-Zoster virus infection in patients with chronic myelogenous leukemia treated with imatinib mesylate. Clin Cancer Res 9(3):976–980

Mazza JJ, Yale SH, Arrowood JR et al (2005) Efficacy of the influenza vaccine in patients with malignant lymphoma. Clin Med Res 3(4):214–220

Morton JB, Morrill HJ, LaPlante KL, Caffrey AR (2017) Risk stacking of pneumococcal vaccination indications increases mortality in unvaccinated adults with Streptococcus pneumoniae infections. Vaccine 35(13):1692–1697. https://doi.org/10.1016/j.vaccine.2017.02.026

Natori Y, Humar A, Lipton J et al (2017a) A pilot randomized trial of adjuvanted influenza vaccine in adult allogeneic hematopoietic stem cell transplant recipients. Bone Marrow Transplant 52(7):1016–1021

Natori Y, Shiotsuka M, Slomovic J et al (2017b) A double blind randomized trial of high dose vs. Standard Dose Influenza Vaccine in Adult Solid Organ Transplant Recipients. Clin Infect Dis

Nichols WG, Guthrie KA, Corey L, Boeckh M (2004) Influenza infections after hematopoietic stem cell transplantation: risk factors, mortality, and the effect of antiviral therapy. Clin Infect Dis 39(9):1300–1306

Paules C, Subbarao K (2017) Influenza. *Lancet* 390(10095):697–708

Pentikis HS, Matson M, Atiee G et al (2011) Pharmacokinetics and safety of FV-100, a novel oral anti-herpes zoster nucleoside analogue, administered in single and multiple doses to healthy young adult and elderly adult volunteers. Antimicrob Agents Chemother 55(6):2847–2854

Perrillo RP, Gish R, Falck-Ytter YT (2015) American Gastroenterological Association Institute technical review on prevention and treatment of hepatitis B virus reactivation during immunosuppressive drug therapy. *Gastroenterology* **148**:221–244.e3. https://doi.org/10.1053/j.gastro.2014.10.038

Pletz MW, Welte T (2014) Pneumococcal and influenza vaccination. In: Chalmers J, Pletz MW, Aliberti S (eds) Community-acquired pneumonia. European Respiratory Society, European Respiratory Monographs, pp 266–285

Pletz MW, Maus U, Krug N, Welte T, Lode H (2008) Pneumococcal vaccines: mechanism of action, impact on epidemiology and adaption of the species. Int J Antimicrob Agents 32(3):199–206. https://doi.org/10.1016/j.ijantimicag.2008.01.021

Pletz MW, Welte T, Klugman KP (2010) The paradox in pneumococcal serotypes: highly invasive does not mean highly lethal. Eur Respir J. 36(4):712–713. https://doi.org/10.1183/09031936.00041210

Pletz MW, von Baum H, van der Linden M, Rohde G, Schutte H, Suttorp N et al (2012) The burden of pneumococcal pneumonia - experience of the German competence network CAPNETZ. Pneumologie 66(8):470–475. https://doi.org/10.1055/s-0032-1310103

Poeppl W, Lagler H, Raderer M et al (2015) Influenza vaccination perception and coverage among patients with malignant disease. Vaccine 33(14):1682–1687

Rapezzi D, Sticchi L, Racchi O, Mangerini R, Ferraris AM, Gaetani GF (2003) Influenza vaccine in chronic lymphoproliferative disorders and multiple myeloma. Eur J Haematol 70(4):225–230

Reddy KR, Beavers KL, Hammond SP et al (2015) American gastroenterological association institute guideline on the prevention and treatment of hepatitis B virus reactivation during immunosuppressive drug therapy. Gastroenterology 148:215–219. https://doi.org/10.1053/j.gastro.2014.10.039

Restrepo MI, Reyes LF (2018) Pneumonia as a cardiovascular disease. Respirology 23(3):250–259. https://doi.org/10.1111/resp.13233

Robertson JD, Nagesh K, Jowitt SN et al (2000) Immunogenicity of vaccination against influenza, Streptococcus pneumoniae and Haemophilus influenzae type B in patients with multiple myeloma. Br J Cancer 82(7):1261–1265

Rubin LG, Levin MJ, Ljungman P et al (2014) 2013 IDSA clinical practice guideline for vaccination of the immunocompromised host. Clin Infect Dis 58(3):e44–100

Sandherr M, Hentrich M, von Lilienfeld-Toal M et al (2015) Antiviral prophylaxis in patients with solid tumours and haematological malignancies--update of the guidelines of the infectious diseases working party (AGIHO) of the German Society for Hematology and Medical Oncology (DGHO). Ann Hematol 94(9):1441–1450

Sauerbrei A, Uebe B, Wutzler P (2003) Molecular diagnosis of zoster post varicella vaccination. J Clin Virol 27(2):190–199

Sauerbrei A, Färber I, Brandstädt A, Schacke M, Wutzler P (2004) Immunofluorescence test for sensitive detection of varicella-zoster virus-specific IgG: an alternative to fluorescent antibody to membrane antigen test. J Virol Methods 119(1):25–30

Schmid DS, Jumaan AO (2010) Impact of varicella vaccine on varicella-zoster virus dynamics. Clin Microbiol Rev 23(1):202–217

Schuster MG, Cleveland AA, Dubberke ER et al (2017) Infections in Hematopoietic Cell Transplant Recipients: Results From the Organ Transplant Infection Project, a Multicenter, Prospective, Cohort Study. Open Forum Infect Dis 4(2):ofx050

Schweitzer A, Horn J, Mikolajczyk RT et al (2015) Estimations of worldwide prevalence of chronic hepatitis B virus infection: a systematic review of data published between 1965 and 2013. Lancet 386:1546–1555. https://doi.org/10.1016/S0140-6736(15)61412-X

Shibasaki S, Aoki W, Nomura T, Karasaki M, Sewaki T, Ueda M (2014) Evaluation of Mdh1 protein as an antigenic candidate for a vaccine against candidiasis. Biocontrol Sci 19(1):51–55

Stiver HG, Weinerman BH (1978) Impaired serum antibody response to inactivated influenza A and B vaccine in cancer patients. Can Med Assoc J 119(7):733,-735, 738

Storek J, Viganego F, Dawson MA et al (2003) Factors affecting antibody levels after allogeneic hematopoietic cell transplantation. Blood 101(8):3319–3324

Styczynski J, Reusser P, Einsele H et al (2009) Management of HSV, VZV and EBV infections in patients with hematological malignancies and after SCT: guidelines from the second European conference on infections in leukemia. Bone Marrow Transplant 43(10):757–770

Sweeney CJ, Gilden DH (2001) Ramsay hunt syndrome. J Neurol Neurosurg Psychiatry 71(2):149–154

Terrault NA, Lok ASF, McMahon BJ et al (2018) Update on prevention, diagnosis, and treatment of chronic hepatitis B: AASLD 2018 hepatitis B guidance. Hepatology 67:1560–1599. https://doi.org/10.1002/hep.29800

Theilacker C, Ludewig K, Serr A, Schimpf J, Held J, Bogelein M et al (2016) Overwhelming Postsplenectomy infection: a prospective multicenter cohort study. Clin Infect Dis 62(7):871–878. https://doi.org/10.1093/cid/civ1195

Tomonari A, Iseki T, Takahashi S et al (2003) Varicella-zoster virus infection in adult patients after unrelated cord blood transplantation: a single institute experience in Japan. Br J Haematol 122(5):802–805

Tong S, Revill P (2016) Overview of viral replication and genetic variability. J Hepatol 64:S4–S16. https://doi.org/10.1016/j.jhep.2016.01.027

Torosantucci A, Bromuro C, Chiani P et al (2005) A novel glyco-conjugate vaccine against fungal pathogens. J Exp Med 202(5):597–606

van de Veerdonk FL, Kolwijck E, Lestrade PP et al (2017) Influenza-associated aspergillosis in critically ill patients. Am J Respir Crit Care Med

Vegnente A, Iorio R, Guida S et al (1992) Chronicity rate of hepatitis B virus infection in the families of 60 hepatitis B surface antigen positive chronic carrier children: role of horizontal transmission. Eur J Pediatr 151:188–191. https://doi.org/10.1007/BF01954381

van der Velden AM, Mulder AH, Hartkamp A, Diepersloot RJ, van Velzen-Blad H, Biesma DH (2001) Influenza virus vaccination and booster in B-cell chronic lymphocytic leukaemia patients. Eur J Intern Med 12(5):420–424

Webster RG, Wright SM, Castrucci MR, Bean WJ, Kawaoka Y (1993) Influenza--a model of an emerging virus disease. Intervirology 35(1–4):16–25

Welte T, Pletz M (2017) Pneumonia and the risk of cardiovascular death. Time to change our strategy. Am J Respir Crit Care Med 196(5):541–543. https://doi.org/10.1164/rccm.201707-1421ED

Werle-Lapostolle B, Bowden S, Locarnini S et al (2004) Persistence of cccDNA during the natural history of chronic hepatitis B and decline during adefovir dipivoxil therapy. Gastroenterology 126:1750–1758

Whimbey E, Champlin RE, Couch RB et al (1996) Community respiratory virus infections among hospitalized adult bone marrow transplant recipients. Clin Infect Dis 22(5):778–782

Winthrop KL, Baddley JW, Chen L et al (2013) Association between the initiation of anti-tumor necrosis factor therapy and the risk of herpes zoster. JAMA 309(9):887–895

Xin H, Cutler JE (2011) Vaccine and monoclonal antibody that enhance mouse resistance to candidiasis Clin Vaccine Immunol 18(10):1656–1667

Yalçin SS, Kondolot M, Albayrak N et al (2010) Serological response to influenza vaccine after hematopoetic stem cell transplantation. Ann Hematol 89(9):913–918

Yenikomshian MA, Guignard AP, Haguinet F et al (2015) The epidemiology of herpes zoster and its complications in Medicare cancer patients. BMC Infect Dis 15:106

Yeo W, Chan PKS, Hui P et al (2003) Hepatitis B virus reactivation in breast cancer patients receiving cytotoxic chemotherapy: a prospective study. J Med Virol 70:553–561. https://doi.org/10.1002/jmv.10430

Yri OE, Torfoss D, Hungnes O et al (2011) Rituximab blocks protective serologic response to influenza a (H1N1) 2009 vaccination in lymphoma patients during or within 6 months after treatment. Blood 118(26):6769–6771

Zhang M-Y, Zhu G Q, Zhong J N et al (2017) Nucleos(t) ide analogues for preventing HBV reactivation in immunosuppressed patients with hematological malignancies: a network meta-analysis. Expert Rev Anti-Infect Ther 15:503–513. https://doi.org/10.1080 /14787210.2017.1309291

Vaccination Schedules

7

Benjamin W. Teh

7.1   Introduction

Patients with haematological cancers are at increased risk for a range of vaccine preventable infections (Teh et al. 2014; Morrison 2010; Torda et al. 2014). Higher rates are seen with increasing intensity of treatments such as with allogeneic haematopoietic stem cell transplantation (HSCT) (Kumar et al. 2008; Kyaw et al. 2005). Rates of invasive pneumococcal infection are 50 times higher in allogeneic HSCT (alloHSCT) patients compared to a general population (Kumar et al. 2008). As outlined in the previous chapters, inactivated vaccines for pneumococcus, influenza, meningococcus, *Haemophilus influenza* B, hepatitis B, diphtheria, tetanus, pertussis and polio are available to minimise morbidity and mortality from these infections (Tomblyn et al. 2009; (ATAGI) ATAGoI 2017; Kim et al. 2018). Protection against measles, mumps, rubella and varicella are available in the form of live vaccines (Tomblyn et al. 2009; (ATAGI) ATAGoI 2017; Kim et al. 2018).

Multiple international and national bodies have made recommendations with regards to the type and timing of immunisation for patients with haematological cancers (Tomblyn et al. 2009; Rubin et al. 2014; Ljungman et al. 2009; Tsigrelis and Ljungman 2016; Rieger et al. 2018). Some recommendations have been made on the basis of randomised trials, whilst others have been extrapolated from studies evaluating vaccine responses at various time points following completion of treatment for haematological cancer or HSCT (Cordonnier et al. 2009; Cordonnier et al. 2015a; Cordonnier et al. 2015b; Hinge et al. 2012; Kumar et al. 2007). Most studies in this field have utilised serological endpoints as surrogate markers for clinical protection and efficacy and remain a common outcome used to guide timing of vaccinations (de Lavallade et al. 2011; Cordonnier et al. 2010a).

In this chapter, factors that determine timing of vaccines are discussed and recommendations provided with regard to key vaccine preventable infections across haematology groups; patients with more chronic haematological cancers, acute leukaemia, lymphomas and HSCT.

B. W. Teh (✉)
Department of Infectious Diseases, Peter MacCallum Cancer Centre, Melbourne, VIC, Australia

Sir Peter MacCallum Department of Oncology, University of Melbourne, Melbourne, VIC, Australia

National Centre for Infections in Cancer, Melbourne, VIC, Australia
e-mail: ben.teh@petermac.org

© Springer Nature Switzerland AG 2021
O. A. Cornely, M. Hoenigl (eds.), *Infection Management in Hematology*, Hematologic Malignancies, https://doi.org/10.1007/978-3-030-57317-1_7

7.2   Factors Impacting Timing

Determining optimal timing of vaccination requires careful consideration of several closely interconnected factors. Patients with haematological malignancy are a diverse group of patients receiving a wide range of curative and non-curative treatments, which can be challenging to evaluate. Ideally, vaccination should be timed to be safe with minimal risk for vaccine-related adverse events, cover a period of high risk for infection and occur when patients have sufficient immune capacity to produce a protective response and when haematological treatments do not negatively impact response to vaccination.

7.2.1   Patient Factors

Haematology patients are at increased risk for infection due a combination of patient, disease and treatment-related factors (Teh et al. 2014; Teh et al. 2018). Certain haematological diseases such as chronic lymphocytic leukaemia (CLL) and multiple myeloma (MM) commonly affect older patients who are at increased risk for vaccine-preventable infections such as pneumococcal infection, independent of their malignancy (Teh et al. 2014; Morrison 2007; Jackson et al. 2013). This risk relates to changes to the make-up of immune cells with ageing or immunosenescence (Teh et al. 2014). In addition, other comorbidities such as chronic lung disease, renal impairment, functional or anatomical asplenia maybe present that result in increased risk ((ATAGI) ATAGoI 2017; Kim et al. 2018; Theilacker et al. 2016). As such, for the elderly group of patients, there are vaccinations recommended for their age and comorbidities independent of their haematological malignancy that need to be taken into consideration ((ATAGI) ATAGoI 2017; Kim et al. 2018). Patients who are being treated for haematological diseases will often travel and their intended destination, timing of travel and stage of treatment and related immune suppression will drive timing of vaccination against routine and travel-related infections (Aung et al. 2015).

7.2.2   Disease-Related Factors

7.2.2.1 Disease Burden, Immune Deficiency and Infection Risk Period

Underlying disease-related immune deficiencies such as hypogammaglobulinaemia, defects in complement activity in CLL and monoclonal paraprotein production in MM contribute to the increased risk for encapsulated bacterial infection reported classically for these disease groups (Teh et al. 2014; Morrison 2009; Savage et al. 1982; Blimark et al. 2014). This risk has evolved with the introduction of targeted and immuno-modulatory therapies (Teh et al. 2014; Teh et al. 2017a). However, rates of vaccine-preventable blood stream infections such as with *Streptococcus pneumonia* remain between 14 and 22% of patients with chronic haematological malignancies (Teh et al. 2017a; Andersen et al. 2018). Vaccination targeted to identified periods of increased risk can have a significant impact on reducing morbidity and mortality. Depending on the type of malignancy, the period of increased risk could be early at disease diagnosis or during induction therapy, following consolidation therapy with HSCT or occur late following multiple lines of therapy for relapse disease (Teh et al. 2015a).

For diseases such as CLL and MM, risk is increased during periods of significant burden disease burden (Teh et al. 2014; Sun et al. 2015). With response to treatment, there appears to be a corresponding decline in risk for infection (Sun et al. 2015; Rawstron et al. 1998; Hargreaves et al. 1995). Therefore, an ideal period for vaccination would be prior to commencement of disease-specific therapy when the risks for infection remain high due to burden of disease. Live vaccines remain contraindicated due to ongoing disease-related immune deficiencies, and case fatalities have been reported (Costa et al. 2016).

As the management of these diseases are characterised by cycles of treatment and relapse, cumulative effects of therapy promote ongoing risks for infection (Teh et al. 2014; Teh et al. 2018). Therefore, patients with relapsed and refractory disease are at high risk for infection

(Teh et al. 2015a). MM patients who are not transplant eligible have rates of blood stream infection of up to 14% (Teh et al. 2017a). However, studies evaluating revaccination, new vaccination approaches or use of additional doses in patients with relapse and refractory disease are lacking.

With acute leukaemia and patients undergoing HSCT, the intensity of induction and myeloablative conditioning chemotherapy depletes immune cell numbers and associated immunity to a range of vaccine-preventable infections (Rubin et al. 2014; Shigayeva et al. 2016; Giebink et al. 1986; Witherspoon et al. 1981). Risks for infection are mediated by prolonged neutropenia and delayed immune reconstitution. Vaccination prior to commencement of conditioning chemotherapy has been demonstrated to enhance vaccine responses post HSCT (Locke et al. 2016; Ambati et al. 2015). Chronic graft vs. host disease (GvHD) as a complication of alloHSCT is significantly associated with long-term increased risk for invasive pneumococcal disease (Kulkarni et al. 2000; Engelhard et al. 2002).

7.2.3 Treatment-Related Factors

7.2.3.1 Types of Therapy and Impact on Immunity

When determining timing of vaccination, the impact of treatment for haematological disease on vaccine responses should be carefully considered. Whilst therapies induce control of disease and correspondingly reduce infection risk, some therapies can negatively impact patient response to vaccination. Where possible, concurrent vaccination should be avoided unless the risk for infection is unacceptably high.

Rituximab, an anti CD-20 antibody used in the treatment of CLL and a range of non-Hodgkin's lymphomas (NHL) have been demonstrated to blunt responses to influenza and pneumococcal vaccination (Berglund et al. 2014; Bedognetti et al. 2011; Ide et al. 2014). In observational studies of patients on rituximab therapy or within 6 months of completion, rates of seroprotection following influenza vaccination range from 0% to 25%, and rates of seroconversion remain significantly lower than controls at between 9 and 30% (Berglund et al. 2014; Bedognetti et al. 2011; Ide et al. 2014; Yri et al. 2011). On these reports, deferring vaccination in rituximab-treated patients until 6 months post completion of therapy is generally recommended. The negative effect on vaccine responses has been extrapolated to patients receiving other anti-CD20 antibodies such as ofatumumab. There is also emerging literature of poor vaccination responses in the setting of therapy with Bruton's tyrosine kinase (Btk) inhibitors. Seroprotection rates of 7–26% to influenza vaccination have been reported when patients are receiving ibrutinib therapy whilst in a small study, no patient responded to pneumococcal vaccination (Douglas et al. 2017; Sun et al. 2016; Andrick et al. 2017).

In contrast, immunomodulatory drugs used for the treatment for MM have been shown to potentially enhance response to vaccination, which affords an opportunity for patients to derive more benefit from being vaccinated early during their induction treatment utilising these drugs (Noonan et al. 2012). In addition, the use of live vaccines during maintenance therapy with immunomodulatory drugs, a median of 2 years post HSCT have been shown to be safe (Pandit et al. 2018). However, timing of vaccination post HSCT for safety and optimal is also governed by the type of vaccine and reconstitution of immune cells. In patients post alloHSCT, the occurrence and immune suppressive treatment used for GvHD will impact choice, timing and safety of vaccines (Cordonnier et al. 2015a; Kulkarni et al. 2000).

The use of immune checkpoint inhibitors (ICI) such as PD-1 inhibitor pembrolizumab has revolutionised the treatment of solid tumours, but their use have been associated with immune-related adverse events (Postow et al. 2018). ICI have approved for the management of Hodgkin's lymphoma and has increasingly been trialled for the treatment of a number of acute haematological malignancies (Liu et al. 2018). Patients vaccinated with trivalent inactivated influenza vaccine (IIV) within 2 months of ICI therapy achieved comparable serological responses to health controls (Laubli et al. 2018). However, there has been conflicting data about an association between IIV vaccination and higher than expected incidence of immune-related adverse events (Laubli et al. 2018; Wijn et al. 2018). This has led to some caution around IIV and concurrent ICI therapy and timing of vaccination ((ATAGI) ATAGoI 2017).

7.2.4 Immune Reconstitution

HSCT pose a unique challenge in determining the optimal time for vaccination. Patient's post HSCT can be at increased risk for influenza and invasive pneumococcal infection in the early periods post HSCT, but reconstitution of the immune system in this early period does not support robust response to vaccination. Rates of influenza within 3 months of HSCT can be as high as 15% of symptomatic patients, and up to 15% of invasive pneumococcal infections occur early (Torda et al. 2014; Engelhard et al. 2002; Youssef et al. 2007; Sim et al. 2018). Although overall rates are lower, patients following autologous HSCT (autoHSCT) experience a higher incidence rate of invasive pneumococcal infection in the early post-transplant period (Engelhard et al. 2002). Length of time from HSCT remains a key factor in determining response to influenza vaccination (Karras et al. 2013; Engelhard et al. 1993).

Vaccination is avoided during periods of significant neutropenia from induction or myeloablative conditioning therapy due to likely poor vaccination responses from depleted immune cells and to avoid febrile reaction to vaccines complicating patient management during period of severe neutropenia ((ATAGI) ATAGoI 2017).

Neutrophils recover early post HSCT (Steingrimsdottir et al. 2000). However, immune cells required to effectively respond to vaccines and to control viral infections reconstitute over 12 months. B cells are predominantly responsible for responses to polysaccharide vaccines, whilst responses to conjugate vaccines are dependent on T cells, promoting a more effective response with greater memory (Pletz et al. 2008; Alemu et al.

2016). Generally B cells recover by 6 months, whilst full recovery of CD4 cells can take up to 24 months (Tomblyn et al. 2009; Steingrimsdottir et al. 2000; Schütt et al. 2006). Studies involving multiple inactivated vaccines have focussed on determining the best timing for commencement of revaccination for optimal and durable response, whilst those involving live vaccines have focussed on timing for safety (Cordonnier et al. 2009; Pandit et al. 2018).

7.2.5 Infection Factors

For infections such as influenza, the seasonality of peak transmission and infective periods in winter for temperate countries is an additional factor to be considered for timing of vaccination (Teh et al. 2015b; Azziz Baumgartner et al. 2012). The pandemic spread of influenza such as the H1N1/09 nearly a decade ago may drive the urgent need for vaccination as immunocompromised patients are at significantly higher risk (Tramontana et al. 2010). Outbreaks of vaccine-preventable infection such as measles may require revaccination with live vaccines earlier than anticipated (Machado et al. 2002; Machado et al. 2005a).

Taking all these factors into account (Fig. 7.1), the following sections will discuss timing of vaccination for pneumococcal infection and influenza for HSCT patients and patients with chronic malignancies, acute leukaemia and lymphomas and with recommendations provided.

7.3 Pneumococcal Vaccination

7.3.1 Haematopoietic Stem Cell Transplantation

The largest number of published studies on the timing of vaccination relate to this disease group. Patients following autoHSCT are at higher risk for invasive pneumococcal disease within the first 12 months post-transplant, whilst the risk in alloHSCT patients is later at 14–18 months post-transplant or during periods of GvHD (Torda

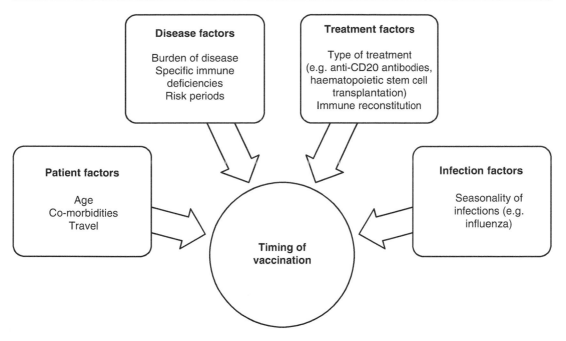

Fig. 7.1 Factors that influence timing of vaccination in patients with haematological malignancy

et al. 2014; Kumar et al. 2008; Youssef et al. 2007). Prior to the availability of pneumococcal conjugate vaccine (PCV), studies evaluating pneumococcal polysaccharide vaccine (PPV) reported poor response rates when delivered at 18–24 months post HSCT (Giebink et al. 1986; Storek et al. 2004; Guinan et al. 1994). Multiple dosing did not significantly improve response rates, with only 19% of vaccinated patients producing a sufficient response to all measured serotypes (Storek et al. 2004; Guinan et al. 1994).

Conjugate vaccines used for vaccination against *Haemophilus influenzae* type B appear to elicit a greater immunological response compared to PPV given concurrently especially with multiple dosing (Guinan et al. 1994). When the pneumococcal conjugate vaccine against 7 serotypes (PCV7) became available, it was evaluated against PPV in a randomised trial with donors vaccinated before transplant and to recipients, 6 months post-transplant (Kumar et al. 2007). Receipt of PCV7 was associated with nearly nine times the odds of achieving a serological response (Kumar et al. 2007). Overall, 90% of patients who received PCV7 achieved a response to at least 1 antigen at 12 months compared to 56% in PPV vaccinated patients and this was significantly different (Kumar et al. 2007). The use of PCV over PPV for initial pneumococcal vaccination started to be established. However, the response with PCV7 was still suboptimal with only a mean of 3 out of the 7 serotypes tested responding (Kumar et al. 2007).

Multiple dosing of PCV7 with different schedules commencing within 12 months of alloHSCT was evaluated in children and adults and produced better responses than single dose of PCV7 (Meisel et al. 2007a; Molrine et al. 2003). In the paediatric study involving alloHSCT from related and unrelated donors, a schedule of three doses of PCV7 delivered monthly commencing at 6–9 months post-transplant reported seroprotection rates against all seven serotypes of 56% following second vaccine dose and 74% after the third dose (Meisel et al. 2007a). In an adult alloHSCT study involving related HSCT, patients received PCV7 at 3, 6 and 12 months (Molrine et al. 2003). Nearly 65% of patients were seroprotected against all 7 serotypes 1 month following third vaccine dose (Molrine et al. 2003). The same study also noted better response rates and higher rates of seroprotection in the early transplant period with PCV7 vaccination in the donor (Molrine et al. 2003).

A large multi-centre randomised trial of myeloablative alloHSCT by Cordonnier et al. comprehensively evaluated timing of a three-dose schedule of PCV7 (monthly) followed by PPV dose 6 months later (Cordonnier et al. 2009). There was no significant difference in the rate of serological response 1 month post third dose between patients who commenced vaccination at 3 months compared to 9 months post alloHSCT (Cordonnier et al. 2009). Rate of serological response to all seven serotypes was 79% if commenced at 3 months vs. 82% if commenced at 9 months (Cordonnier et al. 2009). However, the proportion of patients achieving serological response (PCV7 serotypes) at 1 month post PPV23 was significantly higher in the late vaccination group (Cordonnier et al. 2009). At 24 months post-transplant, the rate of seroprotection appears to be significantly lower in patients vaccinated early (Cordonnier et al. 2009).

In addition to conferring additional protection against more serotypes, PPV23 dosing 6 months later boosts response to PCV7, eliciting serological response from 42% of PCV7 non-responders (Cordonnier et al. 2009). One month post PPV23 vaccination, there was no significant difference in rates of serological response to PPV-specific antigens between early and late vaccination group (Cordonnier et al. 2010b). Both groups achieved response rates above 80% increasing breadth of coverage from PCV7 (Cordonnier et al. 2010b). This study provided the evidence for earlier commencement of pneumococcal vaccination in the HSCT population and the schedule of using three monthly doses of PCV7, followed by PPV23 6 months later. PCV7 provides a robust early response to cover increased risk, and subsequent dose of PPV23 broadens this coverage and potentially rescues non-responders.

Follow-up of 30 survivors from this pivotal study demonstrated retention of immunity to serotypes contained within PCV7 and PPV23 8–11 years post completion of the study

(Cordonnier et al. 2015a). There was no significant decline in serological response rates for both PCV7 and PPV23 antigens, remaining relatively stable at 63–66% (Cordonnier et al. 2015a). Long-term rates of serological response appear to be significantly better in patients who commenced vaccination at 9 months post-transplant (Cordonnier et al. 2015a). Interestingly, an additional dose of PPV23 4 to 9 years post-transplant appears to have limited benefit (Cordonnier et al. 2015a).

A new formulation of PCV with additional serotype coverage (PCV13) was introduced and replaced the use of PCV7. A large multi-centre study in alloHSCT patients evaluated the immunogenicity of three doses, monthly schedule utilising PCV13 commencing 3–6 months post HSCT followed by fourth dose of PCV 6 months later and PPV23 (Cordonnier et al. 2015b). After 3 doses of PCV13 commencing a median of 5 months post HSCT, this schedule resulted in significant increases in geometric mean fold rises in IgG geometric mean concentrations for all vaccine serotypes with 90–98% of patients achieving serological concentrations above defined cut-off (Cordonnier et al. 2015b). An additional dose of PCV13 at 6 months after the third dose resulted in further increases to IgG although this was similar following PPV23. However, rates of local reaction and systemic adverse events were higher (Cordonnier et al. 2015b). In the absence of additional risk factors for invasive pneumococcal infection such as GvHD, it is unclear if the fourth dose of PCV13 offers additional benefits in return for increased side effect profile. As such, additional dose of PCV13 (fourth dose) is only recommended in the setting of additional risk such as GvHD.

The studies previously discussed have largely evaluated alloHSCT following myeloablative conditioned HSCT. In patients post non-myeloablative (reduced intensity conditioning) alloHSCT, serological response rate of 73% was achieved following two doses of PCV commencing 15 months post-transplant (Meerveld-Eggink et al. 2009). There are limited studies evaluating timing and serological response of PCV in autoHSCT patients. Antin et al. evaluated the response of autoHSCT patients to a three-dose schedule of PCV7 delivered at 3, 6 and 12 months following transplantation with or without pre-transplant vaccination (prior to stem cell collection) (Antin et al. 2005). Following completion of this three-dose schedule, more than 60% of patients achieved the defined serological protection for all seven serotypes (Antin et al. 2005). However, patients who received pre-transplant vaccination achieved higher rates of seroprotection earlier and significantly higher geometric mean concentrations against three vaccine serotypes (Antin et al. 2005). A different vaccination schedule consisting of two doses of PCV7 followed by PCV23 at 6, 8 and 14 months post-transplant in a mix population of patients undergoing autoHSCT resulted in serological response rate of 78% to serotypes in the conjugate vaccine (van der Velden et al. 2007). These studies provide supporting evidence for early commencement of vaccination post autoHSCT with multi-dose PCV schedule, PPV23 boosting and consideration of vaccination pre-transplant.

Due to lack of dedicated studies, additional evidence to support scheduling of PCV and the use of PPV23 following PCV in autoHSCT is extrapolated from studies involving alloHSCT.

Overall, the studies discussed have supported commencement of pneumococcal vaccination 3–6 months post alloHSCT and autoHSCT. The most commonly evaluated schedule has been three monthly doses of PCV7, followed by PPV23 6 months post third dose of PCV. Use of PCV13 in place of PCV7 has been evaluated and is now incorporated into recommendations. An additional dose of PCV13 is recommended in the setting of additional risk such as GvHD, whilst the utility long-term boosting with PPV23 remains undefined. Vaccination response and timing in non-myeloablative alloHSCT (e.g. haploidentical or reduced intensity conditioning) remain undefined and currently follow those for myeloablative conditioning. A summary of these recommendations can be found in Table 7.1. Some variation exists between guidelines developed by various international bodies, and these are summarised in Table 7.2.

Table 7.1 Summary of vaccination recommendations made in this chapter

Vaccination	Recommendations—type and timing
Pneumococcal vaccination	
Haematopoietic stem cell transplantation	Allogeneic/autologous: Commence vaccination at 3–6 months post HSCT Three doses of PCV13 (monthly) followed by dose of PPV23, 6 months later In the setting of chronic graft vs. host disease, replace PPV23 with a fourth dose of PCV13
Chronic haematological malignancies	
Multiple myeloma	Where possible, commence vaccination early following disease diagnosis or during induction/maintenance therapy with immunomodulatory drugs as an alternative One dose of PCV13 followed by PPV23, at least 8 weeks later For non-transplant patients, further dose of PPV23 could be considered, but long-term benefits undefined For transplant eligible patients, recommendations as per HSCT
Chronic lymphocytic leukaemia	Commence vaccination early following disease diagnosis, preferably before commencement of treatment especially if anti-CD20 or Btk inhibitor therapy being considered One dose of PCV13 followed by PPV23, at least 8 weeks later Further dose of PPV23 could be considered, but long-term benefits undefined Avoid vaccination during anti-CD20 antibody therapy, vaccinate ≥6 months following completion of anti-CD20 therapy Consider avoidance of vaccination during Btk inhibitor therapy

(continued)

Table 7.1 (continued)

Vaccination	Recommendations—type and timing
Acute leukaemia	If feasible, vaccinate prior to commencement of induction chemotherapy or vaccinate 3–6 months post completion of induction chemotherapy. Vaccination during maintenance chemotherapy appears feasible One dose of PCV13 recommended. Based on non-leukaemic studies, a subsequent dose of PPV23 could improve breadth of response
Lymphomas	If feasible, vaccinate at least 10–14 days prior to commencement of chemotherapy, especially if anti-CD20 or Btk inhibitor therapy being considered One dose of PCV13 followed by PPV23, at least 8 weeks later Avoid vaccination during anti-CD20 antibody therapy, vaccinate ≥6 months following completion of anti-CD20 therapy. Consider avoidance of vaccination during Btk inhibitor therapy
Influenza vaccination	
Haematopoietic stem cell transplantation	Annual inactivated influenza vaccine is recommended Vaccinate at 3–6 months post HSCT Consider vaccination prior to 6 months in the setting of community outbreak of influenza Consider two doses of IIV in patients who are influenza vaccine naïve and in pandemic outbreaks High dose and adjuvant IIV require further study
Chronic haematological malignancies	
Multiple myeloma	Annual inactivated influenza vaccine is recommended Vaccination prior to or whilst not receiving chemotherapy preferable If on chemotherapy, vaccinate between chemotherapy cycles, 7 days prior to start of next cycle If on chemotherapy, consider vaccination early relative to start of influenza transmission season as immunity may take up to 3 months to mature Consider two doses of IIV in patients who are influenza vaccine naïve and in pandemic outbreaks Vaccination during immunomodulatory drug therapy may enhance vaccine response
Chronic lymphocytic leukaemia	Annual inactivated influenza vaccine is recommended Vaccination prior to or whilst not receiving chemotherapy preferable Avoid vaccination during anti-CD20 antibody therapy, vaccinate ≥6 months following completion of anti-CD20 therapy Consider avoidance of vaccination during Btk inhibitor therapy Consider two doses of IIV in patients who are influenza vaccine naïve and in pandemic outbreaks
Acute leukaemia	Annual inactivated influenza vaccine is recommended Vaccination prior to or whilst not receiving chemotherapy preferable Vaccination during maintenance chemotherapy is feasible If on chemotherapy, vaccinate between chemotherapy cycles, 7 days prior to start of next cycle If on chemotherapy, consider vaccination early relative to start of influenza transmission season as immunity may take up to 3 months to mature Consider two doses of IIV in patients who are influenza vaccine naïve and in pandemic outbreaks
Lymphomas	Annual inactivated influenza vaccine is recommended Vaccination prior to or whilst not receiving chemotherapy preferable If on chemotherapy, vaccinate between chemotherapy cycles, 7 days prior to start of next cycle If on chemotherapy, consider vaccination early relative to start of influenza transmission season as immunity may take up to 3 months to mature Avoid vaccination during anti-CD20 antibody therapy, vaccinate ≥6 months following completion of anti-CD20 therapy Consider avoidance of vaccination during Btk inhibitor therapy Consider two doses of IIV in patients who are influenza vaccine naïve and in pandemic outbreaks

HSCT, haematopoietic stem cell transplant; *GvHD*, graft vs. host disease; *Btk*, Bruton's tyrosine kinase; *PCV13*, pneumococcal conjugate vaccine against 13 serotypes; *PPV23*, pneumococcal polysaccharide vaccine against 23 serotypes; *IIV*, inactivated influenza vaccine

Table 7.2 Summary of recommendations by various international bodies and societies, by vaccine-preventable disease

	International groups				
	IDSA 2013 (Rubin et al. 2014)	EBMT/ECIL 2009/2011 (Ljungman et al. 2009; Engelhard et al. 2013)	DGHO 2016/2018 (Rieger et al. 2018; Ullmann et al. 2016)	ATAGI 2017 ((ATAGI) ATAGoI 2017)	HSCT expert group 2009 (Tomblyn et al. 2009)
Pneumococcal vaccination					
Haematopoietic stem cell transplantation	Allogeneic/autologous: Vaccinate 3–6 months post HSCT 3 doses of PCV13 and 1 dose of PPV23 at 12 months post HSCT. Replace PPV23 with additional PCV13 if chronic GvHD present	Allogeneic/autologous: Vaccinatew at 3–6 months post HSCT 3 doses of PCV13 followed by PPV23 Replace PPV23 with additional PCV13 if chronic GvHD present	Allogeneic: Vaccinate 6 months post HSCT 3 doses of PCV13 (monthly) followed by PPV23,12 months later Autologous: Vaccinate 3–6 months post HSCT 3 doses of PCV13 (4–6 weeks apart) followed by PPV23, > 8 weeks later	Allogeneic/autologous: Vaccinated 6 months post HSCT 3 doses of PCV at 6, 8, 12 months post HSCT followed by PPV23, 12 months and 5 years later	Allogeneic/autologous: Vaccinated at 3–6 months post HSCT 3 doses of PCV followed by PPV23 Replace PPV23 with additional PCV if chronic GvHD present
Chronic haematological malignancies (chronic lymphocytic leukaemia, multiple myeloma)	Vaccinate newly diagnosed patients One dose PCV13 followed by PPV23, ≥ 8 weeks later If receiving anti-B cell therapy, vaccination should be delayed to ≥6 months after anti-B cell therapy		If no prior vaccination, PCV13 followed by PPV23, 8–12 weeks later	Vaccinate as early as possible after diagnosis OR Vaccinate if in remission 6 months after chemotherapy If no prior vaccination, PCV13 followed by PPV23, at least 8 weeks later and further dose of PPV23 5 years later	

(continued)

Table 7.2 (continued)

	International groups			
	IDSA 2013 (Rubin et al. 2014)	EBMT/ECIL 2009/2011 (Ljungman et al. 2009; Engelhard et al. 2013)	DGHO 2016/2018 (Rieger et al. 2018; Ullmann et al. 2016)	ATAGI 2017 ((ATAGI) ATAGoI 2017)	HSCT expert group 2009 (Tomblyn et al. 2009)
Acute leukaemia	Vaccinate newly diagnosed patients One dose PCV13 followed by PPV23, ≥8 weeks later 3 months post cancer therapy, patients should be vaccinated according to CDC annual schedule for immunocompetent patients		Vaccinate before commencement of chemotherapy or after first cycle and 3 months after chemotherapy If no prior vaccination, PCV13 followed by PPV23, 8–12 weeks later	Vaccinate as early as possible after diagnosis OR Vaccinate if in remission 6 months after chemotherapy If no prior vaccination, PCV13 followed by PPV23, at least 8 weeks later and further dose of PPV23 5 years later	
Lymphomas	Vaccinate newly diagnosed patients One dose PCV13 followed by PPV23, ≥8 weeks later If receiving anti-B cell therapy, vaccination should be delayed to ≥6 months after anti-B cell therapy		If no prior vaccination, PCV13 followed by PPV23, 8–12 weeks later	Vaccinate as early as possible after diagnosis OR Vaccinate if in remission 6 months after chemotherapy If no prior vaccination, PCV13 followed by PPV23, at least 8 weeks later and further dose of PPV23 5 years later	

	International groups				
	IDSA 2013 (Rubin et al. 2014)	EBMT/ECIL 2009/2011 (Ljungman et al. 2009; Engelhard et al. 2013)	DGHO 2016/2018 (Rieger et al. 2018; Ullmann et al. 2016)	ATAGI 2017 ((ATAGI) ATAGI 2017)	HSCT expert group 2009 (Tomblyn et al. 2009)
Influenza vaccination					
Haematopoietic stem cell transplantation	Allogeneic/autologous: Annual IIV Vaccinate starting at 6 months post HSCT Vaccinate starting at 4 months if there is a community outbreak 2 doses for children (6 months to 8 years)	Allogeneic/autologous: Annual IIV EBMT: Vaccinate 4–6 months post HSCT Consider second dose if first dose given <6 months post HSCT ECIL: Vaccinate at least 3 months post HSCT Give second dose IIV 3–4 weeks later	Allogeneic: Annual IIV Vaccinate at least 3 months post HSCT Consider 2 doses if first dose early post-transplant Autologous: Annual IIV Vaccinate 3–6 months post HSCT Consider 2 doses	Allogeneic/autologous: Annual IIV Timing not specified 2 doses (4 weeks apart) if vaccinated first year post HSCT After, 1 dose annually	Allogeneic/autologous: Annual IIV Vaccinate 4–6 months post HSCT Consider second dose if first dose given <6 months post HSCT Vaccinate starting at 4 months if there is a community outbreak 2 doses for children under 9 years of age
Chronic haematological malignancies (chronic lymphocytic leukaemia, multiple myeloma)	Annual IIV Except patients receiving intensive chemotherapy (e.g. induction, consolidation for acute leukaemia) and anti-B cell therapies. If receiving anti-B cell therapy, vaccination should be delayed to ≥6 months after anti-B cell therapy		Annual IIV Consider 2 doses Vaccinate ≥6 months after anti-CD20 antibody therapy	Annual IIV	
Acute leukaemia	Annual IIV Except patients receiving intensive chemotherapy (induction, consolidation) and anti-B cell therapies If receiving anti-B cell therapy, vaccination should be delayed to ≥6 months after anti-B cell therapy		Annual IIV Consider 2 doses	Annual IIV	

(continued)

Table 7.2 (continued)

	International groups				
	IDSA 2013 (Rubin et al. 2014)	EBMT/ECIL 2009/2011 (Ljungman et al. 2009; Engelhard et al. 2013)	DGHO 2016/2018 (Rieger et al. 2018; Ullmann et al. 2016)	ATAGI 2017 ((ATAGI) ATAGoI 2017)	HSCT expert group 2009 (Tomblyn et al. 2009)
Lymphomas	Annual IIV Except patients receiving intensive chemotherapy (e.g. induction, consolidation for acute leukaemia) and anti-B cell therapies If receiving anti-B cell therapy, vaccination should be delayed to ≥6 months after anti-B cell therapy		Annual IIV Vaccinate ≥6 months after anti-CD20 therapy Consider 2 doses after anti-CD20 therapy	Annual IIV Check with treating doctor if patient receiving immune checkpoint inhibitor	
Notes	Recommendations for patients aged ≥6 months Except for HSCT—3 months post cancer therapy, patients should be vaccinated according to CDC annual schedule for immunocompetent patients Prior to HSCT, patients should receive vaccines indicated for immunocompetent persons based on age, vaccination history, and exposure history and the interval to start of the conditioning regimen is ≥4 weeks for live vaccines and ≥ 2 weeks for inactivated vaccines	Recommendations for patients aged ≥6 months Live attenuated influenza vaccine not recommended	Recommendations for patients aged ≥6 months	Recommendations for patients aged ≥6 months Maximum lifetime dose of one PCV13 and three PPV23	Recommendations for patients aged ≥6 months Consider additional dose of PCV or PPV if patients develop invasive pneumococcal infection after initial vaccination

IDSA, Infectious Diseases Society of America; *EBMT*, European Bone Marrow Transplant Society; *ECIL*, European Congress on Infections in Leukaemia; *DHGO*, German Society for Hematology and Medical Oncology; *ATAGI*, Australian Technical Advisory Group on Immunisation; *HSCT*, haematopoietic stem cell transplant; *GvHD*, graft vs. host disease; *PCV13*, pneumococcal conjugate vaccine against 13 serotypes; *PPV23*, pneumococcal polysaccharide vaccine against 23 serotypes; *IIV*, inactivated influenza vaccine; *CDC*, Centers for Disease Control and Prevention

7.3.2 Chronic Haematological Malignancies

7.3.2.1 Multiple Myeloma

Patients with MM are at increased risk for a range of encapsulated bacterial infection (Teh et al. 2014). Invasive pneumococcal infection remains a significant infection in the era of immunomodulatory drugs and proteasome inhibitor therapy for MM (Teh et al. 2014). *Streptococcus pneumoniae* comprised 18% of blood stream infection isolates during induction therapy, 12% during disease progression and 14% in patients not eligible for autoHSCT (Teh et al. 2017a).

When conventional chemotherapy was the standard of care for MM, vaccination with PPV produced modest responses with 30–60% of patients responding to the vaccine (Chapel et al. 1994; Lazarus et al. 1980). In one of the earliest studies evaluating vaccine responses in MM patients, PPV vaccination in patients with a median of 30 months following diagnosis resulted in a response rate of only 30% (Lazarus et al. 1980). However, prior to vaccination, half the subjects received chemotherapy within 6 weeks, whilst the remainder had chemotherapy more than 12 weeks prior to vaccination (Lazarus et al. 1980). Vaccination with PPV at a median of 15 months post diagnosis resulted in significant increases in antibody concentration in all vaccine serotypes, but these levels waned after 18 months (Birgens et al. 1983). In a later study by Chapel et al., 57% of patients vaccinated 15–18 months following diagnosis, during plateau phase of MM achieved a good serological response (Chapel et al. 1994). When evaluated against serological antibody concentrations achieved by a general population, only 40% of MM patients reached a protective titre following a single dose of PPV delivered very early after chemotherapy or autoHSCT (Robertson et al. 2000).

When it became available, PCV was evaluated in an effort to improve responses in patients with MM. Vaccination responses achieved by a single dose of PCV was compared with PPV in a small cohort of 24 MM patients (Karlsson et al. 2013). Approximately 60% of patients who received PCV7 achieved the serological cut-off for all seven serotypes. Although this was not significantly different from patients who received PPV, the combined antibody fold increases was higher in the PCV-vaccinated patients (Karlsson et al. 2013). In this study, ongoing therapy was associated with poor responses (Karlsson et al. 2013). A single dose of PCV13 at a median of 30 months since MM diagnosis achieves comparable serological response to most vaccine serotypes to normal health control patients (Mustafa et al. 2018). However, a lower proportion of responders maintained responses at 6 months compared to controls, highlighting the likely need for booster dose (Mustafa et al. 2018).

In contrast to vaccination responses during treatment with conventional chemotherapy, two doses of PCV7 given concomitantly with lenalidomide, an immune modulatory drug augments PCV-specific humoral and cellular immune responses (Noonan et al. 2012). Delivery of vaccination concurrently with immune modulatory drug treatment is safe (Pandit et al. 2018; Palazzo et al. 2018). This suggests pneumococcal vaccination could be timed with induction or maintenance therapy with immunomodulatory drugs to enhance expected response to vaccination. The use of PCV13 in three monthly doses with PPV23 boosting, starting at 12 months post autoHSCT in a group of MM patients mostly on lenalidomide maintenance, resulted in a response rate of 58% (Palazzo et al. 2018).

These studies support the observation that response rates to single dose of PPV are modest in patients with MM and not durable. PCV vaccination produces comparable responses to healthy controls but likely require additional doses to maintain responses. Optimal timing of pneumococcal vaccination has not been evaluated in patients with MM. Vaccination in these studies has occurred following a significant duration of disease. Pneumococcal vaccination during a period of stable controlled disease, concurrently with immunomodulatory drugs or with greater time separation from active conventional chemotherapy, may result in a better response. However, this needs to be balanced with the need to cover periods of increased risk.

Patients with MM should receive a dose of PCV13 early following disease diagnosis to ensure mitigation of risk for invasive pneumococcal infection during this period of high disease burden. For non-transplant eligible patients, this should preferably be delivered prior to commencement of therapy, or alternatively during induction or maintenance therapy with immunomodulatory drugs. A subsequent dose of PPV23 should be considered to improve the breadth and duration of response. For transplant eligible patients, an early dose of PCV13 at disease diagnosis or prior to transplant could serve to enhance post-transplant immunity. Following autoHSCT, recommendations should be three doses of PCV13 commencing 3–6 months post-HSCT and a dose of PPV23 6 months later as previously discussed. This approach is supported by international guidelines with variable recommendations with regards to the need for and frequency of PPV23 following PCV13 (Table 7.2). Little guidance is provided by these guidelines with regards to the optimal timing of initial PCV dose.

7.3.3 Chronic Lymphocytic Leukaemia

Patients with CLL are at increased risk for invasive pneumococcal infection with hypogammaglobulinaemia a contributing factor (Morrison 2010). With intravenous immunoglobulin replacement, there is some amelioration of risk (Morrison 2010; Teh et al. 2018). In the era prior to the routine use of chemo-immunotherapeutic regimens incorporating rituximab, the response rates of patients with CLL to PPV23 vaccination ranged from 12 to 20% (Hartkamp et al. 2001; Van der Velden et al. 2007). Varying definitions of serological response were used in these studies. Whilst response rates are low, vaccination with PPV23 resulted in at least 50–60% of patients achieve seroprotection against pneumococcal strains (Hartkamp et al. 2001; Van der Velden et al. 2007). The majority of patients in these studies were not on therapy and had early-stage disease and were vaccinated a median of 40–49 months following disease diagnosis (Hartkamp et al. 2001; Van der Velden et al. 2007).

Conjugate vaccines were evaluated in patients with CLL in hope of achieving better responses. The use of PCV7, a median of 2 years post diagnosis, in a largely untreated CLL patient group resulted in significant increases in antibody concentration against vaccine serotypes but only 29% achieved a significant response to at least six serotypes (Sinisalo et al. 2007). With PCV13, a higher proportion of patients (58%) achieved an adequate response (Pasiarski et al. 2014). In this study, patients have not received treatment for CLL and had early-stage disease (Pasiarski et al. 2014).

When compared head to head, PCV13 produced better and more durable responses. It was evaluated against PPV23 in a randomised trial of untreated CLL patients, stratified for stage of disease and IgG levels (Svensson et al. 2018). Median time from disease diagnosis was 31 months (Svensson et al. 2018). Patients vaccinated with PCV13 achieved significantly higher geometric mean titres against a majority of vaccine serotypes and it remained significantly higher at 6 months post vaccination (Svensson et al. 2018). A significantly higher proportion of patients vaccinated with PCV13 achieved a positive immunological response (41%) compared to PPV23 vaccinated patients (Svensson et al. 2018). Shorter duration of disease and absence of hypogammaglobulinaemia was associated with better vaccination response (Svensson et al. 2018).

As discussed previously, anti-CD20 therapy rituximab negatively impacts response to influenza and pneumococcal vaccination, especially when vaccination occurs within 6 months of rituximab therapy (Berglund et al. 2014; Bedognetti et al. 2011; Ide et al. 2014). Evaluation of PPV23 involving a substantial proportion of CLL patients previously treated with rituximab (more than 12 months previously) reported a low serologic response rate of 10% despite the majority of patients having stable disease or being in remission (Safdar et al. 2008). Patients treated with fludarabine and anti-CD52 (alemtuzumab) within the last 12 months were excluded from this study (Safdar et al. 2008). New targeted therapies such as Btk inhibitors also appear to negatively impact vaccination responses to PCV

(Andrick et al. 2017). Strategies to enhance response to PPV with the use of histamine blocker and granulocyte-macrophage colony-stimulating factor were unsuccessful (Van der Velden et al. 2007; Safdar et al. 2008).

Critically, patients with shorter duration of disease, less advanced stages of CLL, higher IgG levels and less prior lines of therapy had better responses to both PPV and PCV vaccination (Hartkamp et al. 2001; Sinisalo et al. 2007; Pasiarski et al. 2014; Svensson et al. 2018). PCV13 produced better immunological response of longer duration compared to PPV23 (Svensson et al. 2018). Therefore, pneumococcal vaccination with PCV13 in patients with CLL should be delivered early following disease diagnosis, prior to progression of disease, development of hypogammaglobulinaemia and commencement of anti-CD20 antibody therapy. If a patient is currently receiving anti-CD20 antibody-based therapy for CLL or Btk inhibitor, deferring vaccination until 6 months post completion of therapy should be considered. Based on data extrapolated from non-CLL studies, vaccination with PCV13 followed by PPV23 could be considered to boost and broaden breadth of immune response.

7.3.4 Acute Leukaemia and Lymphomas

Patients who are receiving or have completed curative therapy for acute leukaemia, NHL and Hodgkin's lymphoma (HL) are at increased risk for invasive pneumococcal infection with substantial mortality rates due to significantly low levels of pneumococcal serotype-specific antibodies (Meisel et al. 2007b; Lehrnbecher et al. 2009; Wong et al. 2010). This deficiency can persist for up to 9 months (Lehrnbecher et al. 2009). Patients with acute lymphoblastic leukaemia or acute myeloid leukaemia have up to 12 times the risk compared to the general population whilst patients with NHL or HL have about six times the risk (Wong et al. 2010). Splenectomy, if performed for management of HL, contributes additional risk (Theilacker et al. 2016; Cherif et al. 2006).

7.3.5 Acute Leukaemia

Pneumococcal vaccination has been evaluated to reduce risk in these patients. A single dose of PPV produced suboptimal responses of limited duration when used in paediatric patients with ALL, largely delivered within 6 months of induction chemotherapy (Feldman et al. 1985). In contrast, two monthly doses of PCV7 in a cohort consisting mostly of patients with ALL and AML resulted in 86–100% of patients achieving seroprotection against seven vaccine serotypes (Cheng et al. 2012). Half the patients were vaccinated at a median of 6 months post completion of therapy, whilst the remainder were still on maintenance therapy for ALL (Cheng et al. 2012).

The use of a single dose of PCV13 was evaluated in two cohorts of patients consisting mostly of paediatric patients with AML and ALL; one cohort consisted of patients still receiving active immunosuppressive therapy and the other completed immune suppressive therapy within the last 12 months (Hung et al. 2017). Over half the patients in both cohorts had previously received either PCV7 or PCV13. Both groups had more than 70% of patients achieving protective antibody titres, but a significantly higher proportion of patients vaccinated after completing chemotherapy mounted an effective serological response and protective antibody titres to PCV13 serotypes (Hung et al. 2017).

Vaccinating prior to commencement of chemotherapy in patients with acute leukaemia and aggressive NHL is often not feasible due to the urgent need to commence treatment for disease control. Based on these studies, revaccination of patients with AML and ALL with a single dose of PCV13 produces a robust serological response and should be timed at 6–12 months post completion of induction chemotherapy for optimal response. To minimise risk period for infection, revaccination could be delivered as early as 3 months post completion of chemotherapy based on data from studies evaluating vaccination schedules for other conjugate vaccines in the ALL cohort (Lehrnbecher et al. 2011) (Table 7.1).

7.3.6 Lymphomas

PPV vaccination in patients with HL produced serological response comparable to health controls if delivered prior to commencement of treatment including splenectomy (Frederiksen et al. 1989). The interval between vaccination and commencement of chemotherapy correlated with vaccine response and time separation of less than 10–14 days was associated with poorer response (Siber et al. 1986). Multiple dosing of PPV23, guided by antibody levels, achieved serological responses in splenectomised HL patients that were comparable to patients who had trauma-related splenectomies (Landgren et al. 2004). However, 50% of patients with HL received their PPV23 dose before splenectomy, and the majority of these patients were not PPV naïve. A third of patients received one dose of PPV23, whilst the remainder received two or more doses (Landgren et al. 2004). A related study of HL and NHL utilising a similar approach noted a good response in 72% of patients with first vaccine dose, a median of 2 years post chemotherapy (Cherif et al. 2006).

Interestingly, use of PCV7, a median of 9 years, since HL diagnosis was associated with lower geometric mean antibody than PPV23 (Molrine et al. 1995). However, most of the patients have previously received PPV vaccination (Molrine et al. 1995). The same investigators proceeded to evaluate an approach of utilising PCV7 to prime the patient, followed by a dose of PPV23 and compared it to PPV23 vaccination alone (Chan et al. 1996). Patients with HL in this study had completed therapy and remained in remission. Patients who received PCV7 followed by PPV23 had significantly higher levels of geometric mean antibody concentrations for key vaccine serotypes (Chan et al. 1996). This study provided the early evidence for sequencing PCV prior to PPV to prime and improve serologic responses to pneumococcal vaccination.

Available studies of pneumococcal vaccination in patients with HL support vaccination prior to commencement of chemotherapy and the use of PCV13 followed by PPV23. Ideally, this should be at least 10–14 days prior to commencement of chemotherapy. If vaccination prior to chemotherapy is not feasible logistically, vaccination post completion of treatment in the setting of disease remission is a reasonable alternative (Table 7.1).

In a heterogeneous group of solid tumour, NHL and HL patients, the proportion of patients achieving a protective antibody levels was not different to control group following a single dose of PPV23 (Nordoy et al. 2002). Half the patients were not receiving active chemotherapy within the 4 months of vaccination (Nordoy et al. 2002). A single dose of PPV23 in a small group of splenectomised patients with NHL prior to chemotherapy resulted in similar antibody levels with a control group who underwent splenectomy for other reasons (Petrasch et al. 1997). Approximately, 45% of patients achieved a serological response to the single dose of PPV (Petrasch et al. 1997).

However, these studies were conducted in the era prior to the use of rituximab-based therapies. As outlined previously, concurrent use of anti-CD20 antibody rituximab has been shown to negatively impact responses to influenza vaccination, and vaccination within 6 months of completion of rituximab is generally avoided. Therefore, patients with NHL should ideally be vaccinated prior to the commencement of treatment, especially if the use of rituximab-based therapy is being considered. Based on data from HL, vaccination with PCV13 followed by PPV23 would be a reasonable approach for patients with NHL (Table 7.2). Recommendations for patients with high-grade NHL, who proceed to HSCT, are covered under the previous sections.

7.4 Influenza Vaccination

Timing of influenza vaccination is largely driven by the peak periods of infectivity and transmission of influenza, which occurs mainly in winter in temperate countries but more commonly all year-round in tropical countries (Azziz Baumgartner et al. 2012; Englund 2001). Influenza season lasts for an average of 4 months (Azziz Baumgartner et al. 2012). In addition, patients treated for haematological disorders at greater risk during pandemic outbreaks of influenza (Tramontana et al. 2010). Most studies of influenza vaccination in haematology patients have largely focussed on vaccine formulations or approaches to improve overall vaccine responses.

7.4.1 Haematopoietic Stem Cell Transplantation

Infection with influenza virus contributes to significant morbidity and mortality in HSCT patients. Of patients with respiratory symptoms, influenza virus is responsible for up to 30% of cases (Whimbey et al. 1994). Often, they present with lower respiratory tract involvement, and the mortality rate is as high as 25% (Englund 2001). Invasive aspergillosis can be a co-infection or complication of influenza virus infection (Nichols et al. 2004). Vaccination with inactivated influenza vaccine (IIV) has been shown to reduce development of pneumonia and risk for ICU admission (Kumar et al. 2018). Early acquisition of influenza virus infection post HSCT is a risk factor for progression to lower respiratory tract infection (Nichols et al. 2004). However, ongoing immune reconstitution will impact response to influenza vaccination.

Most studies evaluating influenza vaccination in HSCT patients have utilised serological endpoints of seroprotection or seroconversion against strains of influenza as the outcome of interest. There is a significant association between serological response and timing of influenza vaccination with better rates of seroprotection and seroconversion seen with increasing time interval between HSCT and vaccination (Engelhard et al. 1993; Avetisyan et al. 2008; Mohty et al. 2011). The optimal period appears to be more than 6 months post HSCT for alloHSCT patients.

Vaccination at a median of 9 months post-transplant resulted in a significant increase in influenza-specific immune cells, with higher increases seen in patients vaccinated after 6 months (Avetisyan et al. 2008). Overall rate of seroprotection was only 29% to H1N1 and 0% to H3N3 and B strains (Avetisyan et al. 2008). In a mixed group of HSCT patients vaccinated mostly within 4–12 months post HSCT, a similar response rate of 29–34% to different influenza strains was noted (Pauksen et al. 2000). Use of GM-CSF appear to improve response rates for influenza B in the early vaccination group (Pauksen et al. 2000). Vaccination within 6 months of HSCT appears to be ineffective (Engelhard et al. 1993). When delivered 6 months or more following HSCT, influenza vaccine efficacy was high at 80% (Machado et al. 2005b). Seroprotection rates of up to 100% and seroconversion rates ranging from 50 to 60% for three influenza virus strains when patients were vaccinated 6–48 months after HSCT (Yalcin et al. 2010).

During the H1N1 influenza pandemic, a number of studies were conducted to evaluate type, approach and timing of vaccination against the H1N1 strain. Both monovalent ASO3-adjuvanted and non-adjuvanted H1N1/A/09 vaccines were evaluated, and this may limit generalisability of findings to the seasonal trivalent influenza vaccine. However, rates of seroprotection and seroconversion remained significantly associated with duration between vaccination and HSCT with higher responses seen with increasing time separation (Mohty et al. 2011; Issa et al. 2011; Roll et al. 2012). One of the highest rates of seroprotection was seen in patients vaccinated between 6 and 12 months post HSCT (Issa et al. 2011). In some studies, GvHD and use of rituximab were associated with poorer responses (Mohty et al. 2011; Issa et al. 2011; Roll et al. 2012; Villa et al. 2013).

In alloHSCT, a single dose of non-adjuvanted and ASO3-adjuvanted H1N1/A/09 influenza vaccine produced relatively similar rates of seroprotection when vaccination occurred after 6 months post-transplant. A single dose of the non-adjuvanted H1N1/A/09 influenza vaccine was associated with a seroprotection rate of 50% when delivered a median of 9 months following HSCT (Issa et al. 2011). With a single dose of the ASO3-adjuvanted vaccine, seroprotection rates of 42% were noted when alloHSCT patients were vaccinated a median of 15 months following transplant (Roll et al. 2012).

As the pandemic progressed, studies evaluating the utility of multiple dosing to improve vaccine responses started to emerge. In alloHSCT patients, the seroprotection rate was 53% after the first dose of the adjuvanted vaccine and 66% following the second dose (Dhedin et al. 2014). This was similar to the seroprotection rate achieved by patients infected with H1N1/09 influenza (Dhedin et al. 2014). The first dose was delivered a median of 14 months post-transplant (Dhedin et al. 2014).

Discordant results were noted in a mixed group of autoHSCT and alloHSCT patients and were vaccinated with two doses of the ASO3-adjuvanted H1N1/A/09 influenza vaccine separated by 3–4 weeks, at relatively similar time periods. Two doses of the vaccine given 3–4 weeks apart produced a seroprotection rate of 44% after the first dose and 49% after the second dose (Engelhard et al. 2011). Of those that did not response with the first dose, 28% achieved seroprotection after the second dose (Engelhard et al. 2011). AlloHSCT and autoHSCT patients were vaccinated at a median of 34 and 20 months following transplant, respectively (Engelhard et al. 2011). In contrast, two other studies reported much higher rates of seroprotection. Mohty et al. reported rates of seroprotection and seroconversion of 84% following two doses, similar to a single dose in healthy controls when delivered at a median of 30 months following alloHSCT (Mohty et al. 2011). Gueller et al. reported similarly high rates of seroprotection at 53 and 91% after one and two doses of the adjuvant vaccines, respectively (Gueller et al. 2011). Patients were vaccinated with a mean of 20 months following transplant (Gueller et al. 2011).

In the non-pandemic setting, two doses of the standard IIV in alloHSCT achieved seroprotection rate of 19–32% after the first dose with rates relatively unchanged after the second dose (Karras et al. 2013). Patients were immunised at a median of 11 months following transplantation. In line with earlier studies, vaccination responses were better especially against H3N2 strain in patients vaccinated 12 months or more post-transplant (Karras et al. 2013). A similar rate of seroprotection of around 30% was achieved with pre-transplant IIV immunisation, followed by post-transplant IIV immunisation at 6 months (Ambati et al. 2015).

More recently, different formulations of IIV have been evaluated in an effort to improve vaccination responses in HSCT. Halasa et al. evaluated the use of high dose IIV compared to standard dose IIV (Halasa et al. 2016). When delivered at a median of 8 months after HSCT, high dose IIV was associated with a significantly higher seroprotection rate compared to standard dose IIV. Rates of seroprotection for H1N1 were high at 57–69% for both groups and around 40% for influenza B (Halasa et al. 2016). The use of MF59 adjuvanted IIV was evaluated by Natori et al. against standard IIV (Natori et al. 2017). Compared to high dose IIV, vaccination occurred later, at a median of 12 months after transplantation. Seroprotection rates were similar with both vaccine groups and were relatively high at 57–72% depending on influenza strain (Natori et al. 2017). In line with other studies, improved response was associated with increasing duration from transplantation. Interestingly, the MF59 adjuvanted IIV appears to have a greater impact on patients vaccinated later (Natori et al. 2017).

The studies outlined above have utilised serological endpoints of seroprotection or seroconversion against strains of influenza as the outcome of interest. Pinana et al. conducted a prospective study observation study over five seasons evaluating the clinical efficacy of IIV vaccination in alloHSCT (Pinana et al. 2018). Different donor types were evaluated, and patients received vaccination at least 3 months post HSCT (Pinana et al. 2018). A significantly lower rate of proven influenza virus infection, lower progression to lower respiratory tract disease and hospital admission were noted (Pinana et al. 2018).

A major factor in determining timing of vaccination against seasonal influenza is peak transmission period in the year. Improved influenza vaccination responses with increasing duration between HSCT and vaccination need to be balanced with the need for repeated annual influenza vaccination due to regular updates to vaccine strain composition to match antigenic drift (Grohskopf et al. 2018).

Based on the relatively high rates of seroprotection achieved in previously discussed studies, vaccination with single dose of IIV is recommended at least 6 months following HSCT and should be repeated annually. Two doses separated by 3–4 weeks commencing at least 6 months following HSCT should be considered if the patient is influenza vaccine naïve based on data from studies during the H1N1/09 influenza pandemic. Although studies with serological endpoints do not support earlier commencement of vaccination, the observational study by Pinana et al. suggests vaccination at earlier period of 3 months post HSCT is clinically effective (Table 7.1). Recommendations from various international bodies are summarised in Table 7.2.

7.4.2 Haematological Malignancies

Influenza virus is responsible for infection in 15–30% of symptomatic adult patients with leukaemia and other haematological malignancies (Teh et al. 2015b; Yousuf et al. 1997; Elting et al. 1995). It involves the lower respiratory tract in up to 80% of cases and is associated with high mortality rates of 30% (Teh et al. 2015b; Yousuf et al. 1997; Elting et al. 1995).

IIV offers the main protection against influenza virus infection. In a patient group consisting of patients with chronic lymphoproliferative disorders (CLL, MM, NHL, HL), a single dose of trivalent IIV achieved a seroprotection rate of more than 60% against all influenza strains (Rapezzi et al. 2003). Most of the patients with CLL in this study had early-stage disease and were not on treatment (Rapezzi et al. 2003). In contrast, lower rates were reported by Ljungman et al. in a diverse group of patients with disorders that did not include patients with CLL (Ljungman et al. 2005). The seroprotection rates were 16–26% against vaccine strains after a single dose with marginal improvement following a second dose (Ljungman et al. 2005). Our understanding of the efficacy and timing of influenza vaccination in patients with chronic haematological malignancies such as MM, acute leukaemia and lymphoma was advanced by studies conducted during the H1N1/09 influenza pandemic. Due to the novelty of this influenza strain, existing rates of seroprotection were low, and the impact of IIV vaccination could be better assessed.

Mariotti et al. evaluated the impact of a single dose of an MF59-adjuvanted H1N1/09 influenza vaccine in heterogeneous group of patients consisting of patients with MM, lymphoma and leukaemia (Mariotti et al. 2012). A third of patients were on immunomodulatory or proteasome inhibitor therapy, mostly for MM. Overall, the rate of seroprotection 28 days after vaccination was 75%, and it peaked at 86% at 90 days (Mariotti et al. 2012). Higher rate of seroprotection of 93% was seen in patients vaccinated off treatment compared to patients still receiving treatment (Mariotti et al. 2012). For patients on treatment, vaccination occurred between cycles of chemotherapy, 7 days prior to the commencement of the next cycle (Mariotti et al. 2012). Others have also reported higher likelihood of seroconversion when patients are vaccinated between chemotherapy cycles (Mackay et al. 2011).

This study also established the temporal evolution of immunity to influenza vaccination. Rates of seroprotection continued to improve at day 50 and 90 post vaccination, especially in patients still receiving treatment (Mariotti et al. 2012). This reflects delayed development of protective immunity in patients on cancer treatment and suggests that these patients could be vaccinated earlier relative to the start of influenza season. Compared to patients with lymphoma, MM patients achieve better seroprotection rates with vaccination (Mariotti et al. 2012). In line with other studies, this could be aided by concurrent immunomodulatory drug therapy (Noonan et al. 2012).

In contrast, a single dose of ASO3-adjuvanted H1N1/A/09 influenza vaccine in a group of patients with lymphoproliferative disorders (MM, CLL, NHL, HL) including small proportion post autoHSCT resulted in a seroprotection rate of only 35% (Villa et al. 2013). The group that received a second dose 3–4 weeks achieved a marginally higher rate of 40% (Villa et al. 2013).

It should be noted that a third of patients had received three or more lines of chemotherapy, and up to 40% of patients were receiving rituximab-based therapy (Villa et al. 2013). Similar low seroprotection rates after a single dose of this vaccine has been reported (Mackay et al. 2011).

Multiple dosing of this vaccine was evaluated by de Lavallade et al. in patients with B cell malignancies (CLL, NHL, HL), chronic myeloid leukaemia and 6 months post alloHSCT (de Lavallade et al. 2011). Following the first dose, rates of seroprotection were 39%, 85% and 46%, respectively (de Lavallade et al. 2011). This increased significantly to 68% and 73% in patients with B cell malignancies and alloHSCT, respectively, highlighting the benefit of dose of the second vaccine in certain key haematology disease groups (de Lavallade et al. 2011). A slightly higher rate of 81% against H1N1 serotype was noted in a different diverse group of haematological patients including HSCT following two doses of ASO3-adjuvanted H1N1/A/09 influenza vaccine (Cherif et al. 2013). The addition of trivalent IIV following two doses of the adjuvanted IIV resulted in a seroprotection rate of 40–76% for the three influenza strains covered (Cherif et al. 2013).

These studies suggest that during outbreaks of influenza, two doses of adjuvanted IIV specific to the causative strain can result in reasonably high rates of seroprotection for B cell and HSCT patients. It also provides some supportive evidence for consideration of two doses of IIV in influenza vaccine naïve patients with haematological disease. Where possible, patients should be vaccinated whilst off treatment or in between cycles of treatment, 7 days prior to the next cycle. Early vaccination could be considered for patients receiving chemotherapy as immune responses may not fully mature until 2–3 months later (Table 7.1). Annual revaccination is encouraged due to antigenic drift (Grohskopf et al. 2018).

7.4.3 Multiple Myeloma

Over the years, a few studies have focussed on specific diseases such as MM. Patients with MM appear to be at higher risk and experience greater morbidity from influenza virus infection compared to other disease groups (Tramontana et al. 2010). In the era of conventional chemotherapy for MM, serologic responses to trivalent IIV vaccination was poor with only 19% of patients achieving seroprotection (Robertson et al. 2000). Despite the low rates of serological response, vaccination with IIV appears to have a clinical impact with significantly lower rates of respiratory tract infection, hospitalisation and duration of febrile respiratory episodes (Musto and Carotenuto 1997).

The standard of care for patients with MM has shifted to the use of immunomodulatory drugs and proteasome inhibitors (Teh et al. 2014). A recent study demonstrated similarly low seroprotection rate of 15% against all three strains after one dose of trivalent IIV, but this significantly improved to 31% after the second dose (Hahn et al. 2015). MM patients in this study were heavily treated with over half having had two or more autoHSCT (Hahn et al. 2015). Due to associated morbidity and mortality, annual IIV vaccination is recommended for patients with MM prior to commencement of influenza transmission season.

7.4.4 Chronic Lymphocytic Leukaemia

When evaluated in patients with CLL, two doses of the trivalent IIV elicited a seroprotective response in 53% of patients (Bucalossi et al. 1995). A significantly higher response was seen in patients with lower stage disease (Bucalossi et al. 1995). In CLL patients largely with higher stage disease, the seroconversion and seroprotection rates were 30% or lower after two doses (van der Velden et al. 2001). These rates were seen prior to the introduction of anti-CD20-based chemoimmunotherapy and Btk inhibitors. The impact of rituximab on influenza vaccine responses has been seen predominantly in studies involving patients with NHL, but this can be extrapolated to patients with CLL (Ide et al. 2014; Yri et al. 2011; Mackay et al. 2011).

When non-treatment naïve patients with CLL were vaccinated with trivalent IIV whilst on ibrutinib, the rates of seroconversion as low as 7% with relatively little change to rates of seroprotection from pre-vaccination levels for most influenza strains (Douglas et al. 2017; Sun et al. 2016). This is possibly due to the impact of ibrutinib as nearly 90% of patients vaccinated had no previous anti-CD20 antibody therapy in the last 12 months (Douglas et al. 2017). However, these findings will have to be validated in larger studies to fully determine the impact of ibrutinib on vaccination responses in patients with newly diagnosed and previously treated disease and optimal timing of IIV vaccination. As IIV vaccination is associated with low morbidity, its use could still be considered in ibrutinib-treated patients. It should not be relied on in isolation for prevention and management of influenza in CLL patients (Teh et al. 2018).

This suggests that patients with CLL should be vaccinated early prior to commencement of therapy, taking into account influenza transmission season. Whilst IIV vaccination could be considered due to low morbidity associated with this vaccine, patients receiving anti-CD20 monoclonal antibody therapy are unlikely to respond effectively to IIV and other measures such as antiviral prophylaxis in the setting of exposure to proven influenza or early treatment of influenza-like illnesses.

7.4.5 Acute Leukaemia

There are limited studies evaluating the utility of vaccination in patients with acute myeloid leukaemia. In a small study of 10 AML patients vaccinated with a single dose of TIV 9 months following completion of chemotherapy reported a seroconversion rate of 20% to one or more influenza strains (Goswami et al. 2017). Recommendation for annual IIV vaccination 3–6 months post completion of chemotherapy has largely been extrapolated from studies involving high-intensity treatments for haematological diseases and HSCT.

Patients with ALL vaccinated with single dose of trivalent IIV prior to commencement of chemotherapy achieved a significant increase in rates of seroprotection from 43 to 73% (Wong-Chew et al. 2012). Vaccination with single dose of trivalent IIV during ALL maintenance therapy achieved similar rate of seroprotection 43–63% for H1N1 and H3N2 influenza strains and seroconversion rates of 41–56% (Shahgholi et al. 2010) demonstrating maintenance of efficacy if vaccinated during therapy.

During the H1N1/09 pandemic, vaccination of ALL patients on induction or maintenance chemotherapy with two doses of the ASO3-adjuvanted vaccine produced a seroconversion rate of 26% (Leahy et al. 2013). Adult dosing was associated with a better response (Leahy et al. 2013). In contrast, two doses of H1N1/09 vaccine in a mixed group of leukaemia and lymphoma patients during chemotherapy resulted in a higher seroconversion rate of 50% and seroprotection rate of 72% (Hakim et al. 2012). The use of high-dose trivalent IIV did not result in higher responses compared to standard dose trivalent IIV in ALL patients mostly on maintenance therapy (McManus et al. 2014). Both groups achieved seroconversion rates of 25–46% to influenza A vaccine strains (McManus et al. 2014).

To minimise morbidity, mortality and delays to treatment, annual IIV immunisation is recommended in patients with acute leukaemia. Vaccination should be timed prior to commencement of chemotherapy or during maintenance phase of treatment. Based on studies during the H1N1/09 pandemic, two doses of IIV vaccine maybe beneficial.

7.4.6 Lymphomas

The response of patients with NHL and HL to IIV vaccination has been variable across studies. The heterogeneity of time periods, patient population and types of treatment limits direct comparison across studies. During treatment with combination chemotherapy, rate of serologic response of 41–49% across three influenza strains was achieved with two IIV doses (Lo et al. 1993). The level of seroprotection achieved by one dose of IIV was 38% (Nordoy et al. 2002). In contrast, a single dose of IIV in NHL resulted in slightly higher response rates of 47–69% and seroprotection rates of 60–69% (Brydak et al. 2006). The absence of treatment was associated with higher rates of response and protection (Brydak et al. 2006).

In a large multi-centre study across two influenza seasons, patients with NHL were immunised with a single dose of IIV (Centkowski et al. 2007). Half the patients were treatment naïve and very small number of patients received rituximab therapy. Seroresponse and seroprotection rates 1 month following IIV vaccination were 71–94% and 68–84%, respectively, and were comparable to healthy controls (Centkowski et al. 2007). This illustrates a robust response with high rates of protection to IIV is achievable in patients with NHL. Where possible, patients with NHL should be vaccinated prior to commencement of chemotherapy or whilst not on treatment.

With increasing use in NHL management, the negative impact of rituximab-based therapy on responses to influenza vaccination was better understood (Ide et al. 2014; Mackay et al. 2011). This effect appears to be mediated through depletion of memory B cells (Bedognetti et al. 2011). In contrast to rates of seroconversion and seroprotection of 40–70% normally seen in NHL patients following IIV, none of the patients vaccinated with single dose ASO3-adjuvanted IIV vaccine underwent seroconversion if they are receiving rituximab or have received rituximab in the previous 6 months (Mackay et al. 2011). The rate of seroprotection was low at 0–9% (Yri et al. 2011; Mackay et al. 2011).

Similar findings were noted even with the use of two doses of H1N1/09 influenza vaccine with 9% seroconversion rate, and no patients achieved seroprotection (Ide et al. 2014). Patients recently treated with rituximab continued not to respond to vaccination despite employment of a multidose strategy consisting of two doses of ASO3-adjuvanted H1N1/A/09 IIV followed by trivalent IIV (Berglund et al. 2014). After the trivalent IIV, no patients treated with rituximab within last 6 months achieved seroconversion to either the H1N1 or seasonal influenza vaccine strain. In addition, rates of seroprotection remained low at 8–17% (Berglund et al. 2014). However, when NHL patients were mostly vaccinated with trivalent IIV more than 12 months following completion of rituximab, rates of seroconversion and seroprotection were better at up to 30% and 70%, respectively (Bedognetti et al. 2011).

Based on these studies, IIV vaccination during or within 6 months of rituximab-based therapy in patients with NHL results in ineffectual responses and very low rates of seroprotection. Therefore, IIV vaccination should be timed six or more months following completion of rituximab-based therapy. Immunisation in the setting of recent rituximab therapy could be considered in the setting of outbreaks of influenza in the community as it may afford a limited degree of protection, and IIV immunisation is associated with low morbidity.

7.5 Future Directions

Throughout this chapter, the evidence base and rationale for the type of vaccine, vaccination timing and schedule for optimal response has been discussed and recommendations provided. Limitations, in particular lack of robust data for use and timing of additional or booster doses of vaccine to maintain long-term protection, have been highlighted. There is still ongoing debate about broader issues of the use of immunologic endpoints in vaccine studies and their correlation with clinical efficacy. Practical immunological markers of vaccine response that closely correlate with clinical efficacy are required.

Patients with haematological malignancies are living longer with the use of targeted therapies (e.g. Btk inhibitors), new generation monoclonal antibodies, immunomodulatory drugs and increasing use of transplant approaches such as haploidentical HSCT. The impact of these new therapies and treatment approaches on vaccine responses and thus optimal timing of vaccination requires further evaluation in large clinical studies.

In the setting of poor responses due to therapy or disease-related immune deficiency (e.g. GvHD), evaluation of new vaccines such as adjuvanted vaccines and new approaches to scheduling of vaccines will be required.

Some haematological diseases such as CLL and MM remain incurable and disease control is maintained by increasing lines of therapy (Teh et al. 2014). Therefore, patients have long-term risks for preventable infections, and prolonged use of antimicrobial prophylaxis is not feasible. Vaccination would be an effective measure, but there are limited studies evaluating long-term retention of immunity following vaccination. Whilst patients should be vaccinated early at diagnosis or during induction therapy, the use of additional doses (e.g. PPV23) and their timing for optimal response to ensure long-term coverage remain unclear. Together with the need for development of more effective vaccines, these unanswered questions related to vaccination in patients with haematological diseases serve as rich basis for further clinical research.

Despite the wide availability of published literature and guidelines from internal bodies, the uptake of vaccination and compliance with guidelines in patients with haematological diseases remains poor (Ariza-Heredia et al. 2014). To ensure patients derive the most benefit from currently available vaccines, health services research into new models of care, healthcare cost benefits and impact on incidence of preventable infection is required to improve delivery and uptake of vaccination in haematology patients (Teh et al. 2017b).

References

Australian Techinical Advisory Group on Immunisation (ATAGI). The australian immunisation handbook. Australian government department of health, canberra, 2017.

Alemu A, Richards JO, Oaks MK, Thompson MA (2016) Vaccination in multiple myeloma: review of current literature. Clin Lymphoma Myeloma Leuk 16(9):495–502

Ambati A, Boas LS, Ljungman P, Testa L, de Oliveira JF, Aoun M et al (2015) Evaluation of pretransplant influenza vaccination in hematopoietic SCT: a randomized prospective study. Bone Marrow Transplant 50(6):858–864

Andersen MA, Moser CE, Lundgren J, Niemann CU (2018) Epidemiology of bloodstream infections in patients with chronic lymphocytic leukemia: a longitudinal nation-wide cohort study. Leukemia

Andrick B, Alwhaibi A, DL DR, Quershi S, Khan R, Bryan LJ et al (2017) Lack of adequate pneumococcal vaccination response in chronic lymphocytic leukaemia patients receiving ibrutinib. Br J Haematol

Antin JH, Guinan EC, Avigan D, Soiffer RJ, Joyce RM, Martin VJ et al (2005) Protective antibody responses to pneumococcal conjugate vaccine after autologous hematopoietic stem cell transplantation. Biol Blood Marrow Trans 11(3):213–222

Ariza-Heredia EJ, Gulbis AM, Stolar KR, Kebriaei P, Shah DP, McConn KK et al (2014) Vaccination guidelines after hematopoietic stem cell transplantation: practitioners' knowledge, attitudes, and gap between guidelines and clinical practice. Transpl Infect Dis 16(6):878–886

Aung AK, Trubiano JA, Spelman DW (2015) Travel risk assessment, advice and vaccinations in immunocompromised travellers (HIV, solid organ transplant and haematopoeitic stem cell transplant recipients): a review. Travel Med Infect Dis 13(1):31–47

Avetisyan G, Aschan J, Hassan M, Ljungman P (2008) Evaluation of immune responses to seasonal influenza vaccination in healthy volunteers and in patients after stem cell transplantation. Transplantation 86(2):257–263

Azziz Baumgartner E, Dao CN, Nasreen S, Bhuiyan MU, Mah EMS, Al Mamun A et al (2012) Seasonality, timing, and climate drivers of influenza activity worldwide. J Infect Dis 206(6):838–846

Bedognetti D, Zoppoli G, Massucco C, Zanardi E, Zupo S, Bruzzone A et al (2011) Impaired response to influenza vaccine associated with persistent memory B cell depletion in non-Hodgkin's lymphoma patients treated with rituximab-containing regimens. J Immunol 186(10):6044–6055

Berglund A, Willen L, Grodeberg L, Skattum L, Hagberg H, Pauksens K (2014) The response to vaccination against influenza a(H1N1) 2009, seasonal influenza and Streptococcus pneumoniae in adult outpatients with ongoing treatment for cancer with and without rituximab. Acta Oncol 53(9):1212–1220

Birgens HS, Espersen F, Hertz JB, Pedersen FK, Drivsholm A (1983) Antibody response to pneumococcal vaccination in patients with myelomatosis. Scand J Haematol 30(4):324–330

Blimark C, Holmberg E, Mellqvist UH, Landgren O, Bjorkholm M, Hultkrantz ML et al (2014) Multiple myeloma and infections: a population-based study on 9253 multiple myeloma patients. Haematologica

Brydak LB, Machala M, Centkowski P, Warzocha K, Bilinski P (2006) Humoral response to hemagglutinin components of influenza vaccine in patients with non-Hodgkin malignant lymphoma. Vaccine 24(44–46):6620–6623

Bucalossi A, Marotta G, Galieni P, Bigazzi C, Valenzin PE, Dispensa E (1995) Immunological response to influenza virus vaccine in B-cell chronic lymphocytic leukaemia patients. Acta Haematol 93(1):56

Centkowski P, Brydak L, Machala M, Kalinka-Warzocha E, Blasinska-Morawiec M, Federowicz I et al (2007) Immunogenicity of influenza vaccination in patients with non-Hodgkin lymphoma. J Clin Immunol 27(3):339–346

Chan CY, Molrine DC, George S, Tarbell NJ, Mauch P, Diller L et al (1996) Pneumococcal conjugate vaccine primes for antibody responses to polysaccharide pneumococcal vaccine after treatment of Hodgkin's disease. J Infect Dis 173(1):256–258

Chapel H, Lee M, Hargreaves R, Pamphilon D, Prentice A (1994) Randomised trial of intravenous immunoglobulin as prophylaxis against infection in plateau-phase multiple myeloma. Lancet 343(8905):1059–1063

Cheng FW, Ip M, Chu YY, Lin Z, Lee V, Shing MK et al (2012) Humoral response to conjugate pneumococcal vaccine in paediatric oncology patients. Arch Dis Child 97(4):358–360

Cherif H, Landgren O, Konradsen HB, Kalin M, Bjorkholm M (2006) Poor antibody response to pneumococcal polysaccharide vaccination suggests increased susceptibility to pneumococcal infection in splenectomized patients with hematological diseases. Vaccine 24(1):75–81

Cherif H, Hoglund M, Pauksens K (2013) Adjuvanted influenza a (H1N1) 2009 vaccine in patients with hematological diseases: good safety and immunogenicity even in chemotherapy-treated patients. Eur J Haematol 90(5):413–419

Cordonnier C, Labopin M, Chesnel V, Ribaud P, De La Camara R, Martino R et al (2009) Randomized study of early versus late immunization with pneumococcal conjugate vaccine after allogeneic stem cell transplantation. Clin Infect Dis 48(10):1392–1401

Cordonnier C, Labopin M, Jansen KU, Pride M, Chesnel V, Bonnet E et al (2010a) Relationship between IgG titers and opsonocytophagocytic activity of antipneumococcal antibodies after immunization with the 7-valent conjugate vaccine in allogeneic stem cell transplant. Bone Marrow Transplant 45(9):1423–1426

Cordonnier C, Labopin M, Chesnel V, Ribaud P, Camara Rde L, Martino R et al (2010b) Immune response to the 23-valent polysaccharide pneumococcal vaccine after the 7-valent conjugate vaccine in allogeneic stem cell transplant recipients: results from the EBMT IDWP01 trial. Vaccine 28(15):2730–2734

Cordonnier C, Labopin M, Robin C, Ribaud P, Cabanne L, Chadelat C et al (2015a) Long-term persistence of the immune response to antipneumococcal vaccines after Allo-SCT: 10-year follow-up of the EBMT-IDWP01 trial. Bone Marrow Transplant 50(7):978–983

Cordonnier C, Ljungman P, Juergens C, Maertens J, Selleslag D, Sundaraiyer V et al (2015b) Immunogenicity, safety, and tolerability of 13-valent pneumococcal conjugate vaccine followed by 23-valent pneumococcal polysaccharide vaccine in recipients of allogeneic hematopoietic stem cell transplant aged >/=2 years: an open-label study. Clin Infect Dis 61(3):313–323

Costa E, Buxton J, Brown J, Templeton KE, Breuer J, Johannessen I (2016) Fatal disseminated varicella zoster infection following zoster vaccination in an immunocompromised patient. BMJ Case Rep 2016

Dhedin N, Krivine A, Le Corre N, Mallet A, Lioure B, Bay JO et al (2014) Comparable humoral response after two doses of adjuvanted influenza a/H1N1pdm2009 vaccine or natural infection in allogeneic stem cell transplant recipients. Vaccine 32(5):585–591

Douglas AP, Trubiano JA, Barr I, Leung V, Slavin MA, Tam CS (2017) Ibrutinib may impair serological responses to influenza vaccination. Haematologica 102(10):e397–e3e9

Elting LS, Whimbey E, Lo W, Couch R, Andreeff M, Bodey GP (1995) Epidemiology of influenza a virus infection in patients with acute or chronic leukemia. Supp Care Cancer 3(3):198–202

Engelhard D, Nagler A, Hardan I, Morag A, Aker M, Baciu H, et al. Antibody response to a two-dose regimen of influenza vaccine in allogeneic T cell-depleted and autologous BMT recipients. Bone Marrow Transplant 1993;11(1):1–5, 1

Engelhard D, Cordonnier C, Shaw PJ, Parkalli T, Guenther C, Martino R et al (2002) Early and late invasive pneumococcal infection following stem cell transplantation: a European bone marrow transplantation survey. Br J Haematol 117(2):444–450

Engelhard D, Zakay-Rones Z, Shapira MY, Resnick I, Averbuch D, Grisariu S et al (2011) The humoral immune response of hematopoietic stem cell transplantation recipients to AS03-adjuvanted a/California/7/2009 (H1N1)v-like virus vaccine during the 2009 pandemic. Vaccine 29(9):1777–1782

Engelhard D, Mohty B, de la Camara R, Cordonnier C, Ljungman P (2013) European guidelines for prevention and management of influenza in hematopoietic stem cell transplantation and leukemia patients: summary of ECIL-4 (2011), on behalf of ECIL, a joint venture of EBMT, EORTC, ICHS, and ELN. Transpl Infect Dis 15(3):219–232

Englund JA (2001) Diagnosis and epidemiology of community-acquired respiratory virus infections in the immunocompromised host. Biol Blood Marrow Trans 7(Suppl):2S–4S

Feldman S, Malone W, Wilbur R, Schiffman G (1985) Pneumococcal vaccination in children with acute lymphocytic leukemia. Med Pediatr Oncol 13(2):69–72

Frederiksen B, Specht L, Henrichsen J, Pedersen FK, Pedersen-Bjergaard J (1989) Antibody response to pneumococcal vaccine in patients with early stage Hodgkin's disease. Eur J Haematol 43(1):45–49

Giebink GS, Warkentin PI, Ramsay NK, Kersey JH (1986) Titers of antibody to pneumococci in allogeneic bone marrow transplant recipients before and after vaccination with pneumococcal vaccine. J Infect Dis 154(4):590–596

Goswami M, Prince G, Biancotto A, Moir S, Kardava L, Santich BH et al (2017) Impaired B cell immunity in acute myeloid leukemia patients after chemotherapy. J Transl Med 15(1):155

Grohskopf LA, Sokolow LZ, Broder KR, Walter EB, Fry AM, Jernigan DB (2018) Prevention and control of seasonal influenza with vaccines: recommendations of the advisory committee on immunization practices-United States, 2018-19 influenza season. MMWR Recomm Rep 67(3):1–20

Gueller S, Allwinn R, Mousset S, Martin H, Wieters I, Herrmann E et al (2011) Enhanced immune response after a second dose of an AS03-adjuvanted H1N1 influenza a vaccine in patients after hematopoietic stem cell transplantation. Biol Blood Marrow Trans 17(10):1546–1550

Guinan EC, Molrine DC, Antin JH, Lee MC, Weinstein HJ, Sallan SE et al (1994) Polysaccharide conjugate vaccine responses in bone marrow transplant patients. Transplantation 57(5):677–684

Hahn M, Schnitzler P, Schweiger B, Kunz C, Ho AD, Goldschmidt H et al (2015) Efficacy of single versus boost vaccination against influenza virus in patients with multiple myeloma. Haematologica 100(7):e285–e288

Hakim H, Allison KJ, Van De Velde LA, Li Y, Flynn PM, McCullers JA (2012) Immunogenicity and safety of inactivated monovalent 2009 H1N1 influenza a vaccine in immunocompromised children and young adults. Vaccine 30(5):879–885

Halasa NB, Savani BN, Asokan I, Kassim A, Simons R, Summers C et al (2016) Randomized double-blind study of the safety and immunogenicity of standard-dose trivalent inactivated influenza vaccine versus high-dose trivalent inactivated influenza vaccine in adult hematopoietic stem cell transplantation patients. Biol Blood Marrow Trans 22(3):528–535

Hargreaves R, Lea J, Griffiths H, Faux J, Holt J, Reid C et al (1995) Immunological factors and risk of infection in plateau phase myeloma. J Clin Pathol 48(3):260–266

Hartkamp A, Mulder AH, Rijkers GT, van Velzen-Blad H, Biesma DH (2001) Antibody responses to pneumococcal and haemophilus vaccinations in patients with B-cell chronic lymphocytic leukaemia. Vaccine 19(13–14):1671–1677

Hinge M, Ingels HA, Slotved HC, Molle I (2012) Serologic response to a 23-valent pneumococcal vaccine administered prior to autologous stem cell transplantation in patients with multiple myeloma. APMIS 120(11):935–940

Hung TY, Kotecha RS, Blyth CC, Steed SK, Thornton RB, Ryan AL et al (2017) Immunogenicity and safety of single-dose, 13-valent pneumococcal conjugate vaccine in pediatric and adolescent oncology patients. Cancer 123(21):4215–4223

Ide Y, Imamura Y, Ohfuji S, Fukushima W, Ide S, Tsutsumi C et al (2014) Immunogenicity of a monovalent influenza A(H1N1)pdm09 vaccine in patients with hematological malignancies. Hum Vaccin Immunother 10(8):2387–2394

Issa NC, Marty FM, Gagne LS, Koo S, Verrill KA, Alyea EP et al (2011) Seroprotective titers against 2009 H1N1 influenza a virus after vaccination in allogeneic hematopoietic stem cell transplantation recipients. Biol Blood Marrow Trans 17(3):434–438

Jackson LA, Gurtman A, van Cleeff M, Jansen KU, Jayawardene D, Devlin C et al (2013) Immunogenicity and safety of a 13-valent pneumococcal conjugate vaccine compared to a 23-valent pneumococcal polysaccharide vaccine in pneumococcal vaccine-naive adults. Vaccine 31(35):3577–3584

Karlsson JHH, Andersson K, Roshani L, Andréasson B, Wennerås C (2013) Pneumococcal vaccine responses in elderly patients with multiple myeloma, Waldenstrom's macroglobulinemia, and monoclonal gammopathy of undetermined significance. Trials Vaccinol 2:31–38

Karras NA, Weeres M, Sessions W, Xu X, Defor T, Young JA et al (2013) A randomized trial of one versus two doses of influenza vaccine after allogeneic transplantation. Biol Blood Marrow Trans 19(1):109–116

Kim DK, Riley LE, Hunter P (2018) Advisory committee on immunization practices recommended immunization schedule for adults aged 19 years or older - United States, 2018. MMWR Morb Mortal Wkly Rep 67(5):158–160

Kulkarni S, Powles R, Treleaven J, Riley U, Singhal S, Horton C et al (2000) Chronic graft versus host disease is associated with long-term risk for pneumococcal infections in recipients of bone marrow transplants. Blood 95(12):3683–3686

Kumar D, Chen MH, Welsh B, Siegal D, Cobos I, Messner HA et al (2007) A randomized, double-blind trial of pneumococcal vaccination in adult allogeneic stem cell transplant donors and recipients. Clin Infect Dis 45(12):1576–1582

Kumar D, Humar A, Plevneshi A, Siegal D, Franke N, Green K et al (2008) Invasive pneumococcal disease in adult hematopoietic stem cell transplant recipients: a decade of prospective population-based surveillance. Bone Marrow Transplant 41(8):743–747

Kumar D, Ferreira VH, Blumberg E, Silveira F, Cordero E, Perez-Romero P et al (2018) A 5-year prospective multicenter evaluation of influenza infection in transplant recipients. Clin Infect Dis 67(9):1322–1329

Kyaw MH, Rose CE Jr, Fry AM, Singleton JA, Moore Z, Zell ER et al (2005) The influence of chronic illnesses on the incidence of invasive pneumococcal disease in adults. J Infect Dis 192(3):377–386

Landgren O, Bjorkholm M, Konradsen HB, Soderqvist M, Nilsson B, Gustavsson A et al (2004) A prospective study on antibody response to repeated vaccinations with pneumococcal capsular polysaccharide in splenectomized individuals with special reference to Hodgkin's lymphoma. J Intern Med 255(6):664–673

Laubli H, Balmelli C, Kaufmann L, Stanczak M, Syedbasha M, Vogt D et al (2018) Influenza vaccination of cancer patients during PD-1 blockade induces serological protection but may raise the risk for immune-related adverse events. J Immunother Cancer 6(1):40

de Lavallade H, Garland P, Sekine T, Hoschler K, Marin D, Stringaris K et al (2011) Repeated vaccination is required to optimize seroprotection against H1N1 in the immunocompromised host. Haematologica 96(2):307–314

Lazarus HM, Lederman M, Lubin A, Herzig RH, Schiffman G, Jones P et al (1980) Pneumococcal vaccination: the response of patients with multiple myeloma. Am J Med 69(3):419–423

Leahy TR, Smith OP, Bacon CL, Storey L, Lynam P, Gavin PJ et al (2013) Does vaccine dose predict response to the monovalent pandemic H1N1 influenza a vaccine in children with acute lymphoblastic leukemia? A single-Centre study. Pediatr Blood Cancer 60(10):1656–1661

Lehrnbecher T, Schubert R, Behl M, Koenig M, Rose MA, Koehl U et al (2009) Impaired pneumococcal immunity in children after treatment for acute lymphoblastic leukaemia. Br J Haematol 147(5):700–705

Lehrnbecher T, Schubert R, Allwinn R, Dogan K, Koehl U, Gruttner HP (2011) Revaccination of children after completion of standard chemotherapy for acute lymphoblastic leukaemia: a pilot study comparing different schedules. Br J Haematol 152(6):754–757

Liu Y, Bewersdorf JP, Stahl M, Zeidan AM (2018) Immunotherapy in acute myeloid leukemia and myelodysplastic syndromes: the dawn of a new era? Blood Rev

Ljungman P, Nahi H, Linde A (2005) Vaccination of patients with haematological malignancies with one or two doses of influenza vaccine: a randomised study. Br J Haematol 130(1):96–98

Ljungman P, Cordonnier C, Einsele H, Englund J, Machado CM, Storek J et al (2009) Vaccination of hematopoietic cell transplant recipients. Bone Marrow Transplant 44(8):521–526

Lo W, Whimbey E, Elting L, Couch R, Cabanillas F, Bodey G (1993) Antibody response to a two-dose influenza vaccine regimen in adult lymphoma patients on chemotherapy. Eur J Clin Microbiol Infect Dis 12(10):778–782

Locke FL, Menges M, Nishihori T, Nwoga C, Alsina M, Anasetti C (2016) Boosting humoral and cellular immunity to pneumococcus by vaccination before and just after autologous transplant for myeloma. Bone Marrow Transplant 51(2):291–294

Machado CM, Goncalves FB, Pannuti CS, Dulley FL, de Souza VA (2002) Measles in bone marrow transplant recipients during an outbreak in Sao Paulo. Brazil Blood 99(1):83–87

Machado CM, de Souza VA, Sumita LM, da Rocha IF, Dulley FL, Pannuti CS (2005a) Early measles vaccination in bone marrow transplant recipients. Bone Marrow Transplant 35(8):787–791

Machado CM, Cardoso MR, da Rocha IF, Boas LS, Dulley FL, Pannuti CS (2005b) The benefit of influenza vaccination after bone marrow transplantation. Bone Marrow Transplant 36(10):897–900

Mackay HJ, McGee J, Villa D, Gubbay JB, Tinker LM, Shi L et al (2011) Evaluation of pandemic H1N1 (2009) influenza vaccine in adults with solid tumor and hematological malignancies on active systemic treatment. J Clin Virol 50(3):212–216

Mariotti J, Spina F, Carniti C, Anselmi G, Lucini D, Vendramin A et al (2012) Long-term patterns of humoral and cellular response after vaccination against influenza a (H1N1) in patients with hematologic malignancies. Eur J Haematol 89(2):111–119

McManus M, Frangoul H, McCullers JA, Wang L, O'Shea A, Halasa N (2014) Safety of high dose trivalent inactivated influenza vaccine in pediatric patients with acute lymphoblastic leukemia. Pediatr Blood Cancer 61(5):815–820

Meerveld-Egginkk A, van der Velden AM, Ossenkoppele GJ, van de Loosdrecht AA, Biesma DH, Rijkers GT (2009) Antibody response to polysaccharide conjugate vaccines after nonmyeloablative allogeneic stem cell transplantation. Biol Blood Marrow Trans 15(12):1523–1530

Meisel R, Kuypers L, Dirksen U, Schubert R, Gruhn B, Strauss G et al (2007a) Pneumococcal conjugate vaccine provides early protective antibody responses in children after related and unrelated allogeneic hematopoietic stem cell transplantation. Blood 109(6):2322–2326

Meisel R, Toschke AM, Heiligensetzer C, Dilloo D, Laws HJ, von Kries R (2007b) Increased risk for invasive pneumococcal diseases in children with acute lymphoblastic leukaemia. Br J Haematol 137(5):457–460

Mohty B, Bel M, Vukicevic M, Nagy M, Levrat E, Meier S et al (2011) Graft-versus-host disease is the major determinant of humoral responses to the AS03-adjuvanted influenza a/09/H1N1 vaccine in allogeneic hematopoietic stem cell transplant recipients. Haematologica 96(6):896–904

Molrine DC, George S, Tarbell N, Mauch P, Diller L, Neuberg D et al (1995) Antibody responses to polysaccharide and polysaccharide-conjugate vaccines after treatment of Hodgkin disease. Ann Intern Med 123(11):828–834

Molrine DC, Antin JH, Guinan EC, Soiffer RJ, MacDonald K, Malley R et al (2003) Donor immunization with pneumococcal conjugate vaccine and early protective antibody responses following allogeneic hematopoietic cell transplantation. Blood 101(3):831–836

Morrison VA (2007) Management of infectious complications in patients with chronic lymphocytic leukemia. Hematology Am Soc Hematol Educ Program 2007:332–338

Morrison VA (2009) Infectious complications in patients with chronic lymphocytic leukemia: pathogenesis, spectrum of infection, and approaches to prophylaxis. Clin Lymphoma Myeloma 9(5):365–370

Morrison VA (2010) Infectious complications of chronic lymphocytic leukaemia: pathogenesis, spectrum of infection, preventive approaches. Best Pract Res Clin Haematol 23(1):145–153

Mustafa SS, Shah D, Bress J, Jamshed S (2018) Response to PCV13 vaccination in patients with multiple myeloma versus healthy controls. Hum Vaccin Immunother:1–3

Musto P, Carotenuto M (1997) Vaccination against influenza in multiple myeloma. Br J Haematol 97(2):505–506

Natori Y, Humar A, Lipton J, Kim DD, Ashton P, Hoschler K et al (2017) A pilot randomized trial of adjuvanted influenza vaccine in adult allogeneic hematopoietic stem cell transplant recipients. Bone Marrow Transplant 52(7):1016–1021

Nichols WG, Guthrie KA, Corey L, Boeckh M (2004) Influenza infections after hematopoietic stem cell transplantation: risk factors, mortality, and the effect of antiviral therapy. Clin Infect Dis 39(9):1300–1306

Noonan K, Rudraraju L, Ferguson A, Emerling A, Pasetti MF, Huff CA et al (2012) Lenalidomide-induced immunomodulation in multiple myeloma: impact on vaccines and antitumor responses. Clin Cancer Res 18(5):1426–1434

Nordoy T, Aaberge IS, Husebekk A, Samdal HH, Steinert S, Melby H et al (2002) Cancer patients undergoing chemotherapy show adequate serological response to vaccinations against influenza virus and Streptococcus pneumoniae. Med Oncol 19(2):71–78

Palazzo M, Shah GL, Copelan O, Seier K, Devlin SM, Maloy M et al (2018) Revaccination after autologous hematopoietic stem cell transplantation is safe and effective in patients with multiple myeloma receiving Lenalidomide maintenance. Biol Blood Marrow Trans 24(4):871–876

Pandit A, Leblebjian H, Hammond SP, Laubach JP, Richardson PG, Baden LR et al (2018) Safety of live-attenuated measles-mumps-rubella and herpes zoster vaccination in multiple myeloma patients on maintenance lenalidomide or bortezomib after autologous hematopoietic cell transplantation. Bone Marrow Transplant 53(7):942–945

Pasiarski M, Rolinski J, Grywalska E, Stelmach-Goldys A, Korona-Glowniak I, Gozdz S et al (2014) Antibody and plasmablast response to 13-valent pneumococcal conjugate vaccine in chronic lymphocytic leukemia patients--preliminary report. PLoS One 9(12):e114966

Pauksen K, Linde A, Hammarstrom V, Sjolin J, Carneskog J, Jonsson G et al (2000) Granulocyte-macrophage colony-stimulating factor as immunomodulating factor together with influenza vaccination in stem cell transplant patients. Clin Infect Dis 30(2):342–348

Petrasch S, Kuhnemund O, Reinacher A, Uppenkamp M, Reinert R, Schmiegel W et al (1997) Antibody responses of splenectomized patients with non-Hodgkin's lymphoma to immunization with polyvalent pneumococcal vaccines. Clin Diagn Lab Immunol 4(6):635–638

Pinana JL, Perez A, Montoro J, Gimenez E, Dolores Gomez M, Lorenzo I et al (2018) Clinical effectiveness of influenza vaccination after allogeneic hematopoietic stem cell transplantation: a cross-sectional prospective observational study. Clin Infect Dis

Pletz MW, Maus U, Krug N, Welte T, Lode H (2008) Pneumococcal vaccines: mechanism of action, impact on epidemiology and adaption of the species. Int J Antimicrob Agents 32(3):199–206

Postow MA, Sidlow R, Hellmann MD (2018) Immune-related adverse events associated with immune checkpoint blockade. N Engl J Med 378(2):158–168

Rapezzi D, Sticchi L, Racchi O, Mangerini R, Ferraris AM, Gaetani GF (2003) Influenza vaccine in chronic lymphoproliferative disorders and multiple myeloma. Eur J Haematol 70(4):225–230

Rawstron AC, Davies FE, Owen RG, English A, Pratt G, Child JA et al (1998) B-lymphocyte suppression in multiple myeloma is a reversible phenomenon specific to normal B-cell progenitors and plasma cell precursors. Br J Haematol 100(1):176–183

Rieger CT, Liss B, Mellinghoff S, Buchheidt D, Cornely OA, Egerer G et al (2018) Anti-infective vaccination strategies in patients with hematologic malignancies or solid tumors-guideline of the infectious diseases working party (AGIHO) of the German Society for Hematology and Medical Oncology (DGHO). Ann Oncol 29(6):1354–1365

Robertson JD, Nagesh K, Jowitt SN, Dougal M, Anderson H, Mutton K et al (2000) Immunogenicity of vaccination against influenza, Streptococcus pneumoniae and Haemophilus influenzae type B in patients with multiple myeloma. Br J Cancer 82(7):1261–1265

Roll D, Ammer J, Holler B, Salzberger B, Schweiger B, Jilg W et al (2012) Vaccination against pandemic H1N1 (2009) in patients after allogeneic hematopoietic stem cell transplantation: a retrospective analysis. Infection 40(2):153–161

Rubin LG, Levin MJ, Ljungman P, Davies EG, Avery R, Tomblyn M et al (2014) 2013 IDSA clinical practice guideline for vaccination of the immunocompromised host. Clin Infect Dis 58(3):e44–100

Safdar A, Rodriguez GH, Rueda AM, Wierda WG, Ferrajoli A, Musher DM et al (2008) Multiple-dose granulocyte-macrophage-colony-stimulating factor plus 23-valent polysaccharide pneumococcal vaccine in patients with chronic lymphocytic leukemia: a prospective, randomized trial of safety and immunogenicity. Cancer 113(2):383–387

Savage DG, Lindenbaum J, Garrett T (1982) Biphasic pattern of bacterial infection in multiple myeloma. Ann Intern Med 96(1):47–50

Schütt P, Brandhorst D, Stellberg W, Poser M, Ebeling P, Müller S et al (2006) Immune parameters in multiple myeloma patients: influence of treatment and correlation with opportunistic infections. Leuk Lymphoma 47(8):1570–1582

Shahgholi E, Ehsani MA, Salamati P, Maysamie A, Sotoudeh K, Mokhtariazad T (2010) Immunogenicity of trivalent influenza vaccine in children with acute lymphoblastic leukemia during maintenance therapy. Pediatr Blood Cancer 54(5):716–720

Shigayeva A, Rudnick W, Green K, Chen DK, Demczuk W, Gold WL et al (2016) Invasive pneumococcal disease among immunocompromised persons: implications for vaccination programs. Clin Infect Dis 62(2):139–147

Siber GR, Gorham C, Martin P, Corkery JC, Schiffman G (1986) Antibody response to pretreatment immunization and post-treatment boosting with bacterial polysaccharide vaccines in patients with Hodgkin's disease. Ann Intern Med 104(4):467–475

Sim SA, Leung VKY, Ritchie D, Slavin MA, Sullivan SG, Teh BW (2018) Viral respiratory tract infections in allogeneic hematopoietic stem cell transplantation recipients in the era of molecular testing. Biol Blood Marrow Trans 24(7):1490–1496

Sinisalo M, Vilpo J, Itala M, Vakevainen M, Taurio J, Aittoniemi J (2007) Antibody response to 7-valent conjugated pneumococcal vaccine in patients with chronic lymphocytic leukaemia. Vaccine 26(1):82–87

Steingrimsdottir H, Gruber A, Bjorkholm M, Svensson A, Hansson M (2000) Immune reconstitution after autologous hematopoietic stem cell transplantation in relation to underlying disease, type of high-dose therapy and infectious complications. Haematologica 85(8):832–838

Storek J, Dawson MA, Lim LC, Burman BE, Stevens-Ayers T, Viganego F et al (2004) Efficacy of donor vaccination before hematopoietic cell transplantation and recipient vaccination both before and early after transplantation. Bone Marrow Transplant 33(3):337–346

Sun C, Tian X, Lee YS, Gunti S, Lipsky A, Herman SE et al (2015) Partial reconstitution of humoral immunity and fewer infections in patients with chronic lymphocytic leukemia treated with ibrutinib. Blood 126(19):2213–2219

Sun C, Gao J, Couzens L, Tian X, Farooqui MZ, Eichelberger MC et al (2016) Seasonal influenza vaccination in patients with chronic lymphocytic leukemia treated with Ibrutinib. JAMA Oncol 2(12):1656–1657

Svensson T, Kattstrom M, Hammarlund Y, Roth D, Andersson PO, Svensson M et al (2018) Pneumococcal conjugate vaccine triggers a better immune response than pneumococcal polysaccharide vaccine in patients with chronic lymphocytic leukemia a randomized study by the Swedish CLL group. Vaccine 36(25):3701–3707

Teh BW, Harrison SJ, Pellegrini M, Thursky KA, Worth LJ, Slavin MA (2014) Changing treatment paradigms for patients with plasma cell myeloma: impact upon immune determinants of infection. Blood Rev 28(2):75–86

Teh BW, Harrison SJ, Worth LJ, Spelman T, Thursky KA, Slavin MA (2015a) Risks, severity and timing of infections in patients with multiple myeloma: a longitudinal cohort study in the era of immunomodulatory drug therapy. Br J Haematol 171(1):100–108

Teh BW, Worth LJ, Harrison SJ, Thursky KA, Slavin MA (2015b) Risks and burden of viral respiratory tract infections in patients with multiple myeloma in the era of immunomodulatory drugs and bortezomib: experience at an Australian Cancer hospital. Supp Care Cancer 23(7):1901–1906

Teh BW, Harrison SJ, Slavin MA, Worth LJ (2017a) Epidemiology of bloodstream infections in patients with myeloma receiving current era therapy. Eur J Haematol 98(2):149–153

Teh BW, Joyce T, Slavin MA, Thursky KA, Worth LJ (2017b) Impact of a dedicated post-transplant vaccination service at an Australian cancer centre. Bone Marrow Transplant 52(12):1681–1683

Teh BW, Tam CS, Handunnetti S, Worth LJ, Slavin MA (2018) Infections in patients with chronic lymphocytic leukaemia: mitigating risk in the era of targeted therapies. Blood Rev 32(6):499–507

Theilacker C, Ludewig K, Serr A, Schimpf J, Held J, Bogelein M et al (2016) Overwhelming

Postsplenectomy infection: a prospective multicenter cohort study. Clin Infect Dis 62(7):871–878

Tomblyn M, Chiller T, Einsele H, Gress R, Sepkowitz K, Storek J et al (2009) Guidelines for preventing infectious complications among hematopoietic cell transplantation recipients: a global perspective. Biol Blood Marrow Trans 15(10):1143–1238

Torda A, Chong Q, Lee A, Chen S, Dodds A, Greenwood M et al (2014) Invasive pneumococcal disease following adult allogeneic hematopoietic stem cell transplantation. Transpl Infect Dis 16(5):751–759

Tramontana AR, George B, Hurt AC, Doyle JS, Langan K, Reid AB et al (2010) Oseltamivir resistance in adult oncology and hematology patients infected with pandemic (H1N1) 2009 virus. Australia Emerg Infect Dis 16(7):1068–1075

Tsigrelis C, Ljungman P (2016) Vaccinations in patients with hematological malignancies. Blood Rev 30(2):139–147

Ullmann AJ, Schmidt-Hieber M, Bertz H, Heinz WJ, Kiehl M, Kruger W et al (2016) Infectious diseases in allogeneic haematopoietic stem cell transplantation: prevention and prophylaxis strategy guidelines 2016. Ann Hematol 95(9):1435–1455

Van der Velden AM, Van Velzen-Blad H, Claessen AM, Van der Griend R, Oltmans R, Rijkers GT et al (2007) The effect of ranitidine on antibody responses to polysaccharide vaccines in patients with B-cell chronic lymphocytic leukaemia. Eur J Haematol 79(1):47–52

van der Velden AM, Mulder AH, Hartkamp A, Diepersloot RJ, van Velzen-Blad H, Biesma DH (2001) Influenza virus vaccination and booster in B-cell chronic lymphocytic leukaemia patients. Eur J Intern Med 12(5):420–424

van der Velden AM, Claessen AM, van Velzen-Blad H, de Groot MR, Kramer MH, Biesma DH et al (2007) Vaccination responses and lymphocyte subsets after autologous stem cell transplantation. Vaccine 25(51):8512–8517

Villa D, Gubbay J, Sutherland DR, Laister R, McGeer A, Cooper C et al (2013) Evaluation of 2009 pandemic H1N1 influenza vaccination in adults with lymphoid malignancies receiving chemotherapy or following autologous stem cell transplant. Leuk Lymphoma 54(7):1387–1395

Whimbey E, Elting LS, Couch RB, Lo W, Williams L, Champlin RE et al (1994) Influenza a virus infections among hospitalized adult bone marrow transplant recipients. Bone Marrow Transplant 13(4):437–440

Wijn DH, Groeneveld GH, Vollaard AM, Muller M, Wallinga J, Gelderblom H et al (2018) Influenza vaccination in patients with lung cancer receiving anti-programmed death receptor 1 immunotherapy does not induce immune-related adverse events. Eur J Cancer 104:182–187

Witherspoon RP, Storb R, Ochs HD, Fluornoy N, Kopecky KJ, Sullivan KM et al (1981) Recovery of antibody production in human allogeneic marrow graft recipients: influence of time posttransplantation, the presence or absence of chronic graft-versus-host disease, and antithymocyte globulin treatment. Blood 58(2):360–368

Wong A, Marrie TJ, Garg S, Kellner JD, Tyrrell GJ, Group S (2010) Increased risk of invasive pneumococcal disease in haematological and solid-organ malignancies. Epidemiol Infect 138(12):1804–1810

Wong-Chew RM, Frias MN, Garcia-Leon ML, Arriaga-Pizano L, Sanson AM, Lopez-Macias C et al (2012) Humoral and cellular immune responses to influenza vaccination in children with cancer receiving chemotherapy. Oncol Lett 4(2):329–333

Talcii SS, Kondolot M, Albayrak N, Altas AB, Karacan Y, Kuskonmaz B et al (2010) Serological response to influenza vaccine after hematopoetic stem cell transplantation. Ann Hematol 89(9):913–918

Youssef S, Rodriguez G, Rolston KV, Champlin RE, Raad II, Safdar A (2007) Streptococcus pneumoniae infections in 47 hematopoietic stem cell transplantation recipients: clinical characteristics of infections and vaccine-breakthrough infections, 1989-2005. Medicine (Baltimore) 86(2):69–77

Yousuf HM, Englund J, Couch R, Rolston K, Luna M, Goodrich J et al (1997) Influenza among hospitalized adults with leukemia. Clin Infect Dis 24(6):1095–1099

Yri OE, Torfoss D, Hungnes O, Tierens A, Waalen K, Nordoy T et al (2011) Rituximab blocks protective serologic response to influenza A (H1N1) 2009 vaccination in lymphoma patients during or within 6 months after treatment. Blood 118(26):6769–6771

Parasitic Infections

8

Stéphane Bretagne and Nikolai Klimko

8.1 Introduction

Among the numerous parasitic species described in humans, only a few have been reported in patients with hematological malignancies (HM), mainly after hematopoietic stem cell transplantation (HSCT) and more specifically after allogeneic HSCT (allo-HSCT) (Gea-Banacloche et al. 2009; Ljungman et al. 2016; Fabiani et al. 2017). A possible bias is that parasites are mainly prevalent in developing countries and therefore not reported in association with HM knowing that these countries perform a limited number of HSCT. Another possibility is the lack of easy diagnostic means with a subsequent lack of definite diagnosis. A third possibility is a true rarity because the immune balance deregulation needed to allow a parasite to express pathogenicity is simply not present in these settings. For instance, treatment of lymphoid cancer with ibrutinib is reported to be associated with an increase of bacterial and fungal infections but not with parasite infections (Varughese et al. 2018). Whatever the explanation is, the consequence is that, with few exceptions (e.g., toxoplasmosis), knowledge on parasitic infection in hematological malignancies is mostly based on random case reports or small cohorts, mainly in allo-HSCT, which is the major condition favoring the occurrence of parasitic infections (Gea-Banacloche et al. 2009).

However, when parasitic infections occur, they can have a huge impact on the prognosis in patients with HM. It is therefore necessary to be aware of the risk, especially when managing patients referred from an endemic country/area. From the biological point of view, one must separate three main mechanisms to explain occurrence of parasitic diseases in immunocompromised patients: (1) reactivation of dormant infections, (2) de novo infection after/during immunosuppressive treatment, and (33) infections transmitted by transfusion of blood products. In the first possibility, the patient kept the parasite under a dormant form, and no infection occurs as long as the immune system controlling the parasite growth is efficient. If such infection is known, preventive measures can be proposed before the onset of full-blown disease. The second possibility is the occurrence of de novo infection during the immunodeficiency phase. The best way of prevention is avoiding exposure. The third possibility refers to safety of blood transfusion and graft donation with few case reports in nonendemic countries,

S. Bretagne (✉)
Parasitology-Mycology Laboratory, Lariboisière, Saint-Louis, Fernand Widal Hospitals, Assistance Publique-Hôpitaux de Paris (AP-HP), Paris, France

Université de Paris, Paris, France
e-mail: stephane.bretagne@aphp.fr

N. Klimko (✉)
Department of Clinical Mycology, Allergy and Immunology, North Western State Medical University, Saint Petersburg, Russia

© Springer Nature Switzerland AG 2021
O. A. Cornely, M. Hoenigl (eds.), *Infection Management in Hematology*, Hematologic Malignancies, https://doi.org/10.1007/978-3-030-57317-1_8

both with malaria (Abdelkefi et al. 2004; Mejia et al. 2012) and Chagas disease (Forés et al. 2007). This issue remains a challenge in not only developing countries (Gopal et al. 2012) but also, see for instance, *Babesia* spp. infections in North America (Tonnetti et al. 2019). However, challenges in endemic countries are expected when management of HM will expand, both because of safety blood constrains and constant reinfections. These last issues are not part of this chapter.

This chapter focuses on parasites possibly present before any treatment for hematology malignancy for which prophylactic or diagnostic screening could be implemented. The two main parasitic diseases in this case are toxoplasmosis and strongyloidiasis for which strong recommendations exist for preventing them. Other parasites are also possibly present before any therapeutic procedure, but there is no recommendation due to the rarity of the reported cases. The best way to prevent these parasitic diseases is a careful report of the different residencies and/or travel in endemic areas. The second part presents rare pathogens diagnosed after therapy initiation; evidence is often postmortem underlining the need to improve their diagnosis.

8.2 Parasitic Infections Possibly Present Before Treatment of Hematological Malignancies

8.2.1 *Toxoplasma gondii*

Toxoplasma gondii is a ubiquitous coccidian parasite of which the definite host (harboring the sexual stage) is the cat, and which is able to contaminate a variety of intermediate hosts, from mammals to birds. Two routes of contamination are possible: either the ingestion of oocysts shed by cats in the environment or the ingestion of undercooked meat containing cysts, the main contaminating route at least in Europe (Cook et al. 2000). Once infected, humans develop a strong immunity able to control the parasite growth. Toxoplasmosis is therefore seen only in immuno-

compromised host such as fetuses upon maternal infection during pregnancy, or HIV-positive patients, and solid organ transplant or HSCT recipients. This is by far the most studied parasitic infection in this latter setting, and more specifically after allo-HSCT than after auto-HSCT, with a higher incidence in cord blood HSCT (Martino et al. 2005) and with haploidentical and unrelated mismatched donor HSCT (Gajurel et al. 2015).

In HSCT patients, the main mechanism explaining the occurrence of toxoplasmosis is reactivation of tissue cysts. The currently accepted hypothesis is that these cysts are living in a dormant form, mainly in muscles or brain, which allows a constant immune stimulation. This would explain the lifelong persistence of detectable antibodies. Therefore, the recommendation in HSCT is to perform pretreatment tests for the presence of antibodies. There are numerous commercially available assays providing IgG titers. If anti-*Toxoplasma* IgGs are detected, the interpretation is that latent cysts are present and can potentially multiply after HSCT. Seroprevalence depends on several factors, of which the culinary habits are probably major but also the socioeconomic environment, explaining the differences between counties (Pappas et al. 2009). Of note, decline in seroprevalence is observed in several countries, and more specifically in France, a country known to have a high seroprevalence several decades ago (Guigue et al. 2018). The reason for this decline is probably the lower parasitism of consumed meat. This means that the risk of reactivation for young patients is probably lower than it used to be, although always present (Decembrino et al. 2017). On the contrary, the seroprevalence remains high in older patients with still a high risk of reactivation (Guigue et al. 2018).

The observation of full-blown toxoplasmosis is a rather late complication of HSCT occurring after a median of 45 days although a positive quantitative real-time polymerase chain reaction (qPCR) result has been reported as soon as 2 days after allo-HSCT (Martino et al. 2005). Encephalitis is the main clinical manifestation, but pneumonia and myocarditis are also frequent findings, although often diagnosed at autopsy

(Gajurel et al. 2015). However, before the onset of encephalitis, several studies using quantitative real-time polymerase chain reaction (qPCR) have shown the presence of circulating parasites (strictly speaking, circulating DNA of the parasite) and the progressive increase of the parasite load (Costa et al. 2000; Bretagne et al. 2000; Martino et al. 2005). Hence, the creation of the concept of "*Toxoplasma* infection" as defined by fever and a positive PCR finding for *T. gondii* in blood (Martino et al. 2000). Therefore, due to this risk of *Toxoplasma*-related life-threatening events, the usual recommendations when the expected resultant immunosuppression is high are to screen patients for the presence of IgG and to provide prophylaxis in seropositive recipients (Gea-Banacloche et al. 2009; Ullmann et al. 2016). When prophylaxis is not possible because of allergies or toxicities, posttransplant monitoring with qPCR in unexplained fevers in seropositive patients can also be proposed (Martino et al. 2005; Conrad et al. 2016). For the donor in allo-HSCT, serology is designed to estimate the risk, which is higher in case of donor−/recipient+, which should increase the suspicion index of *Toxoplasma* reactivation (Martino et al. 2005). The transmission through blood or bone marrow transfusion, although theoretically possible, has never been firmly documented after HSCT, and no specific screening of blood product using qPCR is recommended (Gajurel et al. 2015).

Despite these recommendations for prophylaxis in seropositive patients, in a review including 259 seropositive recipients after allo-HSCT, at least 67% were not given anti-*Toxoplasma* prophylaxis (Gajurel et al. 2015). As a result, toxoplasmosis remains a reality after allogeneic allo-HSCT. In a recent case–control study of 23 cases in a single French center, the risk factors identified were indeed the absence of effective anti-*Toxoplasma* prophylaxis, to a lesser extent high-grade acute graft-versus-host disease, and receipt of the TNF-a blocker etanercept (Conrad et al. 2016). The attributable mortality was 43.5%. In this study, 87% of the patients with toxoplasmosis were seropositive, but only 85% of them were receiving effective anti-*Toxoplasma* prophylaxis because of concerns about adverse effects of trimethoprim–sulfamethoxazole or atovaquone. Consequently, the authors recommend, as others (Gajurel et al. 2015), prescribing effective prophylactic drug regimens or adopting a *T. gondii* PCR-driven preemptive approach (Conrad et al. 2016). The main measures and strategies to avoid toxoplasmosis are listed in Table 8.1.

8.2.2 *Strongyloides stercoralis*

Among the soil-transmitted helminths or geohelminths, which comprise *Ascaris lumbricoides*, hookworms (*Ancylostoma duodenale* and *Necator americanus*), *Trichuris trichiura*, and *Strongyloides stercoralis*, only the latter owns a specificity explaining the risk of infection in immunocompromised patients (Greaves et al. 2013). The female worm sheds eggs of which some immediately convert into infecting larvae before shed in stools. Thus, in contrast to other geohelminths, which need obligatory maturation in the environment before re-entering a new host, *S. stercoralis* is able to maintain a constant cycle in a given individual. The usual route of infection is the transdermal route, although ingestion is also major as a source of infection (Zeehaida et al. 2011). The notion that a person can remain infected for decades, even the whole life, has been established for long (Mansfield et al. 1996; Prendki et al. 2011). The regular migration of larvae, more or less synchronic, explains the oscillating hypereosinophilia characteristic with this helminth. This also explains why life-threatening hyperinfection syndrome (HS), or malignant strongyloidiasis, can occur in some immunocompromised patients (Keiser and Nutman 2004; Nutman 2017).

The HS is known as case reports in both auto-HSCT and allo-HSCT with a high mortality above 80% (Wirk and Wingard 2009). Therefore, the same screening precautions proposed in allo-HSCT should be used among autologous recipients as well (Gea-Banacloche et al. 2009). Unfortunately, allo-HSCT recipients still decease of HS with a lack of preventive treatment (Malki Al and Song 2016; Alpern et al. 2017).

Screening for strongyloidiasis is therefore strongly recommended before starting any immu-

Table 8.1 Parasites possibly present as dormant/asymptomatic infections before hematological malignancy (HM) treatment

Parasites	Screening before HM treatment	Prophylaxis or preventive treatment	Main clinical forms after HM treatment	Lab diagnosis after HM treatment	Therapy
Toxoplasma gondii	*Toxoplasma* IgG test	Trimethoprim/sulfamethoxazole (TMP/SMX)[a] 1 double-strength tablet (160/800 mg)/d, 4 days x week, or 2 double-strength tablets (160/800 mg)/d, 3 days x week, or 1 standard-dose tablet (80/400 mg)/d, or pyrimethamine and sulfadiazine 2–3 tables per week or dapsone[a] 100 mg/d or atovaquone[a] 1500 mg/d	Encephalitis, pneumonia, myocarditis, chorioretinitis (rare)	qPCR, histopathology	Pyrimethamine 200 mg loading dose, then 50–75 mg/d plus folic acid, oral or IV, 10–15 mg/d plus sulfadiazine 1 g if <60 kg; 1.5 g if ≥60 kg, q6h or clindamycin oral or IV, 600 mg q6h
Strongyloides stercoralis	Patients from endemic area or with unexplained eosinophilia: Multiple stool microscopy, *Strongyloides* IgG test	Patients from endemic area or screening test+: Ivermectin 200 µg/kg/d for 2 days, or albendazole 800 mg/d for 7 days	Gastroenteritis, disseminated strongyloidiasis (DS), hyperinfection syndrome (HS)	Multiple stool microscopy, *Strongyloides* IgG, in DS/HS patients— Respiratory secretions, urine, ascites fluid, and CSF examination	Asymptomatic or intestinal Disease: Ivermectin 200 µg/kg/d for 2 days DS or HS: Ivermectin 200 µg/kg/d per day until lab tests are negative for 2 weeks
Leishmania infantum	None	None	Fever with pancytopenia	Bone marrow aspirate microscopy, *Leishmania* qPCR	Liposomal amphotericin B 4 mg/kg/d on days 1–5, 10, 17, 24, 31, and 38 (total dose 40 mg/kg)
Trypanosoma cruzi	Patient from endemic countries: *T. cruzi* Serum IgG test	Patient from endemic countries: *T. cruzi* serum IgG test+: Benznidazole or nifurtimox	Acute: Fever, rash, lymphadenopathy, hepatosplenomegaly, myocarditis, meningoencephalitisChronic: Cardiomegaly, megaesophagus, and megacolon	Blood microscopy and culture, *T. cruzi* serum IgG, qPCR, RT-PCR	Benznidazole 10–14 mg/kg/d for 60 days OR nifurtimox 8–10 mg/kg/d in 3 divided doses for 90 days

Parasites	Screening before HM treatment	Prophylaxis or preventive treatment	Main clinical forms after HM treatment	Lab diagnosis after HM treatment	Therapy
Plasmodium falciparum, P. vivax and P. *ovale, P. malariae*	None	None	Fever, respiratory distress syndrome, cardiomyopathy, renal and liver failure, etc.	Thick blood films microscopy, qPCR	Artesunate IV 2.4 mg/kg, repeat at 12, 24, and then once daily for 6 days plus clindamycin IV 20 mg/kg/d daily, divided every 8 h, for 7 days OR quinine dihydrochloride IV 20 mg/kg/d for 7 days

qPCR, quantitative polymerase chain reaction
[a]Dose can be reduced in patients with mild renal insufficiency

nosuppressive treatments in patients coming from endemic areas (Gea-Banacloche et al. 2009; Greaves et al. 2013). While the risk of potential infection is easily suspected in patients coming from tropical and subtropical countries and the endemic zones of this parasitic disease (Schär et al. 2013), the risk is often underappreciated in patients from Western countries. It is therefore of utmost importance to obtain histories from all patients to identify potential exposure through remote residence or travel in risk areas (Gea-Banacloche et al. 2009). The suspicion also includes unexplained peripheral eosinophilia (Gea-Banacloche et al. 2009).

The diagnosis of strongyloidiasis is historically based on stool examination with concentration methods (Baermann technique or agar culture), but the sensitivity is below 90% even if several consecutive samples are examined (Luvira et al. 2014). Indeed, three consecutive samples are recommended because of intermittent larval output in stools. Other options available for screening are serological tests developed to increase the diagnostic sensitivity. The sensitivity of these tests is nevertheless lower in patients with hematological malignancies or HTLV-1 infection (Levenhagen and Costa-Cruz 2014). Unfortunately, false negative results exist and can be falsely reassuring (Alpern et al. 2017). The main pitfall is nevertheless the low specificity of these tests because of the cross-reactivity with other nematodes. This lack of specificity could be disregarded when the treatment is well tolerated and the goal is to prevent deadly hyperinfection. Thus, given the high seroprevalence in endemic countries (Gómez-Junyent et al. 2018), the wisest decision should be to consider every patient coming from endemic areas as potentially infected and act accordingly. Molecular diagnostic techniques are under development and evaluation, and one of the most interesting features would be to identify relapse after treatment (Nutman 2017).

Prevention of strongyloidiasis is, thus, indicated for all patients from endemic areas regardless of the microbiological confirmation, even if the latter is of course useful to evaluate the load and therefore to follow the treatment efficacy and identify potential relapse (Table 8.1). Prevention

is also indicated when candidates for chemotherapy or HSCT not coming from an endemic area have a history of residency in endemic areas and, even more so, when pretreatment screening tests are positive for *Strongyloides* or in case of unexplained eosinophilia (Keiser and Nutman 2004).

The first choice for prophylactic treatment consists of ivermectin 200 mg daily for 2 days, preferred to albendazole 400 mg bid for 7 days, given its better efficacy and good tolerance (Henriquez-Camacho et al. 2016). For patients with pretreatment positive screening tests, parasite clearance after therapy should be verified to prevent recurrence (Gea-Banacloche et al. 2009). There are no data available to recommend iterative treatment to prevent reoccurrence although careful clinical and parasitological monitoring is recommended (Gea-Banacloche et al. 2009). This is particularly true for hematological conditions associated with HTLV-1 where decreasing treatment efficacy is observed. Indeed, the infection with HTLV-1 is associated with specific immune defects against *S. stercoralis*, and iterative treatments with different drugs regimens are often necessary (Carvalho and Da Fonseca 2004).

8.2.3 Leishmaniasis

Leishmaniasis comprises different clinical pictures of zoonotic diseases transmitted by the bites of sandflies. They have a worldwide geographical distribution in India, Africa, South-America, and the Mediterranean basin in Europe (Alvar et al. 2012). Leishmaniases are also very diverse both by their clinical presentation and the microorganism responsible (Alvar et al. 2012). One distinguishes cutaneous leishmaniasis, mucocutaneous leishmaniasis, and the visceral form. Although cutaneous and mucosal leishmaniasis have been reported in solid organ transplant, visceral leishmaniasis due to *Leishmania infantum* is the most reported clinical form in hematology (Ljungman et al. 2016). Infection with *L. infantum* is usually asymptomatic and, as for *Toxoplasma gondii*, living parasites could persist lifelong in immunocompetent hosts (Bogdan 2008). Therefore, the most probable explanation for leishmaniasis in hematology patients is reactivation of latent infection although primary infection by insect bites or by blood transfusion may occur, too.

Even in endemic countries with diagnostic capabilities, visceral leishmaniasis is rarely reported. A recent review has collected only 12 cases, 10 after allo-HSCT and 2 after autologous HSCT (Tatarelli et al. 2018). This seems strange if the hypothesis of persistent infection is true once the patient is infected because of the wide geographical distribution of the parasites (Alvar et al. 2012). One can hypothesize that some patients control the infection upon immune recovery to explain the rarity of the disease in endemic areas (Mouri et al. 2015). One can also consider the effect of frequent antifungal treatments in HM patients knowing that amphotericin B is very effective against the parasite (Meyerhoff 1999). The clinical presentation was fever with pancytopenia, and the diagnosis is based on examination of bone marrow aspirate (Tatarelli et al. 2018). Out of the 12 reported patients, 9 were diagnosed 12 weeks after HSCT, others until more than 4 years, showing that it is a late complication or that the diagnosis was not established earlier, although most of the patients lived or had traveled in endemic areas. More systematic use of qPCR with species identification in case of unexplained fever or engraftment failure in patients having lived in endemic areas should detect the parasite earlier, before the onset of full-blown disease (Foulet et al. 2007). The above 12 patients were treated with liposomal amphotericin B as recommended (Meyerhoff 1999), and out of 11 patients with known outcome, only two died. In case of unresponsiveness to liposomal amphotericin B, pentavalent antimony can be used (Morizot et al. 2016).

For possible preventive measures (Table 8.1), there is no anti-*Leishmania* antibody screening proposed, given the high prevalence of the population in endemic areas (Antinori et al. 2008), and there is no proposal of treating asymptomatic patients to eradicate the parasite (Meeting World Health Organization 2010). Only prevention of sandfly bites can be recommended to patients living or traveling to endemic areas (Pavli and Maltezou 2010).

8.3 Chagas Disease or American Trypanosomiasis

Trypanosoma cruzi is a hemoflagellate protozoan close to *Leishmania* spp. transmitted through dejections on skin of blood-sucking triatomine insects, also known as kissing bugs. Itching caused by the insect bites allows the transdermal inoculation of the parasite. Infection results in Chagas disease, regarded as a neglected tropical disease with sociocultural impacts (Pérez-Molina and Molina 2018). The initial phase of infection is (oligo-)symptomatic and usually resolves spontaneously within 8–12 weeks although severe acute myocarditis or meningoencephalitis can occur. In the chronic phase, the parasite can invade macrophages and different organs (heart, skin, and brain) and stay alive for 10–30 years or even lifelong (Pérez-Molina and Molina 2018). This chronic infection results in up to 30–40% of cases in several organ dysfunctions, dominated by cardiomegaly and megaesophagus (Pérez-Molina and Molina 2018). Sustained health programs have resulted in limitation of the geographical zone of the parasite (Pérez-Molina and Molina 2018). Beside the vector-borne transmission, the infection can also be acquired by contaminated blood transfusion and solid organ transplantation and, like toxoplasmosis, by maternal transmission during pregnancy (Forés et al. 2007; Pérez-Molina and Molina 2018). The transmission is limited to Central and South America, but immigration, first from rural to urban communities and from endemic to nonendemic countries, has led to an increase in Chagas disease reports in endemic and nonendemic countries in solid organ transplantation (Ison and Nalesnik 2011). The risk of Chagas disease through organ donation is well known and has led to specific recommendations (Pierrotti et al. 2018).

After HSCT, the risk of reactivation has been reported as high as 17–40% in Latin America (Altclas et al. 2005). However, very few cases occurred in nonendemic countries in patients from Latin America. One case has been documented in Italy in a 9-year-old Argentinian girl with acute myeloid leukemia after allo-HSCT (Angheben et al. 2012). The diagnosis was performed on microscopic visualization of the parasite on a blood smear 3 days before death (Angheben et al. 2012). A second case was reported in an adult from San Salvador who underwent auto-HSCT for myeloma in California (Guiang et al. 2013). The diagnosis of reactivation was ascertained by using PCR on blood (Guiang et al. 2013). In another adult patient from a rural area in Bolivia treated in Spain for Hodgkin lymphoma, the parasitic disease reactivated as confirmed by PCR (Pérez-Molina et al. 2015). This patient had been treated for chronic Chagas disease (benznidazole 5 mg/kg per day for 60 days) more than 1 year before chemotherapy for Hodgkin lymphoma. Thus, even in endemic countries such as Argentina, where donors and recipients have been tested for Chagas disease from the beginning of HSCT (Pinazo et al. 2011), there are surprisingly few reports on reactivation of Chagas disease after HSCT. Therefore, if preemptive therapy can be envisaged in endemic countries (Altclas et al. 2005), no such recommendations should be followed in nonendemic countries (Gea-Banacloche et al. 2009).

While diagnosis in the acute phase or in the full-blown disease after reactivation can be established by direct identification of the parasites in blood (blood smears or after concentration methods), in the chronic phase, diagnosis relies on the detection of circulating antibodies against *T. cruzi* (Pérez-Molina and Molina 2018). Low-level parasitemia should be better detected using qPCR for monitoring clinical reactivation and for treatment monitoring (Duffy et al. 2009). However, commercial ELISA tests have a better performance than qPCR for the diagnosis of the chronic phase (Brasil et al. 2010).

Only two drugs are licensed for treating Chagas disease, benznidazole and nifurtimox (Pérez-Molina and Molina 2018). While the need for treatment of the acute phase is consense (Pérez-Molina and Molina 2018), the treatment of the chronic phase has shown little benefit, if any, compared with placebo (Pérez-Molina et al. 2009).

In conclusion, history of donors and recipients born or ever lived for at least 6 months in endemic areas should be recorded and a serological test for anti-*T. cruzi* serum IgG antibody can be proposed (Table 8.1). After HSCT, in case of any doubt about reactivation, the most sensitive method for establishing the diagnosis should be a qPCR assay as proposed for solid organ transplant recipients (Pérez-Molina and Molina 2018).

8.4 Dormant Forms of *Plasmodium* Parasites

Plasmodium falciparum is by far the most common in tropical countries and associated with a high mortality in children. In contrast to *P. falciparum*, the other species *Plasmodium vivax*, *Plasmodium ovale*, and *Plasmodium malariae* can persist in humans for years either under a hypnozoite form for *P. vivax* and *P. ovale* or an unknown form for *P. malariae*. Therefore, after a unspecific febrile episode, the parasite remains quiescent in liver (*P. vivax* and *P. ovale*) or in an unknown location (*P. malariae*) and can be the source of late relapses up to 2 years for *P. vivax*, and possibly up to several decades for *P. malariae* (Vinetz et al. 1998).

Despite the number of people harboring *Plasmodium* spp., only two cases of *P. vivax* infection in the setting of HSCT have been reported (Raina et al. 1998; Inoue et al. 2010) and none for *P. malariae*. The risk of reactivation of a latent *Plasmodium* seems very low, and should not promote specific measures except careful history taking (Table 8.1). Upon suspicion, thin and thick blood films can be repeatedly done to exclude malaria. A sensitive qPCR can be added (Farrugia et al. 2011). If reactivation of latent *Plasmodium* seems rare, this is not the case for *Plasmodium* infection during hematological treatment which raises concerns about safety of blood products and derivatives where malaria is endemic (Gopal et al. 2012).

8.5 Parasitic Infections Acquired After Treatment of Hematological Malignancies

Given the immunosuppression acquired after treatment for hematological malignancy, the patients are more susceptible to any de novo infection and more specifically to some parasitic diseases. Among these parasites are the species able to reactivate latent infection but also to develop de novo infection such as the parasites described above. Knowing the mode of contamination, the best way to prevent them is avoid exposure as much as possible by following protective measures, most of them belonging to general hygiene, in particular, access to clean water and handwashing (Table 8.2), and chemotherapy for malaria. Unfortunately, while these preventive measures are easy to follow for travelers, because the duration of the journey is limited, these measures can be impracticable for people with low incomes in endemic countries.

For preventing toxoplasmosis, avoiding undercooked meat and washing salads before consumption are recommended (Gea-Banacloche et al. 2009). For strongyloidiasis, the recommendation is not to walk barefoot on soil in endemic areas possibly contaminated with human feces (Gea-Banacloche et al. 2009), and should be completed by avoidance of raw vegetables (Greaves et al. 2013). For leishmaniasis, the only way is to protect against sandfly bites using repellents and bed nets. For preventing Chagas disease, one should avoid dwellings with possible niches for vectors such as houses with mud walls or a thatched roof (Gea-Banacloche et al. 2009). Table 8.1 displays the main methods of diagnosis

Table 8.2 Parasitic infections acquired after treatment of hematological malignancies

Parasites	Prophylaxis	Main clinical forms	Lab diagnosis	Therapy
Cryptosporidium spp.	General hygiene, avoiding childcare while diarrheic, visit of farms, and swimming in public pools or recreational water pounds	Acute or chronic diarrhea	Stool smears microscopy with specific staining (auramine, Ziehl–Neelsen), qPCR	Azithromycin 500–1000 mg on day 1, then 250–1000 mg/d, nitazoxanide 1000 mg/d
Other intestinal protozoan parasites (*Blastocystis hominis, Cystoisospora belli, Cyclospora cayetanensis, Entamoeba* spp., *Giardia intestinalis*	General hygiene	Acute or chronic diarrhea	Stool microscopy, qPCR	Metronidazole 750–1500 mg/d or Cotrimoxazole (800/160) bid
Microsporidia (*Enterocytozoon bieneusi, Encephalitozoon* spp.)	Unknown	Diarrhea, disseminated infection	Stool smears and material from extraintestinal sites microscopy with specific staining (weber chrome, Calcofluor white), qPCR	*Encephalitozoon* spp.: Albendazole 800 mg/d
Babesia spp.	Avoiding woods where ticks and deer thrive	Fever and hemolytic anemia	Blood film microscopy, qPCR	Atovaquone 1500 mg/d plus azithromycin 500–1000 mg on day 1, then 250–1000 mg/d
Acanthamoeba spp.	General hygiene for lens wearers, avoiding swimming in recreational water pounds	Encephalitis, pneumonia, cutaneous, disseminated infection	Microscopy, histopathology, qPCR	Liposomal amphotericin B 5 mg/kg/d

qPCR, quantitative polymerase chain reaction

and treatment of these diseases. Of course, it is of utmost importance to avoid blood supplies possibly contaminated with *Plasmodium* spp. (Abdelkefi et al. 2004; Mejia et al. 2012), *Trypanosoma cruzi* (Forés et al. 2007), but also *Babesia* spp. (Tonnetti et al. 2019).

8.6 Intestinal Protozoa

There are several parasites causing diarrhea in hematological patients. Often, they are considered when other etiologies, viral or bacterial, have been excluded. More importantly, they have to be excluded when facing diarrhea in the context of intestinal graft-versus-host disease because the therapeutic attitude is radically different: increase versus decrease of immunosuppressive therapy (Müller et al. 2004; Legrand et al. 2011). These parasites have their own biology and treatment. They often warrant specific diagnostic methods, which can be realized only if they are specifically requested. The emergence of syndromic multiplex PCR assays designed for symptoms, here diarrhea, is probably revolutionizing diagnosis, once the issue of quantification can be solved (Van Lint et al. 2013). Indeed, detection of low nucleic acid loads may not be related to a specific disease. Thresholds of positivity will be probably necessary to initiate treatment in immunocompromised patients.

8.7 Cryptosporidiosis

Cryptosporidium is a protozoan parasite responsible for cryptosporidiosis, a leading cause of waterborne disease. Cryptosporidiosis results in self-limited diarrhea in immunocompetent hosts but can cause life-threatening wasting in immunocompromised individuals (Checkley et al. 2015). *Cryptosporidium* spp. belong to the coccidian taxon (as *Toxoplasma gondii*), and they multiply inside the enterocytes of the targeted host. Seventeen of the 40 species described have been found in humans (Feng et al. 2018). Their transmission is fecal–oral, and human contamination occurs after drinking contaminated water, or food, or after contact with infected individuals (children) or animals (calves). They are regularly mentioned in headlines because of the continuous observation of outbreaks (Gharpure et al. 2019). The success of this parasite is due to oocysts directly contaminating without the need of maturation in the environment, huge numbers of oocysts shed by an infected individual, a long period of at least 7 days of survival in the environment, and high tolerance to chlorine, the main agent used for obtaining safe drinkable water. The supply of the potable water (surface versus dwelling) is probably important to estimate the risk of contamination, knowing that surface waters are more easily contaminated with cattle manure (Checkley et al. 2015).

Cryptosporidiosis has been reported as case reports in the context of allo-HSCT (Manivel et al. 1985; Rio et al. 1986; Müller et al. 2004; Faraci et al. 2007; Schiller et al. 2018). More informative are the prospective studies on the incidence in this population. In a systematic follow-up of 52 patients with diarrhea after HSCT, 5 were found *Cryptosporidium* in a stool sample at a median of 503 days (range 20–790) post HSCT (Legrand et al. 2011). Diarrhea disappeared after 5 weeks of azithromycin and nitazoxanide combination treatment in three patients. The other two died of invasive fungal infection. The authors concluded on the need to improve surveillance and to conduct additional studies delineating the efficacy of treatment (Legrand et al. 2011). Indeed, in children undergoing HSCT for primary immune deficiency, some can harbor *Cryptosporidium* sp. during the follow-up of HSCT, whereas they remained asymptomatic (Davies et al. 2017). The authors concluded that asymptomatic carriage could be more common than currently believed (Davies et al. 2017).

Thus, cryptosporidiosis should be searched in all transplant recipients with acute or chronic diarrhea. The usual diagnostic means for cryptosporidiosis is the microscopic observation of oocysts after specific staining (auramine, Ziehl–Neelsen) of stools smears (Checkley et al. 2015). PCR assays are expected to be more sensitive, hence the issue of threshold raised above (Checkley et al. 2015). More specifically, qPCR can remain positive long after the microscopy has become negative (Fig. 8.1). Species identification

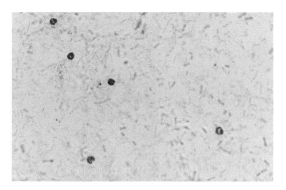

Fig. 8.1 Cryptosporidiosis in an 18-year-old man 15 days after allo-HSCT for acute lymphocytic leukemia receiving cyclosporine and methotrexate for graft-versus-host disease prevention. *Cryptosporidium* sp. (*Cryptosporidium cuniculus* upon DNA sequencing) appears as brilliant pink corpuscles (6–7 μm in diameter) with irregular content upon Ziehl–Neelsen staining of thin fecal smears. The patient was prescribed nitazoxanide 500 mg twice a day for 10 days. The diarrhea lasted 7 days. Subsequent fecal smears were microscopy positive after 30 days, then negative although qPCR remained positive for at least one additional month

and genotyping are mandatory for deciphering the possible routes of infection (Feng et al. 2018).

There is no indisputably effective treatment, except immunosuppression recovery. The most prescribed are azithromycin with or without nitazoxanide (licensed in this indication only in the United States) with no obvious parasitological clearance (Legrand et al. 2011; Davies et al. 2017). Hence, the importance of prevention includes avoidance of childcare while diarrheic, visit of farms, and swimming in public pools or recreational water pounds (Table 8.2). Of note, alcohol-based handwashing may not be sufficient to kill this resistant parasite when hands are dirty or greasy (https://www.cdc.gov/handwashing/index.html). Potentially contaminated surfaces should be cleaned with hydrogen peroxide (https://www.cdc.gov/parasites/crypto/childcare/outbreak.html).

8.8 Other Intestinal Protozoan Parasites

Beside *Cryptosporidium* spp., there are other coccidian parasites possibly pathogenic for humans. *Cyclospora cayetanensis* and *Cystoisospora belli* (previously *Isospora belli*) are more and more fre-

quently reported because of multiplication of travels abroad, in countries with unsafe drinking water (Giangaspero and Gasser 2019). There are also outbreaks traced to food sources (Legua and Seas 2013). There is no report of these common enteric pathogens in HSCT patients. One explanation might be the actual rarity of these parasites in hematology patients. Another explanation could be the efficiency of cotrimoxazole for treating *Cyclospora* and *Cystoisospora* (and administrated for other purposes in HM patients), which does not justify reporting in the literature.

Coccidian parasites are not the only intestinal protozoans associated with diarrhea. *Giardia intestinalis* (Ajumobi et al. 2014), *Entamoeba* spp., and *Blastocystis hominis* infections are frequent but easily amenable to metronidazole therapy (Table 8.2). They could be treated without warranting publication.

The diagnosis of these intestinal protozoans still relies on microscopy by skilled technicians and is more effective when specific requests are clearly notified by clinicians (Cama and Mathison 2015). The way multiplex PCR is changing this approach is currently unknown.

8.9 Microsporidiosis

Microsporidia are a group of unicellular parasites with a very specific biology, historically considered as parasite but now related to fungi, and with a major importance in veterinary medicine (Han and Weiss 2017). They are characterized by the presence of a polar tube, which allows entry into eukaryotic cells according to a mechanism completely different from the one used by protozoan parasites. Few species have been reported in humans: *Enterocytozoon bieneusi* is well documented in HIV-positive patients with low CD4 count and in solid organ—mainly kidney—recipients (Metge et al. 2000; Hocevar et al. 2014); and *Encephalitozoon* spp. are much less reported in humans. *Enterocytozoon bieneusi* is responsible for protracted wasting diarrhea but has not been reported in HSCT in the literature, although asymptomatic or paucisymptomatic cases are probable (Fig. 8.2). *Encephalitozoon* spp. are responsible for disseminated infections with

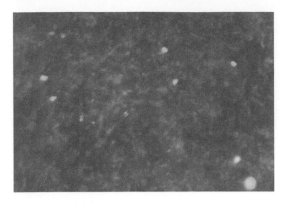

Fig. 8.2 Presence of *Enterocytozoon bieneusi* (identification confirmed by PCR) on a fecal smear (Calcofluor white staining) in a 56-year-old woman 15 days after allo-HSCT for myelodysplasia. The parasite appears as fluorescent blue bacilliform corpuscles (1 × 3 μm) due to the presence of chitin in the cell wall. The patient was receiving cyclosporine and methotrexate for graft-versus-host disease prevention. The diarrhea lasted only a few days. Subsequent fecal smears were microscopy negative, although the qPCR remained positive for 40 days reflecting a decreasing parasitic load. The patient did not receive specific therapy and died 3 months later of her underlying disease

microsporidia identified in respiratory specimens with very few cases reported in HSCT (Kelkar et al. 1997; Teachey et al. 2004; Orenstein et al. 2005; Meissner et al. 2012; Sıvgın et al. 2013).

Microsporidia cannot grow on usual media, and they are identified by microscopy using specific stains (Weber chrome, Calcofluor white). The precise identification of the species needs electron microscopy and DNA sequencing (Orenstein et al. 2005; Meissner et al. 2012).

Whereas *Enterocytozoon bieneusi* is not susceptible to albendazole (but to fumagillin), albendazole (400 mg twice daily) can be proposed to treat *Encephalitozoon* spp. There is no recommendation for the duration of the treatment. However, this treatment could not be evaluated in four of the five cases reported since the diagnosis was made at autopsy (Kelkar et al. 1997; Teachey et al. 2004; Orenstein et al. 2005; Meissner et al. 2012). The last case mentioned specifically hepatotoxicity due to albendazole, not to the microorganism (Sıvgın et al. 2013). In the absence of clear source of contamination, no prevention guidelines have been established (Table 8.2).

8.10 Babesiosis

Human babesiosis is caused by a protozoan parasite close to *Plasmodium* spp. for their morphology and the intraerythrocytic localization, although the vectors are not insects but ticks. The vast majority of cases in the United States are due to *Babesia microti*, transmitted by *Ixodes scapularis*, also called the deer tick, hence the expansion of deer advocated for explaining the increase of incidence in some northeastern states of the United States (Vannier and Krause 2012). *Babesia divergens* is rather reported in Europe and mainly in asplenic patients (Vannier and Krause 2012). However, babesiosis is present worldwide, and the diagnosis is probably underestimated in malaria-endemic countries because of diagnostic confusion (Vannier and Krause 2012).

There are very few cases reported in HSCT patients. The diagnosis was generally unexpected and made by systematic blood thin-film examination in patients with unexplained fever and a mild-to-moderate hemolytic anemia. The rare cases reported in HSCT were transfusion transmitted (Cirino et al. 2008; Bade and Yared 2016; LeBel et al. 2017). Another case occurred 3 years post allo-HSCT for CML and was suspected therefore to be acquired far after the HSCT procedure in a *Babesia*-endemic region of the United States (Lubin et al. 2011). If screening in endemic areas using qPCR develops, one can expect more diagnoses because of the higher sensitivity of qPCR over microscopic examination (Primus et al. 2018). Indeed, the issue is to improve the safety of blood transfusion in endemic areas (Tonnetti et al. 2019).

Due to the rarity of babesiosis in HSCT, no systematic guidelines can be provided. Only a careful history taking to know whether the patient had lived or traveled in endemic areas can increase the suspicion index. The history of tick bites is probably not relevant given their frequency. The most effective way to detect babesiosis remains a careful examination of blood films, which is the rule in hematology (Table 8.2).

The proposed treatment is a combination of atovaquone and azithromycin, a combination as effective as clindamycin and quinine but with less adverse effects. Immunocompromised patients are prone to relapse, and the treatment can require at least 4 weeks of therapy, plus 2 weeks after disappearance of the parasite on blood film. Preventive measures consist of avoiding woods where ticks and deer thrive (Vannier and Krause 2012).

8.11 Free-Living Amoebae

Free-living amoebae are ubiquitous in the environment and thrive in mud. They are also frequently present in tap water (but also bottled water) and air-conditioning systems (Thomas and Ashbolt 2011). They present as a dormant cyst stage or an active infective trophozoite stage. In contrast to their counterpart *Entamoeba histolytica*, they do not behave as human parasite (Król-Turmińska and Olender 2017). Several species are known to be responsible for central nervous system infections such as granulomatous amoebic encephalitis, and for acute eye infections, mainly in contact lens wearers (Król-Turmińska and Olender 2017).

There are very few cases reported in the setting of hematological diseases, all with *Acanthamoeba* spp. After inhalation, the most probable portal of entry along with damaged skin, the patients developed encephalitis (Anderlini et al. 1994; Feingold et al. 1998; Pemán et al. 2008; Kaul et al. 2008; Abd et al. 2009; Akpek et al. 2011; Epperla et al. 2016; Coven et al. 2017). All the patients died and mostly diagnosis was established by histopathological examination of infected tissues at autopsy only (Abd et al. 2009). There is also a description of cutaneous infection due to *Acanthamoeba castellanii* with secondary dissemination in a patient treated for lymphoma (Sells et al. 2016). The patient died 10 weeks later despite different consecutive treatment with azoles, clarithromycin, and liposomal amphotericin B (Sells et al. 2016). Interestingly, *Acanthamoeba* was identified in the humidifier of the continuous positive airway pressure device used for the patient, underlining the need of proper maintenance and cleaning procedures of equipment (Sells et al. 2016). Another case reported a successful treatment (liposomal amphotericin 5 mg/kg daily) of *Acanthamoeba* sinusitis in a child after allo-HSCT (Juan et al. 2016). Whether identification of *Acanthamoeba* in sinuses is frequent in children and whether this carriage can disappear after treatment is unknown. Obviously, prevalence studies on the carriage of free-living amoebae are necessary to understand the biology of these parasites, the risk of secondary invasion, and to propose preventive measures (Table 8.2).

8.12 Conclusion

The development of immunosuppressive therapy in hematology raises several concerns about the risk of parasitic infections. First, when diagnosed late, they are associated with high morbidity and mortality. Second, their diagnosis often is delayed, hence the poor prognosis cited above, because of the lack of sensitive and specific diagnostic tools but also because of the low suspicion index of clinicians. Third, several of them are known as case reports or small series only, precluding strong therapeutic recommendations, often transferred from other patient populations.

All these reasons underline the need to anticipate the diagnosis. To manage parasitic diseases, one must consider the phases before and after immunosuppressive therapy. Before treatment, the main risk is reactivation of latent parasites. A comprehensive reporting of travel and residency history, even remote, should be performed to maintain a high index of suspicion (Table 8.1). For the parasites for which no efficient treatment of the latent forms exists (*Toxoplasma gondii*, *Leishmania infantum*, *Trypanosoma cruzi*), the best way is to propose prophylaxis against the active forms (*Toxoplasma gondii*) or to adopt a qPCR-driven surveillance (*Toxoplasma gondii*, *Leishmania* spp., *Trypanosoma cruzi*), or simply ask for specific research on blood in any doubt (*Plasmodium vivax*, *Babesia* spp.).

After immunosuppressive therapy and until immune defense recovery, the best way to prevent infection is by protective measures intervening with contamination routes of parasites. This can be included in travel counseling for patients who absolutely want to go to tropical endemic areas. One should reassure comprehension of risks and adherence to preventive measures. For patients originating from these endemic areas, the best is to screen and treat before starting any immunosuppressive therapy (Sánchez-Montalvá et al. 2016). However, some parasites are acquired in temperate climates, such as *Toxoplasma gondii, Leishmania infantum, Trypanosoma cruzi, Babesia* spp., or free-living amoebae. Each of these parasites requires specific prevention according to their respective biology (Tables 8.1 and 8.2).

Acknowledgments The authors thank Dr. Samia Hamane (Saint Louis Hospital Parasitology and Mycology Laboratory) for providing photography of *Cryptosporidium* sp. and *Enterocytozoon bieneusi* of allo-HSCT patients.

References

Abd H, Saeed A, Jalal S et al (2009) Ante mortem diagnosis of amoebic encephalitis in a haematopoietic stem cell transplanted patient. Scand J Infect Dis 41:619–622. https://doi.org/10.1080/00365540903015117

Abdelkefi A, Ben Othman T, Torjman L et al (2004) Plasmodium falciparum causing hemophagocytic syndrome after allogeneic blood stem cell transplantation. Hematol J 5:449–450. https://doi.org/10.1038/sj.thj.6200531

Ajumobi AB, Daniels JA, Sostre CF, Trevino HH (2014) Giardiasis in a hematopoietic stem cell transplant patient. Transpl Infect Dis 16:984–987. https://doi.org/10.1111/tid.12272

Akpek G, Uslu A, Huebner T et al (2011) Granulomatous amebic encephalitis: an under-recognized cause of infectious mortality after hematopoietic stem cell transplantation. Transpl Infect Dis 13:366–373. https://doi.org/10.1111/j.1399-3062.2011.00612.x

Alpern JD, Arbefeville SS, Vercellotti G et al (2017) Strongyloides hyperinfection following hematopoietic stem cell transplant in a patient with HTLV-1-associated T-cell leukemia. Transpl Infect Dis 19:e12638. https://doi.org/10.1111/tid.12638

Altclas J, Sinagra A, Dictar M et al (2005) Chagas disease in bone marrow transplantation: an approach to preemptive therapy. Bone Marrow Transplant 36:123–129. https://doi.org/10.1038/sj.bmt.1705006

Alvar J, Vélez ID, Bern C et al (2012) Leishmaniasis worldwide and global estimates of its incidence. PLoS One 7:e35671. https://doi.org/10.1371/journal.pone.0035671

Anderlini P, Przepiorka D, Luna M et al (1994) Acanthamoeba meningoencephalitis after bone marrow transplantation. Bone Marrow Transplant 14:459–461

Angheben A, Giaconi E, Menconi M et al (2012) Reactivation of Chagas disease after a bone marrow transplant in Italy: first case report. Blood Transfus 10:542–544. https://doi.org/10.2450/2012.0015-12

Antinori S, Cascio A, Parravicini C et al (2008) Leishmaniasis among organ transplant recipients. Lancet Infect Dis 8:191–199. https://doi.org/10.1016/S1473-3099(08)70043-4

Bade NA, Yared JA (2016) Unexpected babesiosis in a patient with worsening anemia after allogeneic hematopoietic stem cell transplantation. Blood 128:1019–1019. https://doi.org/10.1182/blood-2016-05-717900

Bogdan C (2008) Mechanisms and consequences of persistence of intracellular pathogens: leishmaniasis as an example. Cell Microbiol 10:1221–1234. https://doi.org/10.1111/j.1462-5822.2008.01146.x

Brasil PEAA, De Castro L, Hasslocher-Moreno AM et al (2010) ELISA versus PCR for diagnosis of chronic Chagas disease: systematic review and meta-analysis. BMC Infect Dis 10:337. https://doi.org/10.1186/1471-2334-10-337

Bretagne S, Costa JM, Foulet F et al (2000) Prospective study of toxoplasma reactivation by polymerase chain reaction in allogeneic stem-cell transplant recipients. Transpl Infect Dis 2:127–132

Cama VA, Mathison BA (2015) Infections by intestinal Coccidia and Giardia duodenalis. Clin Lab Med 35:423–444. https://doi.org/10.1016/j.cll.2015.02.010

Carvalho EM, Da Fonseca PA (2004) Epidemiological and clinical interaction between HTLV-1 and Strongyloides stercoralis. Parasite Immunol 26:487–497. https://doi.org/10.1111/j.0141-9838.2004.00726.x

Checkley W, White AC, Jaganath D et al (2015) A review of the global burden, novel diagnostics, therapeutics, and vaccine targets for cryptosporidium. Lancet Infect Dis 15:85–94. https://doi.org/10.1016/S1473-3099(14)70772-8

Cirino CM, Leitman SF, Williams E et al (2008) Transfusion-associated babesiosis with an atypical time course after nonmyeloablative transplantation for sickle cell disease. Ann Intern Med 148:794–795. https://doi.org/10.7326/0003-4819-148-10-200805200-00018

Conrad A, Le Maréchal M, Dupont D et al (2016) A matched case-control study of toxoplasmosis after allogeneic haematopoietic stem cell transplantation: still a devastating complication. Clin Microbiol Infect 22:636–641. https://doi.org/10.1016/j.cmi.2016.04.025

Cook AJ, Gilbert RE, Buffolano W et al (2000) Sources of toxoplasma infection in pregnant women: European multicentre case-control study. European Research Network on Congenital Toxoplasmosis. BMJ 321:142–147

Costa JM, Pautas C, Ernault P et al (2000) Real-time PCR for diagnosis and follow-up of toxoplasma reactivation after allogeneic stem cell transplantation using fluorescence resonance energy transfer hybridization probes. J Clin Microbiol 38:2929–2932

Coven SL, Song E, Steward S et al (2017) Acanthamoeba granulomatous amoebic encephalitis after pediatric hematopoietic stem cell transplant. Pediatr Transplant 21:e13060. https://doi.org/10.1111/petr.13060

Davies AP, Slatter M, Gennery AR et al (2017) Prevalence of Cryptosporidium carriage and disease in children with primary immune deficiencies undergoing hematopoietic stem cell transplant in northern Europe. Pediatr Infect Dis J 36:504–506. https://doi.org/10.1097/INF.0000000000001517

Decembrino N, Comelli A, Genco F et al (2017) Toxoplasmosis disease in paediatric hematopoietic stem cell transplantation: do not forget it still exists. Bone Marrow Transplant 52:1326–1329. https://doi.org/10.1038/bmt.2017.117

Duffy T, Bisio M, Altcheh J et al (2009) Accurate real-time PCR strategy for monitoring bloodstream parasitic loads in Chagas disease patients. PLoS Negl Trop Dis 3:e419. https://doi.org/10.1371/journal.pntd.0000419

Epperla N, Olteanu H, Hamadani M (2016) Think outside the box: Acanthamoeba encephalitis following autologous haematopoietic stem cell transplantation. Br J Haematol 175:758–758. https://doi.org/10.1111/bjh.14329

Fabiani S, Fortunato S, Petrini M, Bruschi F (2017) Allogeneic hematopoietic stem cell transplant recipients and parasitic diseases: a review of the literature of clinical cases and perspectives to screen and follow-up active and latent chronic infections. Transpl Infect Dis 19:e12669. https://doi.org/10.1111/tid.12669

Faraci M, Cappelli B, Morreale G et al (2007) Nitazoxanide or CD3+/CD4+ lymphocytes for recovery from severe Cryptosporidium infection after allogeneic bone marrow transplant? Pediatr Transplant 11:113–116. https://doi.org/10.1111/j.1399-3046.2006.00622.x

Farrugia C, Cabaret O, Botterel F et al (2011) Cytochrome b gene quantitative PCR for diagnosing Plasmodium falciparum infection in travelers. J Clin Microbiol 49:2191–2195. https://doi.org/10.1128/JCM.02156-10

Feingold JM, Abraham J, Bilgrami S et al (1998) Acanthamoeba meningoencephalitis following autologous peripheral stem cell transplantation. Bone Marrow Transplant 22:297–300. https://doi.org/10.1038/sj.bmt.1701320

Feng Y, Ryan UM, Xiao L (2018) Genetic diversity and population structure of Cryptosporidium. Trends Parasitol 34:997–1011. https://doi.org/10.1016/j.pt.2018.07.009

Forés R, Sanjuán I, Portero F et al (2007) Chagas disease in a recipient of cord blood transplantation. Bone Marrow Transplant 39:127–128. https://doi.org/10.1038/sj.bmt.1705551

Foulet F, Botterel F, Buffet P et al (2007) Detection and identification of Leishmania species from clinical specimens by using a real-time PCR assay and sequencing of the cytochrome B gene. J Clin Microbiol 45:2110–2115. https://doi.org/10.1128/JCM.02555-06

Gajurel K, Dhakal R, Montoya JG (2015) Toxoplasma prophylaxis in haematopoietic cell transplant recipients: a review of the literature and recommendations. Curr Opin Infect Dis 28:283–292. https://doi.org/10.1097/QCO.0000000000000169

Gea-Banacloche J, Masur H, Arns da Cunha C et al (2009) Regionally limited or rare infections: prevention after hematopoietic cell transplantation. Bone Marrow Transplant 44:489–494

Gharpure R, Perez A, Miller AD et al (2019) Cryptosporidiosis outbreaks - United States, 2009-2017. MMWR Morb Mortal Wkly Rep 68:568–572. https://doi.org/10.15585/mmwr.mm6825a3

Giangaspero A, Gasser RB (2019) Human cyclosporiasis. Lancet Infect Dis 19:e226–e236. https://doi.org/10.1016/S1473-3099(18)30789-8

Gómez-Junyent J, Paredes D, Hurtado JC et al (2018) High seroprevalence of Strongyloides stercoralis among individuals from endemic areas considered for solid organ transplant donation: a retrospective serum-bank based study. PLoS Negl Trop Dis 12:e0007010. https://doi.org/10.1371/journal.pntd.0007010

Gopal S, Wood WA, Lee SJ et al (2012) Meeting the challenge of hematologic malignancies in sub-Saharan Africa. Blood 119:5078–5087. https://doi.org/10.1182/blood-2012-02-387092

Greaves D, Coggle S, Pollard C et al (2013) Strongyloides stercoralis infection. BMJ 347:f4610–f4610. https://doi.org/10.1136/bmj.f4610

Guiang KMU, Cantey P, Montgomery SP et al (2013) Reactivation of Chagas disease in a bone marrow transplant patient: case report and review of screening and management. Transpl Infect Dis 15:E264–E267. https://doi.org/10.1111/tid.12157

Guigue N, Léon L, Hamane S et al (2018) Continuous decline of toxoplasma gondii Seroprevalence in hospital: a 1997-2014 longitudinal study in Paris, France. Front Microbiol 9:2369. https://doi.org/10.3389/fmicb.2018.02369

Han B, Weiss LM (2017) Microsporidia: obligate intracellular pathogens within the fungal kingdom. Microbiol Spectr 5:97–113. https://doi.org/10.1128/microbiolspec.FUNK-0018-2016

Henriquez-Camacho C, Gotuzzo E, Echevarria J et al (2016) Ivermectin versus albendazole or thiabendazole for Strongyloides stercoralis infection. Cochrane Database Syst Rev 2:CD007745. https://doi.org/10.1002/14651858.CD007745.pub3

Hocevar SN, Paddock CD, Spak CW et al (2014) Microsporidiosis acquired through solid organ transplantation: a public health investigation. Ann Intern Med 160:213–220. https://doi.org/10.7326/M13-2226

Inoue J, Machado CM, Lima GFM d C et al (2010) The monitoring of hematopoietic stem cell transplant donors and recipients from endemic areas for malaria. Rev Inst Med Trop Sao Paulo 52:281–284. https://doi.org/10.1590/s0036-46652010000500012

Ison MG, Nalesnik MA (2011) An update on donor-derived disease transmission in organ transplantation. Am J Transplant 11:1123–1130. https://doi.org/10.1111/j.1600-6143.2011.03493.x

Juan A, Alonso L, Olivé T et al (2016) Successful treatment of sinusitis by Acanthamoeba in a pediatric patient after allogeneic stem cell transplantation. Pediatr Infect Dis J 35:1350–1351. https://doi.org/10.1097/INF.0000000000001329

Kaul DR, Lowe L, Visvesvara GS et al (2008) Acanthamoeba infection in a patient with chronic graft-versus-host disease occurring during treatment with voriconazole. Transpl Infect Dis 10:437–441. https://doi.org/10.1111/j.1399-3062.2008.00335.x

Keiser PB, Nutman TB (2004) Strongyloides stercoralis in the immunocompromised population. Clin Microbiol Rev 17:208–217. https://doi.org/10.1128/cmr.17.1.208-217.2004

Kelkar R, Sastry PS, Kulkarni SS et al (1997) Pulmonary microsporidial infection in a patient with CML undergoing allogeneic marrow transplant. Bone Marrow Transplant 19:179–182. https://doi.org/10.1038/sj.bmt.1700536

Król-Turmińska K, Olender A (2017) Human infections caused by free-living amoebae. Ann Agric Environ Med 24:254–260. https://doi.org/10.5604/12321966.1233568

LeBel DP, Moritz ED, O'Brien JJ et al (2017) Cases of transfusion-transmitted babesiosis occurring in non-endemic areas: a diagnostic dilemma. Transfusion 57:2348–2354. https://doi.org/10.1111/trf.14246

Legrand F, Grenouillet F, Larosa F et al (2011) Diagnosis and treatment of digestive cryptosporidiosis in allogeneic haematopoietic stem cell transplant recipients: a prospective single Centre study. Bone Marrow Transplant 46:858–862. https://doi.org/10.1038/bmt.2010.200

Legua P, Seas C (2013) Cystoisospora and cyclospora. Curr Opin Infect Dis 26:479–483. https://doi.org/10.1097/01.qco.0000433320.90241.60

Levenhagen MA, Costa-Cruz JM (2014) Update on immunologic and molecular diagnosis of human strongyloidiasis. Acta Trop 135:33–43. https://doi.org/10.1016/j.actatropica.2014.03.015

Ljungman P, Snydman D, Boeckh M (2016) Transplant infections. Springer, Cham

Lubin AS, Snydman DR, Miller KB (2011) Persistent babesiosis in a stem cell transplant recipient. Leuk Res 35:e77–e78. https://doi.org/10.1016/j.leukres.2010.11.029

Luvira V, Watthanakulpanich D, Pittisuttithum P (2014) Management of Strongyloides stercoralis: a puzzling parasite. Int Health 6:273–281. https://doi.org/10.1093/inthealth/ihu058

Malki Al MM, Song JY (2016) Strongyloides hyperinfection syndrome following haematopoietic stem cell transplantation. Br J Haematol 172:496–496. https://doi.org/10.1111/bjh.13814

Manivel C, Filipovich A, Snover DC (1985) Cryptosporidiosis as a cause of diarrhea following bone marrow transplantation. Dis Colon Rectum 28:741–742

Mansfield LS, Niamatali S, Bhopale V et al (1996) Strongyloides stercoralis: maintenance of exceedingly chronic infections. Am J Trop Med Hyg 55:617–624. https://doi.org/10.4269/ajtmh.1996.55.617

Martino R, Maertens J, Bretagne S et al (2000) Toxoplasmosis after hematopoietic stem cell transplantation. Clin Infect Dis 31:1188–1195. https://doi.org/10.1086/317471

Martino R, Bretagne S, Einsele H et al (2005) Early detection of toxoplasma infection by molecular monitoring of toxoplasma gondii in peripheral blood samples after allogeneic stem cell transplantation. Clin Infect Dis 40:67–78. https://doi.org/10.1086/426447

Meeting WECOTCOTL, World Health Organization (2010) Control of the Leishmaniases (2010) Report of a meeting of the WHO Expert Committee on the Control of Leishmaniases, Geneva, 22–26 March 2010. WHO technical report series 949 (2010). WHO, Geneva

Meissner EG, Bennett JE, Qvarnstrom Y et al (2012) Disseminated microsporidiosis in an immunosuppressed patient. Emerging Infect Dis 18:1155–1158. https://doi.org/10.3201/eid1807.120047

Mejia R, Booth GS, Fedorko DP et al (2012) Peripheral blood stem cell transplant-related Plasmodium falciparum infection in a patient with sickle cell disease. Transfusion 52:2677–2682. https://doi.org/10.1111/j.1537-2995.2012.03673.x

Metge S, Van Nhieu JT, Dahmane D et al (2000) A case of Enterocytozoon bieneusi infection in an HIV-negative renal transplant recipient. Eur J Clin Microbiol Infect Dis 19:221–223

Meyerhoff A (1999) U.S. Food and Drug Administration approval of AmBisome (liposomal amphotericin B) for treatment of visceral leishmaniasis. Clin Infect Dis 28:42–48. discussion 49–51. https://doi.org/10.1086/515085

Morizot G, Jouffroy R, Faye A et al (2016) Antimony to cure visceral Leishmaniasis unresponsive to liposomal amphotericin B. PLoS Negl Trop Dis 10:e0004304. https://doi.org/10.1371/journal.pntd.0004304

Mouri O, Benhamou M, Leroux G et al (2015) Spontaneous remission of fully symptomatic visceral leishmaniasis. BMC Infect Dis 15:445. https://doi.org/10.1186/s12879-015-1191-6

Müller CI, Zeiser R, Grüllich C et al (2004) Intestinal cryptosporidiosis mimicking acute graft-versus-host disease following matched unrelated hematopoietic stem cell transplantation. Transplantation 77:1478–1479

Nutman TB (2017) Human infection with Strongyloides stercoralis and other related Strongyloides species. Parasitology 144:263–273. https://doi.org/10.1017/S0031182016000834

Orenstein JM, Russo P, Didier ES et al (2005) Fatal pulmonary microsporidiosis due to encephalitozoon cuniculi following allogeneic bone marrow transplantation for acute myelogenous leukemia. Ultrastruct Pathol 29:269–276. https://doi.org/10.1080/01913120590951257

Pappas G, Roussos N, Falagas ME (2009) Toxoplasmosis snapshots: global status of toxoplasma gondii seroprevalence and implications for pregnancy and congenital toxoplasmosis. Int J Parasitol 39:1385–1394. https://doi.org/10.1016/j.ijpara.2009.04.003

Pavli A, Maltezou HC (2010) Leishmaniasis, an emerging infection in travelers. Int J Infect Dis 14:e1032–e1039. https://doi.org/10.1016/j.ijid.2010.06.019

Pemán J, Jarque I, Frasquet J et al (2008) Unexpected postmortem diagnosis of Acanthamoeba meningoencephalitis following allogeneic peripheral blood stem cell transplantation. Am J Transplant 8:1562–1566. https://doi.org/10.1111/j.1600-6143.2008.02270.x

Pérez-Molina JA, Molina I (2018) Chagas disease. Lancet 391:82–94. https://doi.org/10.1016/S0140-6736(17)31612-4

Pérez-Molina JA, Pérez-Ayala A, Moreno S et al (2009) Use of benznidazole to treat chronic Chagas' disease: a systematic review with a meta-analysis. J Antimicrob Chemother 64:1139–1147. https://doi.org/10.1093/jac/dkp357

Pérez-Molina JA, Perez AM, Norman FF et al (2015) Old and new challenges in Chagas disease. Lancet Infect Dis 15:1347–1356. https://doi.org/10.1016/S1473-3099(15)00243-1

Pierrotti LC, Carvalho NB, Amorin JP et al (2018) Chagas disease recommendations for solid-organ transplant recipients and donors. Transplantation 102:S1–S7. https://doi.org/10.1097/TP.0000000000002019

Pinazo M-J, Miranda B, Rodríguez-Villar C et al (2011) Recommendations for management of Chagas disease in organ and hematopoietic tissue transplantation programs in nonendemic areas. Transplant Rev (Orlando) 25:91–101

Prendki V, Fenaux P, Durand R et al (2011) Strongyloidiasis in man 75 years after initial exposure. Emerging Infect Dis 17:931–932. https://doi.org/10.3201/eid1705.100490

Primus S, Akoolo L, Schlachter S et al (2018) Efficient detection of symptomatic and asymptomatic patient samples for Babesia microti and Borrelia burgdorferi infection by multiplex qPCR. PLoS One 13:e0196748. https://doi.org/10.1371/journal.pone.0196748

Raina V, Sharma A, Gujral S, Kumar R (1998) Plasmodium vivax causing pancytopenia after allogeneic blood stem cell transplantation in CML. Bone Marrow Transplant 22:205–206. https://doi.org/10.1038/sj.bmt.1701299

Rio B, Le Tourneau A, Sobahni I et al (1986) Cryptosporidiosis in grafting of allogeneic bone marrow. Presse Med 15:1414–1416

Sánchez-Montalvá A, Salvador F, Ruiz-Camps I et al (2016) Imported disease screening prior to chemotherapy and bone marrow transplantation for Oncohematological malignancies. Am J Trop Med Hyg 95:1463–1468. https://doi.org/10.4269/ajtmh.16-0458

Schär F, Trostdorf U, Giardina F et al (2013) Strongyloides stercoralis: global distribution and risk factors. PLoS Negl Trop Dis 7:e2288. https://doi.org/10.1371/journal.pntd.0002288

Schiller J, Klein S, Engels M et al (2018) Case report: a Cryptosporidium infection in a patient with relapsed T-lymphoblastic lymphoma undergoing allogeneic stem cell transplantation. Eur J Haematol 100:383–385. https://doi.org/10.1111/ejh.12998

Sells RF, Chen CA, Wong MT et al (2016) Continuous positive airway pressure-associated cutaneous amoebiasis in an immunosuppressed patient. Br J Dermatol 174:625–628. https://doi.org/10.1111/bjd.14231

Sıvgın S, Eser B, Kaynar L et al (2013) Encephalitozoon intestinalis: a rare cause of diarrhea in an allogeneic hematopoietic stem cell transplantation (HSCT) recipient complicated by Albendazole-related hepatotoxicity. Turk J Haematol 30:204–208. https://doi.org/10.4274/Tjh.90692

Tatarelli P, Fornaro G, Del Bono V et al (2018) Visceral leishmaniasis in hematopoietic cell transplantation: case report and review of the literature. J Infect Chemother 24:990–994. https://doi.org/10.1016/j.jiac.2018.05.008

Teachey DT, Russo P, Orenstein JM et al (2004) Pulmonary infection with microsporidia after allogeneic bone marrow transplantation. Bone Marrow Transplant 33:299–302. https://doi.org/10.1038/sj.bmt.1704327

Thomas JM, Ashbolt NJ (2011) Do free-living amoebae in treated drinking water systems present an emerging health risk? Environ Sci Technol 45:860–869. https://doi.org/10.1021/es102876y

Tonnetti L, Townsend RL, Dodd RY, Stramer SL (2019) Characteristics of transfusion-transmitted Babesia microti, American red Cross 2010-2017. Transfusion 67:496. https://doi.org/10.1111/trf.15425

Ullmann AJ, Schmidt-Hieber M, Bertz H et al (2016) Infectious diseases in allogeneic haematopoietic stem cell transplantation: prevention and prophylaxis strategy guidelines 2016. Ann Hematol 95:1435–1455. https://doi.org/10.1007/s00277-016-2711-1

Van Lint P, Rossen JW, Vermeiren S et al (2013) Detection of Giardia lamblia, Cryptosporidium spp. and Entamoeba histolytica in clinical stool samples by using multiplex real-time PCR after automated DNA isolation. Acta Clin Belg 68:188–192. https://doi.org/10.2143/ACB.3170

Vannier E, Krause PJ (2012) Human babesiosis. N Engl J Med 366:2397–2407. https://doi.org/10.1056/NEJMra1202018

Varughese T, Taur Y, Cohen N et al (2018) Serious infections in patients receiving Ibrutinib for treatment of lymphoid Cancer. Clin Infect Dis 67:687–692. https://doi.org/10.1093/cid/ciy175

Vinetz JM, Li J, McCutchan TF, Kaslow DC (1998) Plasmodium malariae infection in an asymptomatic 74-year-old Greek woman with splenomegaly. N Engl J Med 338:367–371. https://doi.org/10.1056/NEJM199802053380605

Wirk B, Wingard JR (2009) Strongyloides stercoralis hyperinfection in hematopoietic stem cell transplantation. Transpl Infect Dis 11:143–148. https://doi.org/10.1111/j.1399-3062.2008.00360.x

Zeehaida M, Zairi NZ, Rahmah N et al (2011) Strongyloides stercoralis in common vegetables and herbs in Kota Bharu, Kelantan, Malaysia. Trop Biomed 28:188–193

Antimicrobial Stewardship

9

Patricia Muñoz and Ana Fernández-Cruz

9.1   Introduction

Antimicrobial stewardship programs are becoming more common, but the experience specifically in hematologic neutropenic patients is scarce. Concerns about poor outcomes due to immune deficiency, and lack of specific data have prevented so far a comprehensive implementation of antimicrobial stewardship in this population. Neutropenia is the most important risk factor for infection and the most frequent reason for broad-spectrum antimicrobial long-term use in hematologic malignancy patients. Infections caused by multidrug-resistant (MDR) microorganisms are a relevant issue in this scenario. In the ever-growing emergence of multidrug-resistant microorganisms which hampers the early administration of targeted small spectrum therapy, antimicrobial stewardship is becoming an urgent necessity. Limited but increasing favorable data show that application of antimicrobial stewardship principles to immunocompromised hosts is feasible.

Antimicrobial stewardship is a term that does not have an exact equivalent in many languages, and may be understood as "responsible use of antibiotics." A current broad definition of antimicrobial stewardship is the one provided by Dyar et al. "Antimicrobial stewardship is a coherent set of actions which promote using antimicrobials in ways that ensure sustainable access to effective therapy for all who need them" (Dyar et al. 2017; Barlam et al. 2016). This definition encompasses both the individual and the social perspective of rational use of antimicrobials. Its aim is to optimize antimicrobial use so that the need of an individual to get the best possible antimicrobial is balanced to the preservation of active antimicrobials for all who need them.

The alarming increase in resistance to antimicrobials has led to the development of antimicrobial stewardship in an effort to prevent and control this epidemic. As stated by the ESGAP (European Study Group for Antimicrobial Stewardship) in their "Mission and Objectives," the link between antibiotic use and resistance is

P. Muñoz (✉)
Clinical Microbiology and Infectious Diseases Department, Hospital General Universitario Gregorio Marañón, Universidad Complutense de Madrid, Madrid, Spain

Instituto de Investigación Sanitaria del Hospital Gregorio Marañón, Madrid, Spain

Medicine Department, School of Medicine, Universidad Complutense de Madrid, Madrid, Spain

CIBER de Enfermedades Respiratorias (CIBERES CB06/06/0058), Madrid, Spain
e-mail: pmunoz@hggm.es

A. Fernández-Cruz (✉)
Infectious Diseases Unit, Internal Medicine Department, Hospital Universitario Puerta de Hierro-Majadahonda, Madrid, Spain

Instituto de Investigación Sanitaria Puerta de Hierro - Segovia de Arana, Madrid, Spain

© Springer Nature Switzerland AG 2021
O. A. Cornely, M. Hoenigl (eds.), *Infection Management in Hematology*, Hematologic Malignancies, https://doi.org/10.1007/978-3-030-57317-1_9

clear and reversal of resistance problems is often feasible by changing the patterns of antibiotic use.

In the last 5 years, the rise of citations of antimicrobial stewardship has been exponential. The term was first used in 1996, the first guidelines to include recommendations on antimicrobial stewardship appeared in 1997 (Shlaes et al. 1997) and the ESGAP (former European Study Group for Antibiotic Policies) gained official recognition from the ESCMID Executive Committee in 1999. From then on, programs on antimicrobial stewardship have been progressively implemented in hospitals, and outgrowing to the regional and national level. Intertwined with antimicrobial stewardship are Infection Control and Public Health, but differ in that antimicrobial stewardship concerns specifically how antimicrobials are used, while infection control is aimed to limit the spread of resistant microorganisms. Coordinated efforts between both are essential for curbing emergence and dissemination of multidrug-resistant (MDR) microorganisms (Viale et al. 2015).

Hospital administration must ensure that an antimicrobial stewardship program (AMS) is developed and implemented by means of providing dedicated resources. The antimicrobial stewardship team should be integrated within the hospital's quality improvement and patient safety structure and have clearly defined links with the drug and therapeutics committee and infection prevention and control committee. Multidisciplinary antimicrobial stewardship teams are usually led by specialists in Infectious Diseases or Clinical Microbiology together with pharmacists, and ideally include also prescribers, administrators, infection control experts, and information systems experts. Team members should effectively and measurably optimize antimicrobial use by using interventions customized to fit the institution; the process and outcome indicators of antimicrobial stewardship should be measured and reported to the hospital executive (http://esgap.escmid.org).

AMS have been successful in different categories of patient populations (Timbrook et al. 2016; Katsios et al. 2012). Regarding immunocompro-

mised hosts such as hematologic patients, concerns about poor outcomes due to immune deficiency and lack of specific data have so far prevented a comprehensive implementation of antimicrobial stewardship in this population. However, infections caused by MDR microorganisms are a relevant and increasing issue in this scenario (Baker and Satlin 2016; Bow 2013), and antimicrobial stewardship is becoming an urgent necessity. Limited but increasing favorable data show that the application of antimicrobial stewardship principles to immunocompromised hosts is feasible (Rosa et al. 2014; Robilotti et al. 2017; Madran et al. 2017; Hennig et al. 2018; Ruiz-Ramos et al. 2017; Snyder et al. 2017; Aguilar-Guisado et al. 2017; Abbo and Ariza-Heredia 2014; Gustinetti et al. 2018).

9.1.1 Rationale

9.1.1.1 Antibiotic Stewardship

The collateral damage of broad-spectrum antibiotic use is the selection of resistant bacterial strains, including *Clostridium difficile* (CD) (Gyssens et al. 2013), in addition to potential toxicity, drug–drug interactions, and potential adverse events.

Hematologic malignancy patients are more at risk of acquiring resistant microorganisms because of the need for repeated courses of often empiric broad-spectrum antibiotics due to consecutive episodes of febrile neutropenia (FN) induced by chemotherapy (Gyssens et al. 2013) and also the use of prophylactic antibiotics. Besides, inappropriate antibiotic therapy is more common in infections caused by resistant bacteria in the consequences of inappropriate therapy, are even more severe in these immunosuppressed hosts.

A recent prospective intercontinental study in hematopoietic stem cell transplantation (HSCT) patients (Averbuch et al. 2017) showed a prevalence of 32% MDR among Gram-negative bacilli from bacteremias. Resistance rates were higher in centers providing fluoroquinolone prophylaxis; likewise, in another study, independent risk factors for the acquisition of MDR pathogens in hematologic malignancy patients were prior antibiotic exposure and urinary catheterization (Gudiol et al. 2011). The possible benefits of fluoroquinolones prophylaxis should be weighed against its impact in terms of changes in local ecology, according to the ECIL (European Conference on Infections in Leukemia) critical appraisal of previous guidelines (Mikulska et al. 2018).

In an Italian study, carbapenem-resistant *Klebsiella pneumoniae* colonization was identified in 1% of autologous hematopoietic stem cell transplantation (HSCT) recipients and 2.4% of allogeneic HSCT recipients (Girmenia et al. 2015). According to Cattaneo et al. (Cattaneo et al. 2018), MDR rectal colonization occurs in 6.5% of hematologic inpatients and predicts a 16% probability of MDR-related BSI (bloodstream infection), particularly during neutropenia, as well as a higher probability of unfavorable outcomes in catheter-related BSIs.

Cephalosporins, quinolones, and carbapenems have been associated with ESBL (extended-spectrum beta-lactamase) producing enterobacteriaceae, MDR *Pseudomonas*, and are among the antibiotics with a highest risk for CD (Rodriguez-Baño et al. 2012). Therefore, one of the courses of action of AMS programs is the selection of antibiotics that do not promote the emergence of MDR microorganisms. Moreover, number and duration of prior antibiotics are also risk factors for CD infection. The increase of MDR infections mandates the use of empirical broad-spectrum antibiotics such as carbapenems, oftentimes without any alternative for de-escalation, or without microbiological documentation that provides support for subsequent shift to targeted antibiotics (as bacteriological documentation of the infection in febrile neutropenia is usually obtained in less than 50% of episodes (Le Clech et al. 2018)). In a setting with high rates of resistance, "carbapenem-sparing" regimens are difficult to implement (Viale et al. 2015).

The de-escalation strategy recommended by ECIL-4 guidelines suggests the best possible coverage of resistant pathogens at the onset of infection, followed by subsequent reduction of antibiotic spectrum, if no resistant bacteria are isolated (Averbuch et al. 2013). Furthermore, there is a need for alternatives for treating increasingly resistant microorganisms. The shortage of effective antibiotics is especially alarming in Gram-negative infections. While new antibiotics are developed, some old antibiotics such as Fosfomycin have been repurposed in new indications, in order to preserve the broadest spectrum antibiotics for cases without alternatives ("carbapenem sparing"). Promising new antibiotics are becoming available, though experiences are limited among hematologic malignancy patients (Caston et al. 2017; Fernández-Cruz et al. 2018). Nevertheless, their use is appealing because of the few antibiotic options left to treat MDR infections, which are often toxic (e.g., colistin) and only moderately successful (Mensa et al. 2018; Baker and Satlin 2016). A judicious use of these new antibiotics should be made to avoid further resistance development. The objective of AMS programs is optimizing antibiotic use, mainly to avoid the emergence of even greater resistance, and to foster a more effective and efficient use of available antibiotics.

9.1.1.2 Antifungal Stewardship

Antifungal stewardship has received less attention than its antibacterial counterpart. Invasive fungal infections (IFI) are not as common as bacterial infections, but convey a high health burden and economic cost (des Champs-Bro et al. 2011).

IFI diagnosis is not straightforward. Diagnostic techniques are suboptimal: cultures have a low sensitivity and an early diagnosis is difficult to make, as results are not immediately available (Bouza et al. 2005; Escribano et al. 2015). In most cases, antifungals are used preemptively, based in serological results that lack specificity, or empirically in febrile patients with no evidence of fungal infection, and diagnostic efforts to rule-in or out the diagnosis are challenging. This diagnostic uncertainty, together with the severity of IFI and its high mortality drives the overuse of antifungals and the lack of guidelines fulfilment (Muñoz et al. 2012).

Overuse of antifungals involves high economic costs, development of resistance, risk of toxicity and interactions, and delays in chemotherapy administration. Fungal resistance has been less of a problem compared to bacterial resistance so far (Escribano et al. 2013), but the recent emergence of *C. auris*, the fungal equivalent to carbapenamase-producing bacteria in terms of antimicrobial resistance, underscores the importance of appropriate use of antifungals. Resistance has also developed among *Aspergillus* species, and multi or pan-resistant non-*Aspergillus* mold infections are emerging among hematologic patients. Empiric and prophylactic antifungals are usually effective but apply a selective pressure that allows the emergence of resistant species.

Furthermore, antifungal agents are scarce. Since 2000, no new antifungal class agents have been released (Miller 2018). Therefore, there is a particular need to preserve antifungal activity due to the limited number of agents available.

Prophylaxis encompasses a large proportion of the antifungal use in high-risk patients (Valerio et al. 2014; Valerio et al. 2018). In this context, when breakthrough infections arise, the decision of how to treat is even more complex, and might require empirical combined antifungal therapy in patients with prior exposure to antifungals, due to fear of acquired resistance or selection of intrinsically resistant species.

Although empiric therapy and prophylaxis are effective, audits show frequent deficiencies in antifungal prescription with overprescription and inappropriate use of antifungals. Scores to measure adequacy of therapy are helpful to detect opportunities for stewardship (Valerio et al. 2014). There is room for improvement regarding indication, selection, or duration of antifungal agents (Valerio et al. 2014). Antifungal use requires the input of experts who are knowledgeable of advances in IFI, skilled in the management of the complex patients that need antifungals and aware of local epidemiology and antifungal susceptibilities. Clinical mycology is a complex field justifying the necessity to involve specialists in the clinical management (López-Medrano and Aguado 2015).

Evidence-based guidelines are used as a benchmark to assess appropriate antifungal use. Recent studies analyzing adherence to candidia-sis management guidelines have found surprisingly low compliance, and a worrisome association of this lack of inclusion of the recommendations with poor outcome (Cuervo et al. 2018; Mellinghoff et al. 2018a). These results underline the need for antifungal stewardship (Valerio et al. 2014). The scores used to measure adherence to guidelines in these works, such as the EQUAL Candida score, may be useful to guide antifungal stewardship (Mellinghoff et al. 2018b).

Specifically in patients with hematologic malignancy, in a recent retrospective study performed to assess the need for antifungal stewardship, up to 46.8% of the antifungal prescriptions were considered inappropriate, and another 15.6% were considered debatable (Lachenmayr et al. 2018). The issue of drug–drug interactions is particularly important in patients receiving chemotherapy or immunosuppressors, accounting for 17% of prescriptions considered inadequate.

9.1.2 Implementation of an Antimicrobial Stewardship Program

9.1.2.1 Institutional Level
Institutional support is required to carry out antimicrobial stewardship. In order to be feasible, it should be a priority for the institution. Hospital administration is key for the acceptance of the program and the economic support. Institutional support from pharmacy and infection committees plays a central role (Pulcini et al. 2019).

Creation of a Multidisciplinary Team
The first step is the creation of the antimicrobial stewardship team that will be in charge of the program, including the assessment of the epidemiology of infections, the preventive and therapeutic interventions, and the proposition of standards and local guidelines. Resources should be provided by the institution to incorporate at least an infectious diseases physician and a pharmacist (Valerio et al. 2015a).

Audit of Antimicrobial Use and Development of Guidelines

Audit of antimicrobial use should be the next step. Every hospital and specific departments should establish their own targets regarding their critical objectives determined through previous audits. Comparison of actual use to the guidelines provides an accurate vision of areas of improvement (Lachenmayr et al. 2018) that would be a guide to select the institutional and departmental targets of the antimicrobial stewardship program.

National and international guidelines should be adapted locally and approved by all the stakeholders in order to increase acceptance and subsequently adherence by the providers. Empirical antimicrobial therapy and prophylaxis account for the majority of the antimicrobial prescriptions and should be specifically addressed in local guidelines. Local guidelines should be adapted not only to the institutional patterns of resistance, but also to the hospital-specific targets (López-Medrano et al. 2013a). To further improve acceptance, different thought leaders should collaborate to develop institutional guidelines.

These institutional guidelines should address not only the management of confirmed cases of infection but also specific clinical syndromes that are often associated with infections, such as febrile neutropenia or pulmonary nodules. In the remaining areas of uncertainty, there is also a role for diagnostic stewardship. Both overuse and underuse of diagnostic tests can lead to inappropriate antimicrobial therapy, the role of the steward being to translate this diagnostic information into appropriate treatment (Patel and Fang 2018; Bouza et al. 2018).

Guidelines and protocols should be regularly updated, incorporating changes in epidemiology and newly available diagnostic techniques and antimicrobial resources.

Formulary restriction and prescription approval of antimicrobial drugs usually work better than non-restrictive measures such as education. For practical reasons, antimicrobial medication should be dispensed pending approval in order to avoid potentially harmful delays. Then prescriptions should be reviewed during the first 24–48 h by the members of the antimicrobial stewardship team that would also give feedback to the providers (Ananda-Rajah et al. 2012).

Provider Education

Training is the foundation of antimicrobial stewardship, although relying solely on educational materials for stewardship is not recommended.

Regarding antibiotic use, most critical gaps in knowledge are found about the safety of discontinuing antibiotics in selected febrile neutropenic patients, de-escalating to targeted therapy when an etiologic diagnosis is available, unnecessary combination therapy, inappropriate therapy for multidrug resistant microorganisms, switching to oral route, and indications of restricted antibiotics.

Regarding antifungal therapy, pitfalls include lack of specific knowledge, difficulties in distinguishing colonization from infection, indications for antifungal prophylaxis or empirical therapy, ignoring local azole resistance rates, and the correct dosing of antifungals, among others (Valerio et al. 2015b). When applying a questionnaire about the antifungal knowledge to prescribers, it turned out that lack of awareness of current indications or evidence-based recommendations led to overconsumption of antifungal drugs, as many physicians prescribe antifungal combinations or inappropriate dosages of liposomal amphotericin B (L-AmB), and treat for fungal colonization (Valerio et al. 2015c). Departments with a high rate of inappropriate use require formalized educational programs.

Epidemiologic Surveillance

There are geographical variations in the emergence of resistance that are influenced by local factors. For instance, GNB (Gram negative bacilli) resistance rates are higher in southeast versus North-West Europe (Averbuch et al. 2017). In the Netherlands, the increase of resistance in *Aspergillus* spp. has been associated with the use of antifungals in agriculture. Likewise, at the local level, different patterns of use of antimicrobials in different hospitals, or even departments inside a hospital will yield a distinct resistance profile.

Epidemiological surveillance is of paramount importance to adjust empirical therapy to the expected susceptibility of the local microorganisms. Broad-spectrum antibiotics are necessary in areas with a prevalence of MDR microorganisms above 10%. As for IFI, in areas with a low incidence of resistant *Aspergillus* and non-*Aspergillus* molds, the use of combination therapy for suspected IFI is rarely justified. International guidelines should therefore be adapted locally implementing local epidemiology and antifungal susceptibility patterns.

Digital Support

Clinical decision support systems, combined with computerized physician order entry can improve antimicrobial stewardship by generating individualized recommendations based on combining microbiologic results with patient data on the electronic medical record (López-Medrano et al. 2013a). Digital support facilitates the link between pharmacy and prescribers, and between pharmacists and Infectious Diseases stewards. Alerts about interactions, dose adjustment, reminders for therapeutic drug monitoring or cost are practical examples. Local guidelines should ideally be incorporated to computerized clinical decision support at the time of prescribing, as recommended by IDSA (Infectious Diseases Society of America) guidelines (Barlam et al. 2016). "Point-of-prescription" measures such as the requirement to write an indication for the prescribed antimicrobial can be facilitated by electronic ordering of antimicrobial agents (Hamilton et al. 2015).

Another potential application of new technologies is prospective electronic surveillance. As for IFI, and in particular mold disease, the absence of a consistent and easy to obtain laboratory marker (equivalent to blood culture for *Candida*) complicates surveillance (Ananda-Rajah et al. 2014). The cumbersome detection of cases through personal review of many different results hampers the widespread performance of prospective surveillance. Digital technologies can be useful in easily combining different laboratory results to facilitate mold infection surveillance (Ananda-Rajah et al. 2017).

9.1.2.2 Individual Level

Antibacterial Stewardship

Audits of antibiotic use reveal opportunities for stewardship in the setting of febrile neutropenia. The role of the antimicrobial steward is to ensure patients get the optimal coverage while avoiding the emergence of resistance.

To adjust antibiotic therapy, it is essential to have an etiologic diagnosis. In many occasions, a diagnosis is not thoroughly pursued. Empirical therapy is initiated, and broad-spectrum antibiotics are maintained until resolution, or even blindly escalated if evolution is poor. To overcome this generalized usage of broad-spectrum antibiotics, which in many occasions will prove unnecessary, the diagnostic-driven approach is increasingly popular. An important function of the stewardship program will be to warrant appropriate samples are obtained, and rapid and accurate diagnostic tests are ordered, which may prevent unnecessary initiation and prolonged administration of antimicrobials. Both positive and negative microbiological results are of the utmost importance and will frequently allow de-escalation to reduced spectrum antimicrobials. To that end, the performance of diagnostic tests must be coupled with a stewardship program intervention (Messacar et al. 2017). A tight connection with the Microbiology lab with rapid exchange of information and expert advice is recommended.

When it comes to empirical therapy, it is vital to get it right from the beginning: knowing the local epidemiology will be of great help, but might not be enough, as it is difficult to predict which patients will develop an infection caused by a MDR microorganism. Risk factors for resistance, such as prior antibiotic use or bearing a urinary or intravascular catheter (Gudiol et al. 2011), are common among hematologic malignancy patients.

Recent data suggest that patients with hematologic malignancies who are colonized with MDR *Enterobacteriaceae* have a high risk of developing subsequent infection due to these organisms, in particular during episodes of neutropenia (Cattaneo et al. 2018). The strategy of screening for targeted empiric therapy allows to identify hematologic oncology patients at highest risk of infection with MDR *Enterobacteriaceae* in order to tailor empiric therapy for febrile neutropenia accordingly. This strategy could also spare administration of the broadest-spectrum antibiotics for the treatment of patients who have not been colonized. However, the workload and cost for the laboratory should be considered and screening should only be put in place if proven cost-effective.

Incorrect allergy labeling has been associated with increased inappropriate agent selection and increased use of broad-spectrum agents (Robilotti et al. 2017). Several groups are using Penicillin Skin testing to guide antimicrobial stewardship and to avoid inappropriate diagnoses of antibiotic allergies (Trubiano et al. 2017; Blumenthal et al. 2017; Ramsey and Staicu 2018).

Prospective audit and feedback are the cornerstones of antimicrobial stewardship (Yeo et al. 2012). Based on microbiology results and clinical course, antibiotics will be adjusted to reduce spectrum or enhance activity. Adjustments will include not only de-escalation but also dose adjustments in order to guarantee that the best antibiotic possible in terms of activity and lack of toxicity is administered. These adjustments can be made through a daily restricted antimicrobial agent review. Antibiotics permitted pending approval shall be reevaluated the following day and again after 3–5 days when microbiologic results are available.

To improve the probability for clinical success, dose and schedule of the antimicrobial regimens often need to be optimized (Theuretzbacher 2012). Similar to critically ill patients, hematologic malignancy patients have a low probability of PK/PD target attainment, as the required magnitude of the PK/PD index increases by 50–100% in patients with profound neutropenia resulting in higher required drug exposure.

Bactericidal agents may be critical in neutropenic patients, and preferable over bacteriostatic agents. The applicability of current breakpoints to these patient groups is unclear. For many antibiotics, individualized increased dosages based on therapeutic drug monitoring may be required. For β-lactam and aminoglycoside antibiotics, optimized dosing regimens have been developed based on their mechanism of action (prolonged infusion for time-dependent antibiotics, high isolated doses for concentration-dependent antibiotics). Combination therapy could be necessary when the PK/PD target is beyond clinically achievable drug exposure. Interactions and the possibility of added toxicities in these polymedicated patients should always be taken into consideration for antibiotic selection. The source of the infection should be considered when selecting an antimicrobial. Source control is especially important in patients with impaired immunity and, above all, those infected with MDR that lack optimal antibiotics against them. Source control includes catheter withdrawal, collection draining or surgery. In patients with clinical improvement, consideration to switching to oral route should be given (Aguilar-Guisado et al. 2017).

Recent studies support short-term antibiotic therapy in afebrile or febrile hematologic patients with fever of unknown origin, irrespective of their neutrophil count (Le Clech et al. 2018; Aguilar-Guisado et al. 2017). Traditionally, broad-spectrum antibiotics are maintained until neutrophil recovery, even when symptoms subside, and no clinical or microbiological definite infection has been diagnosed. Last, ECIL guidelines (ECIL-4) advocate to "stop antibiotics in patients with fever of unknown origin (FUO) after apyrexia for 48 h or more, irrespective of neutrophil count or expected duration of neutropenia" (Averbuch et al. 2013; Orasch et al. 2015). The etiologies of persistent unexplained fever in this setting, in many cases, appear not to be related to bacterial infection but caused by malignancy, iatrogenic interventions (drugs – even antibiotics themselves – transfusions), viral (Santolaya et al. 2017) or fungal infections, or others that do not respond to antibiotics (hemorrhage, thrombosis, and mucositis) (Le Clech et al. 2018) so that antibiotics could be safely discontinued early, even if patients remain febrile and neutropenic, once a bacterial infection has been excluded. IDSA 2010 guidelines suggest that stopping intravenous antibiotics after resolution of fever of unknown origin and before neutrophil recovery should be combined with secondary fluoroquinolone prophylaxis (CIII) (Freifeld et al. 2011). However, more recent ECIL-4 guideline avoided recommendations on secondary prophylaxis as a result of the increase of fluoroquinolone resistance (Mikulska et al. 2018). Careful follow-up must be maintained and antimicrobial therapy urgently reinitiated when necessary.

The use of procalcitonin in other settings for antimicrobial stewardship purposes has demonstrated utility, but in immunosuppressed hematologic patients, it failed to reduce the antibiotic duration. Post-transplant physiology and therapies interfere with biomarker levels such as procalcitonin and C- reactive protein.

CD-associated colitis is a consequence of antibiotic use and misuse, and is especially common among hematologic malignancy patients (Callejas-Diaz and Gea-Banacloche 2014). A number of antecedent antibiotics (other than those used to treat CD) have been identified as the most important risk factor for CD recurrence in allogenic stem cell transplant recipients (Mani et al. 2016). Stewardship in this area includes discontinuation of non-essential antibiotics and proton-pump inhibitors, and optimizing therapy to prevent complications and recurrence (McDonald et al. 2018).

State-of-the Art: Experiences in AB Stewardship

Several recent studies on AMS in hematologic malignancy or stem cell transplant recipients focused on checking the safety and efficacy of discontinuing antibiotics in selected patients with febrile neutropenia, regardless of neutrophil counts. Febrile neutropenia is the main reason for antimicrobial use in hematologic malignancy patients, and antibiotics are used empirically in the majority of cases and maintained until neutrophil counts have recovered. A randomized controlled trial showed that in high-risk febrile neutropenic patients, empirical antibiotic therapy can be safely discontinued after 72 h of apyrexia, together with clinical recovery, irrespective of neutrophil counts (Aguilar-Guisado et al. 2017). These results are supported by other retrospective (Gustinetti et al. 2018; Snyder et al. 2017; Ruiz-Ramos et al. 2017; So et al. 2018) and prospective (Madran et al. 2017; Le Clech et al. 2018; Yeo et al. 2012; la Martire et al. 2018) studies that demonstrate a reduction in antibiotic consumption (especially broad-spectrum such as carbapenems) without increase in mortality, ICU admission or relapse of infection. Some of the studies focused specifically on allogenic transplant patients (Snyder et al. 2017; Gustinetti et al. 2018) or critically ill hematologic patients (Ruiz-Ramos et al. 2017) (Table 9.1).

A study of adherence to an antimicrobial stewardship protocol for febrile neutropenia based on the IDSA guidelines showed a decrease in 28-d mortality (Rosa et al. 2014). However, compliance with the protocol was only 53%, and the authors point out the need to develop adherence. In that study, there was no AMS team to implement adherence to the protocol. AMS should be based on specific guidelines, such as ECIL or IDSA guidelines (la Martire et al. 2018).

Antifungal Stewardship

Bedside intervention is the antifungal stewardship scaffold. This intervention would be prompted by the positivity of blood cultures for fungi, initiation of antifungals, or another agreed trigger. Several studies have detected opportunities for improvement in antifungal prescription regarding indication, duration, drug selection, and dosing (Valerio et al. 2014). Antifungal stewardship is key to make sure all these are optimized.

Empirical antifungal use in patients with prolonged neutropenic fever leads to toxicity, risk of antifungal resistance, and increased costs. Limiting antifungal therapy to selected patients has been reported as a reasonable alternative that avoids overtreatment without increasing IFI-related mortality (Aguilar-Guisado et al. 2012; Aguilar-Guisado et al. 2010) and reduces costs (Martin-Pena et al. 2013). The selection of patients for antifungal therapy should be based

Table 9.1 Summary of the main series on antimicrobial stewardship in allogenic transplant or critically ill hematologic patients

Author/journal	Year	Place	Type of study and N	Management	Target population	Compliance rate	Results	Comments
Yeo CL Eur J Clin Microbiol Infect Dis	2012	Singapore	Prospective ITS study 11 month before/after intervention. 556 patients	Prospective audit and feedback ASP	Hematology–oncology unit in a university hospital	86.9%	Significant reversal of prescription trends towards reduced prescription of audited. No other changes were seen for both internal and external controls.	Safe and effective ASPs can be implemented in the complex setting of hematology–oncology inpatients
Rosa RG BMC infectious diseases	2014	Porto allegre (Brazil)	Prospective cohort study 307 FN in 169 subjects	Evaluate whether adherence to an AMS protocol based on IDSA guidelines results in lower rates of mortality in FN	FN in hematology ward single tertiary hospital	53%	Protocol adherence was independently associated with lower 28-d mortality.	There was no AMS team to implement adherence to the protocol
Aguilar-Guisado M Lancet Haematol	2017	Spain	Open-label, randomized, controlled phase 4 trial. 157 episodes	**How long study:** Whether empiric antimicrobial therapy discontinuation driven by a clinical approach regardless of neutrophil recovery would optimize the duration of therapy	Six academic hospitals. Hematologic malignancies or HSCT recipients, with high-risk FN without etiologic diagnosis	N/A	In high-risk patients with hematologic malignancies and febrile neutropenia, empirical therapy can be discontinued after 72 h of apyrexia and clinical recovery irrespective of their neutrophil count.	This clinical approach reduces unnecessary exposure to antimicrobials and is safe.
Ruiz-Ramos J Farmacia Hospitalaria	2017	Valencia (Spain)	Retrospective. 324 antimicrobials in 169 patients	Quasi-experimental pre-post intervention study	Hematologic patients in ICU	Unknown	Compared with the pre-intervention period, there were no significant differences in the variables assessed.	121 modifications were recommended, including 55 treatment discontinuations. No variation was observed in colonization by multi-resistant bacteria.
Madran B Am J Infect Control	2017	Istanbul (Turkey)	Prospective before and after. 152 FN of 95 adult inpatients	Standardized protocol for FN	All adult hematologic and oncologic cancer inpatients. single center	85%	Case fatality rate, bacterial and *Candida* infections decreased among the patients with FN	Appropriate antimicrobial use increased and overall antimicrobial consumption was reduced.

(continued)

Table 9.1 (continued)

Author/journal	Year	Place	Type of study and N	Management	Target population	Compliance rate	Results	Comments
Snyder M Open Forum Infectious Diseases	2017	Florida (US)	Retrospective. 120 patients	A cohort with early de-escalation versus a cohort without early de-escalation	Two groups of Allo-HSCT recipients	N/A (46/110)	Significant reductions in gram-positive broad-spectrum antimicrobial utilization, and trends toward lower use of broad-spectrum gram-negative agents and associated costs and no difference in clinical outcomes.	De-escalating after at least 5 days of broad-spectrum therapy and defervescence did not appear to affect the rate of recurrent fever
La Martire G Eur J Clin Microbiol Infect Dis	2018	Créteil (France)	Prospective. 137 consecutive antibiotic prescriptions (100 for FN)	ITS analysis on antibacterial consumption. Evaluation before and after the implementation of an AS intervention based on ECIL guidelines	High-risk hematology ward in a tertiary referral public university hospital	89%	A significant reduction of the level of carbapenem consumption. Applicability and acceptability of flow charts were high. No differences in terms of intensive care unit transfers, bacteremia incidence, and mortality were found.	Before and after. This should encourage further applications of ECIL guidelines for FN.
Le Clech L Infectious Disease	2018	Brest (France)	20-month prospective observational study. 238 FN in 123 patients	**ANTIBIOSTOP study**: Evaluates the feasibility and safety of short-term antibiotic treatment in afebrile or febrile patients exhibiting FUO, irrespective of their neutrophil count	FN in hematology department	17/82	Neither the composite endpoint, nor each component (in-hospital mortality, intensive care unit admission, relapse of infection 48 h after discontinuation of antibiotics) differed between the two FUO groups	These results suggest that early discontinuation of empirical antibiotics in FUO is safe for afebrile neutropenic patients

Author/journal	Year	Place	Type of study and N	Management	Target population	Compliance rate	Results	Comments
Gustinetti G Biology of Blood and Marrow Transplantation	2018	Genoa (Italy)	Retrospective. 110 consecutive patients	Rates and outcomes of antibiotic de-escalation	Pre-engraftment neutropenia in allogeneic HSCT recipients	25%	Early (<96 h) de-escalation of antibiotic treatment was performed in 25% of the population. Overall de-escalation and discontinuation rate was 55.5%. Failures never represented a recurrence of previous infections bloodstream infections were predictors of early de-escalation	Failure rate of early de-escalation was 15% (4/26). Late de-escalation rate was 30.4% (n = 31) and failure rate 19% (6/31). The rate of de-escalation any time before engraftment was 55.9% (n = 57), including discontinuation in 33 patients (32%). Death at day 60 after HSCT occurred in 3 patients who never underwent de-escalation.
So M Clin Microbiol infect	2018	Canada	Multisite retrospective observational time series study. 1006 patients before/335 after	ASP AB and AF	Leukemia units (HSCT units as controls; also external controls)	Unknown	Antimicrobial utilization and cost decreased in the intervention group, increased in external control but were stable in internal control. Mortality, length of stay and nosocomial C. difficile rate in intervention group remained stable.	The AMS reduced antimicrobial use in leukemia patients without affecting inpatient mortality and length of stay

AMS, antimicrobial stewardship; *ASP*, AMS program; *AB*, Antibiotics; *AF*, antifungals; *HSCT*, hematopoietic stem cell transplant; *FN*, febrile neutropenia; *ITS*, interrupted time series; *FUO*, fever of unknown origin; *ICU*, intensive care unit on risk factors and clinical criteria, and has been specifically evaluated in hematologic malignancy, including high-risk cases such as allogeneic HSCT recipients (Aguilar-Guisado et al. 2012).

Once antifungals have been started, it is important to do all possible diagnostic efforts to confirm or exclude fungal infection in order to adjust antimicrobial therapy accordingly. Trying to reach an etiologic diagnosis is important because IFI diagnosis is elusive, and many etiologies can be confused with fungal disease, whereas empirical antifungals can safely be discontinued based on negative diagnostic tests that convey a very low probability of IFI.

To that end, diagnostic tests for IFI need to be improved. Biomarker-based preemptive strategies in patients receiving anti-mold prophylaxis can be misleading and increase inappropriate antifungal consumption due to a very high proportion of false-positive results (Duarte et al. 2014; Duarte et al. 2017; Vena et al. 2017; Martin-Rabadan et al. 2012). By contrast, they are very useful to help de-escalation in cases of suspected IFI due to their high negative predictive value in this setting, specifically when tested before initiation of antifungals (Duarte et al. 2014).

Knowledge of the local epidemiology helps choosing appropriate empirical antifungals. In settings with a low incidence of azole-resistant *Aspergillus* and non-*Aspergillus* molds, a combined antifungal therapy is rarely required even while awaiting susceptibility results. On the contrary, when facing a breakthrough IFI, it may be reasonable to switch the antifungal class or even add a second antifungal until susceptibility is confirmed. In this scenario, all the efforts to get a confirmed diagnosis are warranted. Penetration of the antifungal into the site of infection needs to be considered. Once a pathogen is identified, antifungal therapy should be de-escalated to the optimal, narrower spectrum drug, and switched to oral therapy when there is an agent with good bioavailability, the patient is stable, and there is no intestinal impairment impacting absoption of oral antifungal agents (i.e., mucositis). The precise moment for de-escalation is still a matter of debate (Vazquez et al. 2014).

Drug–drug interactions should always be considered, in particular, in patients receiving azoles, due to their effect on the cytochrome p450 complex. Many immunosuppressors and chemotherapeutic agents are metabolized through this pathway. For instance, tacrolimus or vincristine toxicity may be enhanced by concomitant use of voriconazole, so these combinations should be avoided, or dose adjustments made. Apparently, commonly used drugs such as proton-pump inhibitors can considerably alter azole bioavailability, increasing or decreasing absorption. Hematologic malignancy patients usually receive many drugs simultaneously, and streamlining therapy while minimizing toxicity and considering interactions can be challenging.

Dose adjustment has its own pitfalls. Liposomal amphotericin B can be nephrotoxic, but does not need dose adjustment in patients with preexisting renal impairment. In fact, nephrotoxicity seems to depend on the accompanying drugs (Stanzani et al. 2017). Though controversial in some cases, TDM (therapeutic drug monitoring) can be very useful to assure adequate levels for efficacy and safety, in particular for azoles, and in critical patients with kidney or liver dysfunction.

Limiting the duration of inappropriate antifungals is one of the main tasks of antifungal stewardship, but also to guarantee that treatment courses are completed, for example, to make sure that candidemia is treated for 14 days after the first negative blood culture, or appropriately longer in cases of metastatic infection.

Just like antibiotic stewardship, antifungal stewardship at the individual level is accomplished through postprescription review and feedback. It requires daily commitment from the multidisciplinary team and of course provider involvement. "Point-of-prescription" implication of the providers documenting indication for antimicrobial use, expected duration of therapy, adherence to empiric treatment guidelines, and reassessment of antimicrobial prescription at 72 hours has shown to improve antimicrobial stewardship (Hamilton et al. 2015). Cases need to

Table 9.2 Summary of the main series on antifungal stewardship programs

Author/Journal	Year	Place	Type of study and N	Management	Target population (% hematologic)	Compliance rate	Results	Comments
Sutepvarnon A Infect Control Hosp Epidemiol	2008	Pratumthani (Thailand)	Prospective Single center 57 patients	Each patient who received AF therapy was visited 3 times	All hospitalized inpatients >15 y-old who were prescribed AF therapy	N/A	Inappropriate antifungal use was 74%. Isolation of Candida species from urine (p 0.004) was a risk factor whereas receipt of an infectious diseases consultation (p 0.004) was protective.	Audit
López-Medrano F Mycology	2012	Madrid (Spain)	Before/after 662 AF prescriptions	Prescriptions of oral or intravenous voriconazole, caspofungin and liposomal amphotericin B were reviewed	Hematology 28.4%	99%	The DDDs of intravenous voriconazole and caspofungin were reduced by 31.4% and 20.2%, respectively. The DDDs of oral voriconazole and dispensed vials of liposomal amphotericin B were increased by 8.2% and 13.9%, respectively. Expenditure on antifungals was reduced	A stewardship program targeting antifungals achieved a reduction in antifungal expenditure without reducing the quality of care provided. Non-compulsory.
Mondain V Infection	2013	Nice (France)	Prospective, single center 6 y. 636 AF prescriptions	Systematic evaluation of all costly AF prescriptions	Hematology 72%	88%	No combination therapies used since 2008. Total antifungal prescriptions (DDD) and their cost were contained between 2003–2010.	AI: Optimal standard of care was achieved for GM testing, performance of CT scan and voriconazole TDM Candidemia: Optimal standard of care was achieved for the timing of AF first-line therapy, duration and removal of CVC (central venous catheter)

(continued)

Table 9.2 (continued)

Author/ Journal	Year	Place	Type of study and N	Management	Target population(% hematologic)	Compliance rate	Results	Comments
Alfandari S Med Mal Infect	2014	Lille (France)	Unknown	ASP for AF	Hematology unit	Unknown	Antifungal consumption decreased by 40%.	A permanent collaboration between hematologists and an infectious diseases physician can improve antifungal prescribing.
Valerio M Mycology	2015	Madrid (Spain)	Quasi-experimental study with a time series design 453 patients	ASP for AF	Hematology 35%	78.4%	The number of DDD decreased from 66.4 to 54.8 per 1000 patient-days. Incidence of candidemia was reduced from 1.49 to 1.14 (p 0.08) and related mortality was reduced from 28% to 16% (p 0.1).	A significant economic impact after the first 12 months of the intervention (p 0.042 at month 13), which was enhanced in the following 24 months (p 0.006 at month 35). Non-compulsory.
Ramos A Rev. Iberoamc Micol	2015	Madrid (Spain)	Prospective study 280 AF prescriptions for 262 patients	Programmed review of restricted AF prescribed in hospitalized patients	Hematology 16%	40%	There was a 42% lower use of AF during the period of the study. Mortality among patients who were treated according to the recommendations of the ASP was 17%, and in whom treatment was not modified, it was 30% (p = 0.393)	Non-compulsory
Molina CID	2017	Seville (Spain)	Quasi-experimental intervention ITS analysis	Peer-to-peer educational interviews between counselors and prescribers from all departments to reinforce the principles of the proper use of antibiotics	All departments	N/A	Effective in decreasing the incidence and mortality rate of hospital-acquired candidemia and MDR BSI through sustained reduction in antibiotic use.	

Author/ Journal	Year	Place	Type of study and N	Management	Target population(% hematologic)	Compliancerate	Results	Comments
Rautemaa-Richardson R JAC	2018	Manchester (UK)	Retrospective 68 patients	AF therapy was stopped following negative biomarker results	ICU All patients prescribed micafungin during 4 month audit	N/A	AF consumption reduced by 49% from 2014 to 2016. Reducing the number of inappropriate initiation of AF by 90%. Concurrently, mortality due to invasive candidiasis was reduced by 58%.	
Whitney L JAC	2019	London (UK)	Prospective 432 patients	Reviewed weekly ID & pharmacist	Adult inpatients receiving AF	84%	Annual antifungal expenditure initially reduced by 30% (£0.98 million to £0.73 million), then increased to 20% above baseline over a 5-year period.	Candida species distribution and rates of resistance were not adversely affected by the intervention

N/A, non-applicable; *AF*, antifungal; *ID*, infectious diseases specialist; *ASP*, antimicrobial stewardship program; *ITS*, interrupted time series be evaluated individually, as there are still uncertainties that need to be addressed in a personalized way. Guidelines are currently very useful to manage confirmed cases of IFI, but there is still a lack of evidence regarding how and when to de-escalate in cases in which IFI is reasonably excluded.

State-of-the Art: Experiences in AF Stewardship (Table 9.2)

Most antifungal stewardship programs have focused on candidiasis (Whitney et al. 2019; Rautemaa-Richardson et al. 2018; Molina et al. 2017), however some include also mold infections. Only a few are centered specifically in hematologic patients (Alfandari et al. 2014), though most of them include them in different proportions (López-Medrano et al. 2013b; Valerio et al. 2015a; Ramos et al. 2015; Mondain et al. 2013), as the hematology department is usually one of the areas with a higher consumption of antifungals.

Antifungal stewardship programs usually achieved a reduction-or at least containment- in cost without reducing the quality of care. Antifungal consumption was reduced, and in particular, the number of inappropriate initiations of antifungals decreased importantly (up to 90% (Rautemaa-Richardson et al. 2018)), and so did the use of antifungal combinations (Mondain et al. 2013). In some cases, candidemia incidence (Valerio et al. 2015a; Molina et al. 2017) and even mortality (Valerio et al. 2015a; Ramos et al. 2015) were diminished. Authors remark that recommendations were non-compulsory, and still, compliance with them was as high as 74–88% (Mondain et al. 2013; Valerio et al. 2015a; Whitney et al. 2019).

In the study focused on hematologic patients (Alfandari et al. 2014), antifungal recommendations were integrated in the decision trees for febrile neutropenia management. A large proportion of the recommendations fall on diagnostic aspects, in particular, related to mold infection suspicion. The implementation of antifungal stewardship in the protected hematology unit resulted in a 40% decrease in costs, in spite of a stable incidence of IFI during the study period.

The authors underline the need for commitment and realistic objectives on the ID side, as well as involvement of the prescribing physicians. Recommendations should be based on acknowledged scientific data to favor acceptance among providers.

9.1.3 Guideline Resources

IDSA (Barlam et al. 2016) guidelines point out a series of recommendations to implement an antimicrobial stewardship program. Recent ESCMID guidelines on global hospital antimicrobial stewardship programs have been developed (Pulcini et al. 2018) that offer a set of core elements and related checklist items for AMS programs. Those are meant to be present in all hospitals, regardless of resources. National guidelines have been developed in different countries (Rodriguez-Baño et al. 2012; de With et al. 2016; Morley and Wacogne 2017).

Online resources to help develop antimicrobial stewardship programs are listed in Paño-Pardo et al. (Paño-Pardo et al. 2013).

9.1.3.1 Other Resources Based on Guidelines

To help tracking of process and outcome measures in order to determine the impact of interventions, several scores of adherence to guidelines have been developed, such as EQUAL score for candidiasis, aspergillosis, cryptococcosis, and others (Mellinghoff et al. 2018b; Cornely et al. 2018; Spec et al. 2018; Cuervo et al. 2018). Interestingly, best scores have been associated with a decrease in mortality (Mellinghoff et al. 2018a; Cuervo et al. 2018).

9.1.4 Next Research Questions

There are still several areas of uncertainty, regarding both diagnosis and therapy. The applicability to immunocompromised hosts of measures such as ruling out nasal colonization by MR *S. aureus* that have proved to be useful in ICU setting to adjust treatment need to be tested in hematologic patients. The utility of new diagnostic techniques in helping antimicrobial stewardship and their effect on outcome must be checked. Issues such as the cost-effectiveness of surveillance cultures to guide empirical therapy have to be confirmed. Knowledge on microbiota and its influence in infection development needs be integrated into antimicrobial stewardship programs.

More translational studies focused specifically in hematologic malignancy patients are needed to establish guidelines on de-escalation and define the safety of de-escalation in different populations, considering different risks: repeated neutropenia episodes versus first, new therapies such as targeted therapies, immunotherapy, CAR-T-cell therapy. There is a need to consider the role of combination therapy in the face of more resistant microorganisms and the role of new antiinfective therapies such as CTL (cytotoxic T lymphocytes) or therapeutic vaccines.

Digital support use needs to be expanded and integrated in everyday care with expert systems that help identify better patients at risk for MDR infections, and help individualize and optimize antibiotic dosing regimens in neutropenic patients. Apps in mobile devices might prove helpful to remind providers reconsidering antimicrobial therapy after a stabilized period.

Furthermore, antimicrobial stewardship programs face the challenge to actively be maintained for long periods of time (López-Medrano et al. 2013a).

References

Abbo LM, Ariza-Heredia EJ (2014) Antimicrobial stewardship in immunocompromised hosts. Infect Dis Clin N Am 28(2):263–279. https://doi.org/10.1016/j.idc.2014.01.008

Aguilar-Guisado M, Espigado I, Cordero E, Noguer M, Parody R, Pachon J, Cisneros JM (2010) Empirical antifungal therapy in selected patients with persistent febrile neutropenia. Bone Marrow Transplant 45(1):159–164. https://doi.org/10.1038/bmt.2009.125

Aguilar-Guisado M, Martin-Peña A, Espigado I, Ruiz Perez de Pipaón M, Falantes J, de la Cruz F, Cisneros JM (2012) Universal antifungal therapy is not needed in persistent febrile neutropenia: a tailored diagnostic and therapeutic approach. Haematologica 97(3):464–471. https://doi.org/10.3324/haematol.2011.049999

Aguilar-Guisado M, Espigado I, Martin-Peña A, Gudiol C, Royo-Cebrecos C, Falantes J, Vázquez-López L, Montero MI, Rosso-Fernández C, de la Luz MM, Parody R, González-Campos J, Garzón-Lopez S, Calderón-Cabrera C, Barba P, Rodríguez N, Rovira M, Montero-Mateos E, Carratala J, Pérez-Simón JA, Cisneros JM (2017) Optimisation of empiricalantimicrobial therapy in patients with haematological malignancies and febrile neutropenia (how long study): an open-label, randomised, controlled phase 4 trial. Lancet Haematol 4(12):e573–e583. https://doi.org/10.1016/S2352-3026(17)30211-9.

Alfandari S, Berthon C, Coiteux V (2014) Antifungal stewardship: implementation in a French teaching hospital. Med Mal Infect 44(4):154–158. https://doi.org/10.1016/j.medmal.2014.01.012

Ananda-Rajah MR, Slavin MA, Thursky KT (2012) The case for antifungal stewardship. Curr Opin Infect Dis 25(1):107–115. https://doi.org/10.1097/QCO.0b013e32834e0680

Ananda-Rajah MR, Martínez D, Slavin MA, Cavedon L, Dooley M, Cheng A, Thursky KA (2014) Facilitating surveillance of pulmonary invasive mold diseases in patients with haematological malignances by screening computed tomography reports using natural language processing. PLoS One 9(9):e107797. https://doi.org/10.1371/journal.pone.0107797.

Ananda-Rajah MR, Bergmeir C, Petitjean F, Slavin MA, Thursky KA, Webb GI (2017) Toward electronic surveillance of invasive Mold diseases in hematology-oncology patients: an expert system combining natural language processing of chest computed tomography reports, microbiology, and antifungal drug data. JCO Clin Cancer Inform 1:1–10. https://doi.org/10.1200/CCI.17.00011.

Averbuch D, Orasch C, Cordonnier C, Livermore DM, Mikulska M, Viscoli C, Gyssens IC, Kern WV, Klyasova G, Marchetti O, Engelhard D, Akova M, Ecil ajvoEEIEE, Eln (2013) European guidelines for empirical antibacterial therapy for febrile neutropenic patients in the era of growing resistance: summary of the 2011 4th European conference on infections in leukemia. Haematologica 98(12):1826–1835. https://doi.org/10.3324/haematol.2013.091025

Averbuch D, Tridello G, Hoek J, Mikulska M, Akan H, Yanez San Segundo L, Pabst T, Ozcelik T, Klyasova G, Donnini I, Wu D, Gulbas Z, Zuckerman T, Botelho de Sousa A, Beguin Y, Xhaard A, Bachy E, Ljungman P, de la Cámara R, Rascon J, Ruiz-Camps I, Vitek A, Patriarca F, Cudillo L, Vrhovac R, Shaw PJ, Wolfs T, O'Brien T, Avni B, Silling G, Al Sabty F, Graphakos S, Sankelo M, Sengeloev H, Pillai S, Matthes S, Melanthiou F, Iacobelli S, Styczynski J, Engelhard D, Cesaro S (2017) Antimicrobial resistance in gram-negative rods causing bacteremia in hematopoietic stem cell transplant recipients: intercontinental prospective study of the infectious diseases working Party of the European Bone Marrow Transplantation Group. Clin Infect Dis 65(11):1819–1828. https://doi.org/10.1093/cid/cix646

Averbuch D, Tridello G, Hoek J, Mikulska M, Akan H, Yanez San Segundo L, Pabst T, Ozcelik T, Klyasova G, Donnini I, Wu D, Gulbas Z, Zuckerman T, Botelho de Sousa A, Beguin Y, Xhaard A, Bachy E, Ljungman P, de la Cámara R, Rascon J, Ruiz-Camps I, Vitek A, Patriarca F, Cudillo L, Vrhovac R, Shaw PJ, Wolfs T, O'Brien T, Avni B, Silling G, Al Sabty F, Graphakos S, Sankelo M, Sengeloev H, Pillai S, Matthes S, Melanthiou F, Iacobelli S, Styczynski J, Engelhard D, Cesaro S (2017) Antimicrobial resistance in gram-negative rods causing bacteremia in hematopoietic stem cell transplant recipients: intercontinental prospective study of the infectious diseases working Party of the European Bone Marrow Transplantation Group. Clin Infect Dis 65(11):1819–1828.. https://doi.org/10.1080/10428194.2016.1193859

Barlam TF, Cosgrove SE, Abbo LM, MacDougall C, Schuetz AN, Septimus EJ, Srinivasan A, Dellit TH, Falck-Ytter YT, Fishman NO, Hamilton CW, Jenkins TC, Lipsett PA, Malani PN, May LS, Moran GJ, Neuhauser MM, Newland JG, Ohl CA, Samore MH, Seo SK, Trivedi KK (2016) Implementing an antibiotic stewardship program: guidelines by the Infectious Diseases Society of America and the Society for Healthcare Epidemiology of America. Clin Infect Dis 62(10):e51–e77. https://doi.org/10.1093/cid/ciw118

Blumenthal KG, Wickner PG, Hurwitz S, Pricco N, Nee AE, Laskowski K, Shenoy ES, Walensky RP (2017) Tackling inpatient penicillin allergies: assessing tools for antimicrobial stewardship. J Allergy Clin Immunol 140(1):154–161. e156. https://doi.org/10.1016/j.jaci.2017.02.005

Bouza E, Guinea J, Pelaez T, Perez-Molina J, Alcala L, Muñoz P (2005) Workload due to Aspergillus fumigatus and significance of the organism in the microbiology laboratory of a general hospital. J Clin Microbiol 43(5):2075–2079. https://doi.org/10.1128/JCM.43.5.2075-2079.2005

Bouza E, Muñoz P, Burillo A (2018) Role of the clinical microbiology Laboratory in Antimicrobial Stewardship. Med Clin North Am 102(5):883–898. https://doi.org/10.1016/j.mcna.2018.05.003

Bow EJ (2013) There should be no ESKAPE for febrile neutropenic cancer patients: the dearth of effective antibacterial drugs threatens anticancer efficacy. J Antimicrob Chemother 68(3):492–495. https://doi.org/10.1093/jac/dks512

Callejas-Díaz A, Gea-Banacloche JC (2014) Clostridium difficile: deleterious impact on hematopoietic stem cell transplantation. Curr Hematol Malig Rep 9(1):85–90. https://doi.org/10.1007/s11899-013-0193-y

Caston JJ, Lacort-Peralta I, Martin-Davila P, Loeches B, Tabares S, Temkin L, Torre-Cisneros J, Paño-Pardo JR (2017) Clinical efficacy of ceftazidime/avibactam versus other active agents for the treatment of bacteremia due to carbapenemase-producing Enterobacteriaceae in hematologic patients. Int J Infect Dis 59:118–123. https://doi.org/10.1016/j.ijid.2017.03.021

Cattaneo C, Di Blasi R, Skert C, Candoni A, Martino B, Di Renzo N, Delia M, Ballanti S, Marchesi F, Mancini V, Orciuolo E, Cesaro S, Prezioso L, Fanci R, Nadali

G, Chierichini A, Facchini L, Picardi M, Malagola M, Orlando V, Trecarichi EM, Tumbarello M, Aversa F, Rossi G, Pagano L, Group S (2018) Bloodstream infections in haematological cancer patients colonized by multidrug-resistant bacteria. Ann Hematol. https://doi.org/10.1007/s00277-018-3341-6

Cornely OA, Koehler P, Arenz D, CM S (2018) EQUAL Aspergillosis score 2018: an ECMM score derived from current guidelines to measure QUALity of the clinical management of invasive pulmonary aspergillosis. Mycoses 61(11):833–836. https://doi.org/10.1111/myc.12820

Cuervo G, García-Vidal C, Puig-Asensio M, Merino P, Vena A, Martin-Peña A, Montejo JM, Ruiz A, Lázaro-Perona F, Fortún J, Fernández-Ruiz M, Suárez AI, Castro C, Cardozo C,

Gudiol C, Aguado JM, Paño JR, Pemán J, Salavert M, Garnacho-Montero J, Cisneros JM, Soriano A, Muñoz P, Almirante B, Carratalá J, Reipi tG, the Spanish C-BG (2018) Usefulness of guideline recommendations for prognosis in patients with candidemia. Med Mycol. https://doi.org/10.1093/mmy/myy118

des Champs-Bro B, Leroy-Cotteau A, Mazingue F, Pasquier F, Francois N, Corm S, Lemaitre L, Poulain D, Yakoub-Agha I, Alfandari S, Sendid B (2011) Invasive fungal infections: epidemiology and analysis of antifungal prescriptions in onco-haematology. J Clin Pharm Ther 36(2):152–160. https://doi.org/10.1111/j.1365-2710.2010.01166.x

Duarte RF, Sánchez-Ortega I, Cuesta I, Arnan M, Patino B, Fernández de Sevilla A, Gudiol C, Ayats J, Cuenca-Estrella M (2014) Serum galactomannan-based early detection of invasive aspergillosis in hematology patients receiving effective antimold prophylaxis. Clin Infect Dis 59(12):1696–1702. https://doi.org/10.1093/cid/ciu673

Duarte RF, Sánchez-Ortega I, Arnan M, Patino B, Ayats J, Sureda A, Cuenca-Estrella M (2017) Serum galactomannan surveillance may be safely withdrawn from antifungal management of hematology patients on effective antimold prophylaxis: a pilot single-center study. Bone Marrow Transplant 52(2):326–329. https://doi.org/10.1038/bmt.2016.279

Dyar OJ, Huttner B, Schouten J, Pulcini C, Esgap (2017) What is antimicrobial stewardship? Clin Microbiol Infect 23(11):793–798. https://doi.org/10.1016/j.cmi.2017.08.026

Escribano P, Peláez T, Muñoz P, Bouza E, Guinea J (2013) Is azole resistance in Aspergillus fumigatus a problem in Spain? Antimicrob Agents Chemother 57(6):2815–2820. https://doi.org/10.1128/AAC.02487-12

Escribano P, Marcos-Zambrano LJ, Peláez T, Muñoz P, Padilla B, Bouza E, Guinea J (2015) Sputum and bronchial secretion samples are equally useful as Broncho alveolar lavage samples for the diagnosis of invasive pulmonary aspergillosis in selected patients. Med Mycol 53(3):235–240. https://doi.org/10.1093/mmy/myu090

Fernández-Cruz A, Alba N, Semiglia-Chong MA, Padilla B, Rodríguez-Macías G, Kwon M, Cercenado E,

Chamorro-de-Vega E, Machado M, Pérez-Lago L, de Vicdma DG, Díez Martín JL, Muñoz P (2018) Real-life experience with ceftolozane/tazobactam in patients with hematologic malignancy and Pseudomonas aeruginosa infection: a case-control study. Antimicrob Agents Chemother. https://doi.org/10.1128/AAC.02340-18

Freifeld AG, Bow EJ, Sepkowitz KA, Boeckh MJ, Ito JI, Mullen CA, Raad II, Rolston KV, Young JA, Wingard JR, Infectious Diseases Society of A (2011) Clinical practice guideline for the use of antimicrobial agents in neutropenic patients with cancer: 2010 update by the Infectious Diseases Society of America. Clin Infect Dis 52(4):427–431. https://doi.org/10.1093/cid/ciq147

Girmenia C, Rossolini GM, Piciocchi A, Bertaina A, Pisapia G, Pastore D, Sica S, Severino A, Cudillo L, Ciceri F, Scime R, Lombardini L, Viscoli C, Rambaldi A, Gruppo Italiano Trapianto Midollo O, Gruppo Italiano Trapianto Midollo Osseo G (2015) Infections by carbapenem-resistant Klebsiella pneumoniae in SCT recipients: a nationwide retrospective survey from Italy. Bone Marrow Transplant 50(2):282–288. https://doi.org/10.1038/bmt.2014.231

Gudiol C, Tubau F, Calatayud L, García-Vidal C, Cisnal M, Sanchez-Ortega I, Duarte R, Calvo M, Carratalá J (2011) Bacteraemia due to multidrug-resistant gram-negative bacilli in cancer patients: risk factors, antibiotic therapy and outcomes. J Antimicrob Chemother 66(3):657–663. https://doi.org/10.1093/jac/dkq494

Gustinetti G, Raiola AM, Varaldo R, Galaverna F, Gualandi F, Del Bono V, Bacigalupo A, Angelucci E, Viscoli C, Mikulska M (2018) De-escalation and discontinuation of empirical antibiotic treatment in a cohort of allogeneic hematopoietic stem cell transplantation recipients during the pre-engraftment period. Biol Blood Marrow Transplant 24(8):1721–1726. https://doi.org/10.1016/j.bbmt.2018.03.018

Gyssens IC, Kern WV, Livermore DM, Ecil ajvoEEI, ESCMID Eo (2013) The role of antibiotic stewardship in limiting antibacterial resistance among hematology patients. Haematologica 98(12):1821–1825. https://doi.org/10.3324/haematol.2013.091769

Hamilton KW, Gerber JS, Moehring R, Anderson DJ, Calderwood MS, Han JH, Mehta JM, Pollack LA, Zaoutis T, Srinivasan A, Camins BC, Schwartz DN, Lautenbach E, Centers for Disease C, Prevention Epicenters P (2015) Point-of-prescription interventions to improve antimicrobial stewardship. Clin Infect Dis 60(8):1252–1258. https://doi.org/10.1093/cid/civ018

Hennig S, Staatz CE, Natanek D, Bialkowski S, Consuelo Llanos Paez C, Lawson R, Clark J (2018) Antimicrobial stewardship in paediatric oncology: impact on optimising gentamicin use in febrile neutropenia. Pediatr Blood Cancer 65(2). https://doi.org/10.1002/pbc.26810

Katsios CM, Burry L, Nelson S, Jivraj T, Lapinsky SE, Wax RS, Christian M, Mehta S, Bell CM, Morris AM (2012) An antimicrobial stewardship program improves antimicrobial treatment by culture site and the quality of antimicrobial prescribing in critically ill patients. Crit Care 16(6):R216. https://doi.org/10.1186/cc11854

Lachenmayr SJ, Berking S, Horns H, Strobeck D, Oysterman H, Berger K (2018) Antifungal treatment in haematological and oncological patients: need for quality assessment in routine care. Mycoses 61(7):464–471. https://doi.org/10.1111/myc.12768

Le Clech L, Talarmin JP, Couturier MA, Ianotto JC, Nicol C, Le Calloch R, Dos Santos S, Hutin P, Tande D, Cogulet V, Berthou C, Guillerm G (2018) Early discontinuation of empirical antibacterial therapy in febrile neutropenia: the ANTIBIOSTOP study. Infect Dis (Lond):1–11. https://doi.org/10.1080/23744235.2018.1438649

López-Medrano F, Aguado JM (2015) Invasive fungal disease: an entity with enough complexity to justify the existence of specialists in its management. Enferm Infecc Microbiol Clin 33(4):219–220. https://doi.org/10.1016/j.eimc.2015.01.001

López-Medrano F, Moreno-Ramos F, de Cueto M, Mora-Rillo M, Salavert M (2013a) How to assist clinicians in improving antimicrobial prescribing: tools and interventions provided by stewardship programs. Enferm Infecc Microbiol Clin 31(Suppl 4):38–44. https://doi.org/10.1016/S0213-005X(13)70131-9

López-Medrano F, Juan RS, Lizasoain M, Catalan M, Ferrari JM, Chaves F, Lumbreras C, Montejo JC, de Tejada AH, Aguado JM (2013b) A non-compulsory stewardship programme for the management of antifungals in a university-affiliated hospital. Clin Microbiol Infect 19(1):56–61. https://doi.org/10.1111/j.1469-0691.2012.03891.x

Madran B, Keske S, Tokca G, Donmez E, Ferhanoglu B, Cetiner M, Mandel NM, Ergonul O (2017) Implementation of an antimicrobial stewardship program for patients with febrile neutropenia. Am J Infect Control. https://doi.org/10.1016/j.ajic.2017.09.030

Mani S, Rybicki L, Jagadeesh D, Mossad SB (2016) Risk factors for recurrent Clostridium difficile infection in allogeneic hematopoietic cell transplant recipients. Bone Marrow Transplant 51(5):713–717. https://doi.org/10.1038/bmt.2015.311

Martin-Peña A, Gil-Navarro MV, Aguilar-Guisado M, Espigado I, de Pipaón MR, Falantes J, Pachón J, Cisneros JM (2013) Cost-effectiveness analysis comparing two approaches for empirical antifungal therapy in hematological patients with persistent febrile neutropenia. Antimicrob Agents Chemother 57(10):4664–4672. https://doi.org/10.1128/AAC.00723-13

Martín-Rabadan P, Gijón P, Alonso Fernásndez R, Ballesteros M, Anguita J, Bouza E (2012) False-positive Aspergillus antigenemia due to blood product conditioning fluids. Clin Infect Dis 55(4):e22–e27. https://doi.org/10.1093/cid/cis493

la Martire G, Robin C, Oubaya N, Lepeule R, Beckerich F, Leclerc M, Barhoumi W, Toma A, Pautas C, Maury S, Akrout W, Cordonnier-Jourdin C, Fihman V,

Venditti M, Cordonnier C (2018) De-escalation and discontinuation strategies in high-risk neutropenic patients: an interrupted time series analyses of antimicrobial consumption and impact on outcome. Eur J Clin Microbiol Infect Dis 37(10):1931–1940. https://doi.org/10.1007/s10096-018-3328-1

McDonald LC, Gerding DN, Johnson S, Bakken JS, Carroll KC, Coffin SE, Dubberke ER, Garey KW, Gould CV, Kelly C, Loo V, Shaklee Sammons J, Sandora TJ, Wilcox MH (2018) Clinical practice guidelines for Clostridium difficile infection in adults and children: 2017 update by the Infectious Diseases Society of America (IDSA) and Society for Healthcare Epidemiology of America (SHEA). Clin Infect Dis 66(7):987–994. https://doi.org/10.1093/cid/ciy149

Mellinghoff SC, Hartmann P, Cornely FB, Knauth L, Kohler F, Kohler P, Krause C, Kronenberg C, Kranz SL, Menon V, Muller H, Naendrup JH, Putzfeld S, Ronge A, Rutz J, Seidel D, Wisplinghoff H, Cornely OA (2018a) Analyzing candidemia guideline adherence identifies opportunities for antifungal stewardship. Eur J Clin Microbiol Infect Dis 37(8):1563–1571. https://doi.org/10.1007/s10096-018-3285-8

Mellinghoff SC, Hoenigl M, Koehler P, Kumar A, Lagrou K, Lass-Florl C, Meis JF, Menon V, Rautemaa-Richardson R, Cornely OA (2018b) EQUAL Candida score: an ECMM score derived from current guidelines to measure QUAlity of clinical Candidaemia management. Mycoses 61(5):326–330. https://doi.org/10.1111/myc.12746

Mensa J, Barberán J, Soriano A, Llinares P, Marco F, Cantón R, Bou G, González Del Castillo J, Maseda E, Azanza JR, Pasquau J, García-Vidal C, Reguera JM, Sousa D, Gomez J, Montejo M, Borges M, Torres A, Álvarez-Lerma F, Salavert M, Zaragoza R, Oliver A (2018) Antibiotic selection in the treatment of acute invasive infections by Pseudomonas aeruginosa: guidelines by the Spanish Society of Chemotherapy. Rev Esp Quimioter 31(1):78–100

Messacar K, Parker SK, Todd JK, Dominguez SR (2017) Implementation of rapid molecular infectious disease diagnostics: the role of diagnostic and antimicrobial stewardship. J Clin Microbiol 55(3):715–723. https://doi.org/10.1128/JCM.02264-16

Mikulska M, Averbuch D, Tissot F, Cordonnier C, Akova M, Calandra T, Ceppi M, Bruzzi P, Viscoli C, European Conference on Infections in L (2018) Fluoroquinolone prophylaxis in haematological cancer patients with neutropenia: ECIL critical appraisal of previous guidelines. J Infect 76(1):20–37. https://doi.org/10.1016/j.jinf.2017.10.009

Miller RA (2018) A case for antifungal stewardship. Curr Fungal Infect Rep 12(33). https://doi.org/10.1007/s12281-018-0307-z

Molina J, Penalva G, Gil-Navarro MV, Praena J, Lepe JA, Pérez-Moreno MA, Ferrándiz C, Aldabo T, Aguilar M, Olbrich P, Jimenez-Mejias ME, Gascon ML, Amaya-Villar R, Neth O, Rodríguez-Hernandez MJ, Gutierrez-Pizarraya A, Garnacho-Montero J, Montero C, Cano J, Palomino J, Valencia R, Álvarez R, Cordero E, Herrero M, Cisneros JM, team P (2017) Long-term impact of an educational antimicrobial stewardship program on hospital-acquired Candidemia and multidrug-resistant bloodstream infections: a quasi-experimental study of interrupted time-series analysis. Clin Infect Dis 65(12):1992–1999. https://doi.org/10.1093/cid/cix692

Mondain V, Lieutier F, Hasseine L, Gari-Toussaint M, Poiree M, Lions C, Pulcini C (2013) A 6-year antifungal stewardship programme in a teaching hospital. Infection 41(3):621–628. https://doi.org/10.1007/s15010-013-0431-1

Morley GL, Wacogne ID (2017) UK recommendations for combating antimicrobial resistance: a review of 'antimicrobial stewardship: systems and processes for effective antimicrobial medicine use' (NICE guideline NG15, 2015) and related guidance. Arch Dis Child Educ Pract Ed. https://doi.org/10.1136/archdischild-2016-311557

Muñoz P, Rojas L, Cervera C, Garrido G, Fariñas MC, Valerio M, Giannella M, Bouza E, Group CS (2012) Poor compliance with antifungal drug use guidelines by transplant physicians: a framework for educational guidelines and an international consensus on patient safety. Clin Transpl 26(1):87–96. https://doi.org/10.1111/j.1399-0012.2011.01405.x

Orasch C, Averbuch D, Mikulska M, Cordonnier C, Livermore DM, Gyssens IC, Klyasova G, Engelhard D, Kern W, Viscoli C, Akova M, Marchetti O, th European Conference on Infections in L, joint venture of Infectious Diseases Working Party of the European Group for B, Marrow T, Infectious Diseases Group of the European Organization for R, Treatment of C, International Immunocompromised Host S, European Leukemia N, European Study Group on Infections in Immunocompromised Hosts of the European Society for Clinical M, Infectious D (2015) Discontinuation of empirical antibiotic therapy in neutropenic leukaemia patients with fever of unknown origin is ethical. Clin Microbiol Infect 21(3):e25–e27. https://doi.org/10.1016/j.cmi.2014.10.014

Paño-Pardo JR, Campos J, Natera Kindelan C, Ramos A (2013) Initiatives and resources to promote antimicrobial stewardship. Enferm Infecc Microbiol Clin 31(Suppl 4):51–55. https://doi.org/10.1016/S0213-005X(13)70133-2

Patel R, Fang FC (2018) Diagnostic stewardship: opportunity for a laboratory-infectious diseases partnership. Clin Infect Dis 67(5):799–801. https://doi.org/10.1093/cid/ciy077

Pulcini C, Binda F, Lamkang AS, Trett A, Charani E, Goff DA, Harbarth S, Hinrichsen SL, Levy-Hara G, Mendelson M, Nathwani D, Gunturu R, Singh S, Srinivasan A, Thamlikitkul V, Thursky K, Vlieghe E, Wertheim H, Zeng M, Gandra S, Laxminarayan R (2018) Developing core elements and checklist items for global hospital antimicrobial stewardship programmes: a consensus approach. Clin Microbiol Infect. https://doi.org/10.1016/j.cmi.2018.03.033

Pulcini C, Binda F, Lamkang AS, Trett A, Charani E, Goff DA, Harbarth S, Hinrichsen SL, Levy-Hara G, Mendelson M, Nathwani D, Gunturu R, Singh S, Srinivasan A, Thamlikitkul V, Thursky K, Vlieghe E, Wertheim H, Zeng M, Gandra S, Laxminarayan R (2019) Developing core elements and checklist items for global hospital antimicrobial stewardship programmes: a consensus approach. Clin Microbiol Infect 25(1):20–25. https://doi.org/10.1016/j.cmi.2018.03.033

Ramos A, Pérez-Velilla C, Asensio A, Ruiz-Antorán B, Folguera C, Cantero M, Orden B, Muñez E (2015) Antifungal stewardship in a tertiary hospital. Rev Iberoam Micol 32(4):209–213. https://doi.org/10.1016/j.riam.2014.11.006

Ramsey A, Staicu ML (2018) Use of a penicillin allergy screening algorithm and penicillin skin testing for transitioning hospitalized patients to first-line antibiotic therapy. J Allergy Clin Immunol Pract 6(4):1349–1355. https://doi.org/10.1016/j.jaip.2017.11.012

Rautemaa-Richardson R, Rautemaa V, Al-Wathiqi F, Moore CB, Craig L, Felton TW, Muldoon EG (2018) Impact of a diagnostics-driven antifungal stewardship programme in a UK tertiary referral teaching hospital. J Antimicrob Chemother 73(12):3488–3495. https://doi.org/10.1093/jac/dky360

Robilotti E, Holubar M, Seo SK, Deresinski S (2017) Feasibility and applicability of antimicrobial stewardship in immunocompromised patients. Curr Opin Infect Dis 30(4):346–353. https://doi.org/10.1097/QCO.0000000000000380

Rodríguez-Baño J, Paño-Pardo JR, Álvarez-Rocha L, Asensio A, Calbo E, Cercenado E, Cisneros JM, Cobo J, Delgado O, Garnacho-Montero J, Grau S, Horcajada JP, Hornero A, Murillas-Angoiti J, Oliver A, Padilla B, Pasquau J, Pujol M, Ruiz-Garbajosa P, San Juan R, Sierra R, Grupo de Estudio de la Infeccion Hospitalaria-Sociedad Espanola de Enfermedades Infecciosas y Microbiologia C, Sociedad Espanola de Farmacia H, Sociedad Espanola de Medicina Preventiva SPeH (2012) Programs for optimizing the use of antibiotics (PROA) in Spanish hospitals: GEIH-SEIMC, SEFH and SEMPSPH consensus document. Enferm Infecc Microbiol Clin 22(1):e21–22 e23. https://doi.org/10.1016/j.eimc.2011.09.018

Rosa RG, Goldani LZ, dos Santos RP (2014) Association between adherence to an antimicrobial stewardship program and mortality among hospitalised cancer patients with febrile neutropaenia: a prospective cohort study. BMC Infect Dis 14:286. https://doi.org/10.1186/1471-2334-14-286

Ruiz-Ramos J, Frasquet J, Poveda-Andres JL, Roma E, Salavert-Lleti M, Castellanos A, Ramírez P (2017) Impact of an antimicrobial stewardship program on critical haematological patients. Farm Hosp 41(4):479–487. https://doi.org/10.7399/fh.2017.41.4.10709

Santolaya ME, Álvarez AM, Acuna M, Avilés CL, Salgado C, Tordecilla J, Varas M, Venegas M, Villarroel M, Zubieta M, Toso A, Bataszew A, Farfán MJ, de la Maza V, Vergara A, Valenzuela R, Torres JP (2017) Efficacy and safety of withholding antimicrobial treatment in children with cancer, fever and neutropenia, with a demonstrated viral respiratory infection: a randomized clinical trial. Clin Microbiol Infect 23(3):173–178. https://doi.org/10.1016/j.cmi.2016.11.001

Shlaes DM, Gerding DN, John JF Jr, Craig WA, Bornstein DL, Duncan RA, Eckman MR, Farrer WE, Greene WH, Lorian V, Levy S, McGowan JE Jr, Paul SM, Ruskin J, Tenover FC, Watanakunakorn C (1997) Society for Healthcare Epidemiology of America and Infectious Diseases Society of America joint committee on the Prevention of antimicrobial resistance: guidelines for the prevention of antimicrobial resistance in hospitals. Clin Infect Dis 25(3):584–599

Snyder M, Pasikhova Y, Baluch A (2017) Early antimicrobial De-escalation and stewardship in adult hematopoietic stem cell transplantation recipients: retrospective review. Open forum. Infect Dis 4(4):ofx226. https://doi.org/10.1093/ofid/ofx226

So M, Mamdani MM, Morris AM, Lau TTY, Broady R, Deotare U, Grant J, Kim D, Schimmer AD, Schuh AC, Shajari S, Steinberg M, Bell CM, Husain S (2018) Effect of an antimicrobial stewardship programme on antimicrobial utilisation and costs in patients with leukaemia: a retrospective controlled study. Clin Microbiol Infect 24(8):882–888. https://doi.org/10.1016/j.cmi.2017.11.009

Spec A, Mejia-Chew C, Powderly WG, Cornely OA (2018) EQUAL Cryptococcus score 2018: a European Confederation of Medical Mycology Score Derived from Current Guidelines to measure QUALity of clinical Cryptococcosis management. Open forum infect dis 5 (11):ofy299. https://doi.org/10.1093/ofid/ofy299

Stanzani M, Vianelli N, Cavo M, Maritati A, Morotti M, Lewis RE (2017) Retrospective cohort analysis of liposomal amphotericin B nephrotoxicity in patients with hematological malignancies. Antimicrob Agents Chemother 61(9). https://doi.org/10.1128/AAC.02651-16

Theuretzbacher U (2012) Pharmacokinetic and pharmacodynamic issues for antimicrobial therapy in patients with cancer. Clin Infect Dis 54(12):1785–1792. https://doi.org/10.1093/cid/cis210

Timbrook TT, Hurst JM, Bosso JA (2016) Impact of an antimicrobial stewardship program on antimicrobial utilization, bacterial susceptibilities, and financial expenditures at an Academic Medical Center. Hosp Pharm 51(9):703–711. https://doi.org/10.1310/hpj5109-703

Trubiano JA, Thursky KA, Stewardson AJ, Urbancic K, Worth LJ, Jackson C, Stevenson W, Sutherland M, Slavin MA, Grayson ML, Phillips EJ (2017) Impact of an integrated antibiotic allergy testing program on antimicrobial stewardship: a multicenter evaluation. Clin Infect Dis 65(1):166–174. https://doi.org/10.1093/cid/cix244

Valerio M, Rodríguez-González CG, Munoz P, Cáliz B, Sanjurjo M, Bouza E, Group CS (2014) Evaluation of antifungal use in a tertiary care institution: antifungal stewardship urgently needed. J Antimicrob Chemother 69(7):1993–1999. https://doi.org/10.1093/jac/dku053

Valerio M, Muñoz P, Rodríguez CG, Caliz B, Padilla B, Fernández-Cruz A, Sánchez-Somolinos M, Gijón P, Peral J, Gayoso J, Frías I, Salcedo M, Sanjurjo M, Bouza E, Mycosis CSGCGo (2015a) Antifungal stewardship in a tertiary-care institution: a bedside intervention. Clin Microbiol Infect 21(5):492 e491–492 e499. https://doi.org/10.1016/j.cmi.2015.01.013

Valerio M, Vena A, Bouza E, Reiter N, Viale P, Hochreiter M, Giannella M, Munoz P, group Cs (2015b) How much European prescribing physicians know about invasive fungal infections management? BMC Infect Dis 15:80. https://doi.org/10.1186/s12879-015-0809-z

Valerio M, Muñoz P, Rodríguez-González C, Sanjurjo M, Guinea J, Bouza E, group Cs (2015c) Training should be the first step toward an antifungal stewardship program. Enferm Infecc Microbiol Clin 33(4):221–227. https://doi.org/10.1016/j.eimc.2014.04.016

Valerio M, Vena A, Rodríguez-González CG, de Vega EC, Mateos M, Sanjurjo M, Bouza E, Muñoz P, Group CS (2018) Repeated antifungal use audits are essential for selecting the targets for intervention in antifungal stewardship. Eur J Clin Microbiol Infect Dis 37(10):1993–2000. https://doi.org/10.1007/s10096-018-3335-2

Vazquez J, Reboli AC, Pappas PG, Patterson TF, Reinhardt J, Chin-Hong P, Tobin E, Kett DH, Biswas P, Swanson R (2014) Evaluation of an early step-down strategy from intravenous anidulafungin to oral azole therapy for the treatment of candidemia and other forms of invasive candidiasis: results from an open-label trial. BMC Infect Dis 14:97. https://doi.org/10.1186/1471-2334-14-97

Vena A, Bouza E, Álvarez-Uría A, Gayoso J, Martín-Rabadán P, Cajuste F, Guinea J, Gomez Castellá J, Alonso R, Muñoz P (2017) The misleading effect of serum galactomannan testing in high-risk haematology patients receiving prophylaxis with micafungin. Clin Microbiol Infect 23(12):1000 e1001–1000 e1004. https://doi.org/10.1016/j.cmi.2017.05.006

Viale P, Giannella M, Bartoletti M, Tedeschi S, Lewis R (2015) Considerations about antimicrobial stewardship in settings with epidemic extended-Spectrum beta-lactamase-producing or Carbapenem-resistant Enterobacteriaceae. Infect Dis Ther 4(Suppl 1):65–83. https://doi.org/10.1007/s40121-015-0081-y

Whitney L, Al-Ghusein H, Glass S, Koh M, Klammer M, Ball J, Youngs J, Wake R, Houston A, Bicanic T (2019) Effectiveness of an antifungal stewardship programme at a London teaching hospital 2010-16. J Antimicrob Chemother 74(1):234–241. https://doi.org/10.1093/jac/dky389

de With K, Allerberger F, Amann S, Apfalter P, Brodt HR, Eckmanns T, Fellhauer M, Geiss HK, Janata O, Krause R, Lemmen S, Meyer E, Mittermayer H, Porsche U, Presterl E, Reuter S, Sinha B, Strauss R, Wechsler-Fordos A, Wenisch C, Kern WV (2016) Strategies to enhance rational use of antibiotics in hospital: a guideline by the German Society for Infectious Diseases. Infection 44(3):395–439. https://doi.org/10.1007/s15010-016-0885-z

Yeo CL, Chan DS, Earnest A, Wu TS, Yeoh SF, Lim R, Jureen R, Fisher D, Hsu LY (2012) Prospective audit and feedback on antibiotic prescription in an adult hematology-oncology unit in Singapore. Eur J Clin Microbiol Infect Dis 31(4):583–590. https://doi.org/10.1007/s10096-011-1351-6

Intensive Care

10

Dimitrios K. Matthaiou and George Dimopoulos

Patients with hematological malignancy are very likely to be in need of intensive care either due to complications of treatment or due to factors related directly to the severity of their disease or their susceptibility to infection. Although the prognosis of such patients was not at all favorable in the beginning, there has been a notable improvement during the last decades due to advances in hematology, oncology, and intensive care. According to a recent meta-analysis (Darmon et al. 2019), there has been a steady decrease in mortality over time in critically ill hematological patients, with the exception of allogeneic stem cell transplant recipients. Thus, there has been a shift from a rather nihilistic approach of no admission to the ICU to a short ICU admission period depending on the severity. In another recent single-center study (Kondakci et al. 2019) comparing ICU survival in hematological patients over two subsequent periods, a distinct increase in survival was noted from 45.2% to 66.7%. This increase was considered to be the result of treatment improvements, but most importantly, to changes of admittance policy, namely timelier admission to the ICU.

Further studies seem to acknowledge this finding. In a recent single-center study (Sauer et al. 2019), the proportion of cancer patients in the ICU increased steadily. However, although 28-day and 1-year mortality were strongly associated with hematological cancers, they both decreased over the 10-year study period. Hematologic patients, compared to solid cancer patients, showed the strongest annual adjusted decrease. In another time trend analysis of long-term outcome in patients with hematological malignancies, an annual decrease in 1-year mortality of 7% was found (de Vries et al. 2018). It should also be noted that, according to this study, the Acute Physiology, Chronic Health Evaluation (APACHE) II score was found to overestimate mortality in this patient population.

This chapter focuses on the following:

(a) When should a patient with hematological malignancy be admitted in the ICU?
(b) What is the prognosis of these patients?
(c) How long should a patient with hematological malignancy be treated in the ICU?
(d) How should a patient with hematological malignancy be treated in the ICU?

10.1 When Should a Patient with Hematological Malignancy Be Admitted in the ICU?

The main reasons for admission of a patient with hematological malignancy in the ICU are complications of treatment for the malignancy or critical illness due to the disease and sepsis, as such patients

D. K. Matthaiou (✉) · G. Dimopoulos (✉)
Department of Critical Care, Attikon University Hospital, University of Athens, Athens, Greece
e-mail: gdimop@med.auth.gr

© Springer Nature Switzerland AG 2021
O. A. Cornely, M. Hoenigl (eds.), *Infection Management in Hematology*, Hematologic Malignancies, https://doi.org/10.1007/978-3-030-57317-1_10

are more susceptible to infectious complications and respiratory failure. The decision of admission to the ICU should be the result of close cooperation between hematologists and intensivists, as there are ethical issues related to end-of-life care for these patients. Thus, a concise decision-making process should be followed (Malak et al. 2014).

First, it is important to assess the hematological status of the patient. Patients with hematological malignancies that have either complete remission after first-line treatment or a good response will mostly benefit from being admitted. In this case, the clinical severity of the patient's condition should be no reason to avoid admission.

However, the deterioration of the hematological status necessitates a careful approach on whether such a patient may benefit from admission. This group includes patients who have either partial response to chemotherapy or relapsed but are still chemosensitive. In this case, other factors should be also taken under consideration including the performance status of the patient, comorbidities, the severity of the disease, age of the patient, as well as the prognosis of the malignancy per se. Also patients with allogeneic bone marrow transplantation as well as patients' high-risk morbidities related to treatment belong to this group. The former have increased mortality compared to overall patient population, while the latter face several ethical issues regarding the potential clinical benefit of treatment contrary to the risks it may pose. In both cases, prognosis assessment may have a crucial role on whether such patients should be transferred in the ICU.

When the underlying disease is irreversible and thus in a palliative stage, then admission to the ICU is futile. The decision not to admit should be clearly explained to the patient and family of the patient, as well as documented in the patient file. In this context, all necessary palliative care should be provided to the patient.

10.2 What Is the Prognosis of These Patients?

Prognosis in patients with hematological malignancies is worse than the general population. There are a number of factors that have been

Table 10.1 Factors associated with mortality in patients with hematological malignancy

Clinical factors	Hematological factors
Simplified acute physiology score II	Neutropenia
Charlson comorbidity index	Performance status (ECOG score > 2)
Sequential organ failure assessment score	Malignant lymphoma
Invasive mechanical ventilation	Hematopoetic stem cell transplantation (HCT-CI score > 2)
Use of vasopressors	Hematological relapse
Hemodialysis	
Prolonged ICU treatment	
Delay in ICU admission	

associated with unfavorable outcomes in patients with hematological malignancy admitted in the ICU, which are either clinical or hematological (Table 10.1.)

Clinical factors include multi-organ failure, high APACHE II or Sequential Organ Failure Assessment (SOFA) or Simplified Acute Physiology Score (SAPS) II score, mechanical ventilation, use of vasopressors, and hemodialysis. Hematological factors include allogeneic hematopoietic stem cell transplantation, performance status>2 as measured by Eastern Cooperative Oncology Group (ECOG) (Zubrod) score, relapse of the disease, malignant lymphoma, and neutropenia.(Al-Zubaidi et al. 2018; Camou et al. 2019; Cornish et al. 2016; Georges et al. 2018; Scheich et al. 2018; Irie et al. 2017; Schuitemaker et al. 2017).

Regarding the use of severity scores in predicting mortality, modifications of the original Sequential Organ Failure Assessment Score (SOFA) have been proposed. The prognostic value of hematological SOFA (SOFAhem), which was defined as the original SOFA score omitting the coagulation and neurological parameters, has been assessed compared to original SOFA score as predictors of mortality in hematological patients (Demandt et al. 2017). Increasing trends in SOFAhem score were independently associated with mortality. Furthermore, it was found to have a stronger relation to mortality compared to the original SOFA score, as it presented higher odds ratios and lower P-values. In another recent study (Greenberg et al. 2016), the prognostic value of a modified SOFA score to account for infection was assessed. The modified score was compared with the original SOFA score, as well as APACHE II score. The modified score had a wider area under the receiver operator characteristic curve. Furthermore, it served as a better discriminator of survivors from non-survivors.

Another very important factor associated with mortality is the increased time from the onset of symptoms to the ICU admission, especially when the patient was admitted more than 24 hours after the onset of symptoms. It was found that in such cases, there was increased use of mechanical ventilation, use of vasopressors, a subsequent prolongation of ICU stay, and increased mortality (Mokart et al. 2013).

The role of bloodstream infections due to multidrug-resistant (MDR) Gram-negative bacteria, especially non-fermenters, as predictor of mortality should be noted. In a recent retrospective single-center study (Scheich et al. 2018), the impact of such infections was assessed. Mortality of patients with MDR Gram-negative bloodstream infection was significantly higher compared to patients with susceptible Gram-negative bloodstream infection. Bloodstream infection due to MDR non-fermentative Gram-negative bacteria and admission in the ICU was independently associated with an increased 30-day mortality.

10.3   How Long Should a Patient with Hematological Malignancy Be Treated in the ICU?

The optimal treatment duration in the ICU in these patients remains unclear. It should be decided depending on patient severity and disease prognosis. In a recent study (Shrime et al. 2016) comparing time-unlimited versus time-limited trials of intensive care assessing 30-day all-cause mortality and mean survival duration, patients with hematological malignancies or less severe illness seemed to benefit from 8 to 12 days

of intensive care. However, regular reassessment every 4–5 days is necessary to decide whether further treatment is beneficial or futile.

Especially for allogeneic stem cell transplantation recipients, early ICU admission should happen as soon as they develop organ failure, as this is associated with decreased mortality. A recent study (Orvain et al. 2018) assessing a score combining the number of organ injuries prior to ICU admission with the time from first organ injury to ICU admission found a significantly higher in-hospital mortality rate even after adjustment for refractory acute graft-versus-host disease (GVHD) and the SOFA score.

10.4   How Should a Patient with Hematological Malignancy Be Treated in the ICU?

A hematologic patient is not essentially different from other patients admitted in the ICU when it comes to infection, with the exception of certain aspects of sepsis management, as well as of respiratory failure. These aspects are the ones this chapter is focusing on, but not in detail, as they are explicitly covered in other chapters.

10.4.1 Respiratory Failure

A major question regarding the respiratory support of such patients is whether non-invasive or invasive ventilation should be used. The etiology is variable including pneumonia, non-infectious diagnoses, and other opportunistic infections. However, in a considerable proportion of around 15%, the etiology of acute respiratory failure may be undetermined and have the higher mortality (Contejean et al. 2016).

It is interesting that non-invasive ventilation at an early stage seems to be associated with lower mortality. However, a high percentage receiving non-invasive ventilation ultimately deteriorate and proceed to intubation (Amado-Rodríguez et al. 2016). A recent study compared non-invasive versus invasive ventilation for acute respiratory failure in patients with hematologic malignancies (Gristina et al. 2011). Although only 20% of the included patients initially received non-invasive mechanical ventilation, almost half of them needed to switch to invasive mechanical ventilation. It is important to note that when non-invasive ventilation was successful, it was associated with improved outcomes, especially in patients with acute lung injury or adult respiratory distress syndrome.

In a recent study (Lee et al. 2015) assessing high-flow nasal cannula oxygen (HFNO) therapy for acute respiratory failure in patients with hematological malignancies, 67% of the recipients failed and needed to change to invasive ventilation. Although no difference was found regarding the severity of the underlying comorbidities, patients who failed with HFNO treatment had a significantly higher percentage of bacterial pneumonia.

Generally, studies report failure of non-invasive ventilation ranging from 40% to over 60%. Even worse patients who switch to invasive ventilation have an increased mortality of up to 80% (Molina et al. 2012). Thus, hematological patients receiving non-invasive ventilation should be very carefully, if at all, selected. Even then, they should be closely monitored and switched to invasive mechanical ventilation as soon as they deteriorate (Schnell et al. 2016; Kusadasi et al. 2017).

A retrospective analysis assessed factors associated with the successful extubation of patients who received invasive mechanical ventilation (Fujiwara et al. 2016). Several factors were identified including respiratory management in an ICU, remission of the hematological disease, female gender, low levels of accompanying non-respiratory organ failure, and the non-use of extracorporeal circulation. However, the only factor independently associated with successful extubation was the respiratory management in an ICU.

The timing of intubation is also an important factor regarding outcome. In a study assessing early predictors of mortality in patients with cancer and acute respiratory failure who were intubated after their admission in the ICU, mortality at day 28 was more than 30%. Factors independently associated with mortality were age, more than one line of chemotherapy, time between respiratory symptoms onset and ICU admission >2 days, oxygen flow at admission, and extra-respiratory symptoms. However, after adjustment for the logistic organ dysfunction score, only time between respiratory symptoms onset and ICU admission more than 2 days and logistic organ dysfunction score were independently associated with mortality (Mokart et al. 2013). These results show the necessity for timely intubation of such patients with acute respiratory failure.

10.4.2 Sepsis/Neutropenia

Sepsis is a very common cause of admission of hematological patients in the ICU. It should be kept in mind that this population may manifest very subtle, if any, signs and symptoms of infection. Such patients are at risk of infection due to conventional as well as opportunistic pathogens. Increased vigilance is necessary for timely intervention. Treatment bundles according to the Surviving Sepsis Campaign (Rhodes et al. 2017) should be followed and the special characteristics of this patient population be taken into account.

Regarding antibiotics, combination therapy should not be used for the routine treatment of sepsis in presence of neutropenia when the etiologic agent is documented. However, combination therapy including aminoglycosides as empirical treatment can be used when the pathogen is unknown and broadening of antimicrobial activity is necessary. It may include antibiotics with activity against Gram-negative pathogens, including anti-pseudomonal agents, as well antibiotics with activity against Gram-positive cocci, especially in suspicion of a catheter-related infection, skin or soft tissue infection or severe mucositis. The presence of opportunistic pathogens, such as yeasts, aspergillus and other molds, and varicella or cytomegalovirus (CMV) should also be actively sought and covered, especially when there is persistent, recurrent fever despite the presence of broad-spectrum antibiotic coverage (Kiehl et al. 2018; Wise et al. 2015; Schnell et al. 2016).

Source control is important. All indwelling catheters should be removed and substituted including central vascular catheters, tunneled catheters, and urinary catheters. Especially for tunneled catheters, if their removal is not possible, prolonged antimicrobial therapy may be administered, when fungemia and septic shock are absent. However, intra-tracheal intubation should not be delayed when neutropenia is present (Schnell et al. 2016; Kiehl et al. 2018; Beed et al. 2010).

Treatment duration may vary. Although antibiotic therapy should be as short as possible to avoid the selection of resistant strains, de-escalation of treatment should not be considered unless the patient is stable with a documented infection due to a pathogen susceptible to the administered antibiotic treatment and neutropenia has remitted. In cases of slow clinical response, undrainable foci of infection, and persistent neutropenia, longer antibiotic courses should be administered (Schnell et al. 2016).

Selective oral decontamination or selective digestive decontamination should be administered upon admission. It is of particular importance in high risk-patients who manifest mucositis, such as recipients of chemotherapy or myeloablation (Schuitemaker et al. 2017).

It is not clear whether granulocyte colony-stimulating factor (G-CSF) is of benefit during neutropenia in the ICU. Prophylactic use may decrease the duration of neutropenia. However, G-CSF administration is of limited benefit in neutropenic patients with sepsis. Furthermore, G-CSF administration is associated with side effects and worsening of the respiratory status. Thus, close monitoring is necessary and G-CSF should be stopped when respiratory deterioration is suspected. The decision of G-CSF administration should be done on a case-by-case-basis, in cooperation with the hematologist (Wise et al. 2015).

10.5   Summary

Patients with hematological malignancy can be in need of intensive care due to various reasons. There has been a steady decrease in mortality, which reflects advances in hematology and intensive care. The decision of admission to the ICU should be the result of a close cooperation between hematologists and intensivists, aiming at addressing various ethical issues, and should be based on a decision-making process. Several factors have been associated with unfavorable outcomes in such patients, which are either clinical or hematological. Hematological patients seem to benefit from 8 to 12 days of intensive care, but regular reassessment every 4 to 5 days is necessary if treatment is to be continued. Regarding treatment, there are certain aspects of sepsis and respiratory support that necessitate a different approach for the hematological patient compared to others. Non-invasive ventilation should be generally avoided, unless patients are carefully selected. Timely intubation is of paramount importance. Sepsis should be treated according to the bundles proposed by Surviving Sepsis Campaign keeping in mind the special characteristics of this patient population.

References

Al-Zubaidi N, Shehada E, Alshabani K, ZazaDitYafawi J, Kingah P, Soubani AO (2018) Predictors of outcome in patients with hematologic malignancies admitted to the intensive care unit. Hematol Oncol Stem Cell Ther 11(4):206–218. https://doi.org/10.1016/j.hemonc.2018.03.003

Amado-Rodríguez L, Bernal T, López-Alonso I, Blázquez-Prieto J, García-Prieto E, Albaiceta GM (2016) Impact of initial Ventilatory strategy in hematological patients with acute respiratory failure: a systematic review and meta-analysis. Crit Care Med 44(7):1406–1413. https://doi.org/10.1097/CCM.0000000000001613

Beed M, Levitt M, WaqasBokhari S (2010) Intensive care management of patients with haematological malignancy, Continuing Education in Anaesthesia. Critical Care & Pain 10(6):167–171. https://doi.org/10.1093/bjaceaccp/mkq034

Camou F, Didier M, Leguay T, Milpied N, Daste A, Ravaud A, Mourissoux G, Guisset O, Issa N (2019) Long-term prognosis of septic shock in cancer patients. Support Care Cancer. https://doi.org/10.1007/s00520-019-04937-4

Contejean A, Lemiale V, Resche-Rigon M, Mokart D, Pène F, Kouatchet A, Mayaux J, Vincent F, Nyunga M, Bruneel F, Rabbat A, Perez P, Meert AP, Benoit D, Hamidfar R, Darmon M, Jourdain M, Renault A, Schlemmer B, Azoulay E (2016) Increased mortality in hematological malignancy patients with acute respiratory failure from undetermined etiology: a Groupe de RechercheenRéanimationRespiratoireen Onco-Hématologique (Grrr-OH) study. Ann Intensive Care 6(1):102. https://doi.org/10.1186/s13613-016-0202-0

Cornish M, Butler MB, Green RS (2016) Predictors of poor outcomes in critically ill adults with hematologic malignancy. Can Respir J 2016:9431385. https://doi.org/10.1155/2016/9431385

Darmon M, Bourmaud A, Georges Q, Soares M, Jeon K, Oeyen S, Rhee CK, Gruber P, Ostermann M, Hill QA, Depuydt P, Ferra C, Toffart AC, Schellongowski P, Müller A, Lemiale V, Mokart D, Azoulay E (2019) Changes in critically ill cancer patients' short-term outcome over the last decades: results of systematic review with meta-analysis on individual data. Intensive Care Med 45(7):977–987. https://doi.org/10.1007/s00134-019-05653-7

Demandt AMP, Geerse DA, Janssen BJP, Winkens B, Schouten HC, van Mook WNKA (2017) The prognostic value of a trend in modified SOFA score for patients with hematological malignancies in the intensive care unit. Eur J Haematol 99(4):315–322. https://doi.org/10.1111/ejh.12919

Fujiwara Y, Yamaguchi H, Kobayashi K, Marumo A, Omori I, Yamanaka S, Yui S, Fukunaga K, Ryotokuji T, Hirakawa T, Okabe M, Wakita S, Tamai H, Okamoto M, Nakayama K, Takeda S, Inokuchi K (2016) The therapeutic outcomes of mechanical ventilation in hematological malignancy patients with respiratory failure. Intern Med 55(12):1537–1545. https://doi.org/10.2169/internalmedicine.55.5822

Georges Q, Azoulay E, Mokart D, Soares M, Jeon K, Oeyen S, Rhee CK, Gruber P, Ostermann M, Hill QA, Depuydt P, Ferra C, Toffart AC, Schellongowski P, Müller A, Lemiale V, Tinquaut F, Bourmaud A, Darmon M (2018) Influence of neutropenia on mortality of critically ill cancer patients: results of a meta-analysis on individual data. Crit Care 22(1):326. https://doi.org/10.1186/s13054-018-2076-z

Gristina, Giuseppe R. MD; Antonelli, Massimo MD; Conti, Giorgio MD; Ciarlone, Alessia MD; Rogante, Silvia MD; Rossi, Carlotta Stat Sci; Bertolini, Guido MD on behalf of the GiViTI (Italian Group for the Evaluation of Interventions in Intensive Care Medicine) Noninvasive versus invasive ventilation for acute respiratory failure in patients with hematologic malignancies: A 5-year multicenter observational survey*, Critical Care Medicine. 2011;39(10):2232–2239 10.1097/CCM.0b013e3182227a27.

Greenberg JA, David MZ, Churpek MM, Pitrak DL, Hall JB, Kress JP (2016) Sequential organ failure assessment score modified for recent infection in patients with hematologic malignant tumors and severe Sepsis. Am J Crit Care 25(5):409–417. https://doi.org/10.4037/ajcc2016281

Irie H, Otake T, Kawai K, Hino M, Namazu A, Shinjo Y, Yamashita S (2017) Prognostic factors in critically ill patients with hematological malignancy admitted to the general intensive care unit: a single-center expe-rience in Japan. J Anesth 31(5):736–743. https://doi.org/10.1007/s00540-017-2390-7

Kiehl MG, Beutel G, Böll B, Buchheidt D, Forkert R, Fuhrmann V, Knöbl P, Kochanek M, Kroschinsky F, La Rosée P, Liebregts T, Lück C, Olgemoeller U, Schalk E, Shimabukuro-Vornhagen A, Sperr WR, Staudinger T, von BergweltBaildon M, Wohlfarth P, Zeremski V, Schellongowski P, Consensus of the German Society of Hematology and Medical Oncology (DGHO), Austrian Society of Hematology and Oncology (OeGHO), German Society for Medical Intensive Care Medicine and Emergency Medicine (DGIIN), and Austrian Society of Medical and General Intensive Care and Emergency Medicine (ÖGIAIN) (2018) Consensus statement for cancer patients requiring intensive care support. Ann Hematol 97(7):1271–1282. https://doi.org/10.1007/s00277-018-3312-y

Kondakci M, Reinbach MC, Germing U, Kobbe G, Fenk R, Schroeder T, Quader J, Zeus T, Rassaf T, Haas R (2019) Interaction of increasing ICU survival and admittance policies in patients with hematologic neoplasms: a single center experience with 304 patients. Eur J Haematol 102(3):265–274. https://doi.org/10.1111/ejh.13206

Kusadasi N, Müller MCA, van Westerloo DJ, Broers AEC, Hilkens MGEC (2017) Blijlevens on behalf of TheHema-Icu study group NMA. The management of critically ill patients with haematological malignancies. Neth J Med 75(7):265–271

Lee HY, Rhee CK, Lee JW (2015) Feasibility of high-flow nasal cannula oxygen therapyfor acute respiratory failure in patients with hematologic malignancies: Aretrospective single-center study. J Crit Care 30(4):773–777. https://doi.org/10.1016/j.jcrc.2015.03.014

Malak S, Sotto JJ, Ceccaldi J, Colombat P, Casassus P, Jaulmes D, Rochant H, Cheminant M, Beaussant Y, Zittoun R, Bordessoule D (2014) Ethical and clinical aspects of intensive care unit admission in patients with hematological malignancies: guidelines of the ethics commission of the French society of hematology. Adv Hematol 2014:704318. https://doi.org/10.1155/2014/704318

Mokart D, Lambert J, Schnell D, Fouché L, Rabbat A, Kouatchet A, Lemiale V, Vincent F, Lengliné E, Bruneel F, Pene F, Chevret S, Azoulay E (2013) Delayed intensive care unit admission is associated with increased mortality in patients with cancer with acute respiratory failure. Leuk Lymphoma 54(8):1724–1729. https://doi.org/10.3109/10428194.2012.753446

Molina R, Bernal T, Borges M, Zaragoza R, Bonastre J, Granada RM, Rodriguez-Borregán JC, Núñez K, Seijas I, Ayestaran I, Albaiceta GM, EMEHU study investigators (2012) Ventilatory support in critically ill hematology patients with respiratory failure. Crit Care 16:R133

Orvain C, Beloncle F, Hamel JF, Del Galy AS, Thépot S, Mercier M, Kouatchet A, Farhi J, Francois S, Ifrah N, Mercat A, Asfar P, Hunault-Berger M, Tanguy-

Schmidt A (2018) Allogeneic stem cell transplantation recipients requiring intensive care: time is of the essence. Ann Hematol 97(9):1601–1609. https://doi.org/10.1007/s00277-018-3320-y

Rhodes A, Evans LE, Alhazzani W, Levy MM, Antonelli M, Ferrer R, Kumar A, Sevransky JE, Sprung CL, Nunnally ME, Rochwerg B, Rubenfeld GD, Angus DC, Annane D, Beale RJ, Bellinghan GJ, Bernard GR, Chiche JD, Coopersmith C, De Backer DP, French CJ, Fujishima S, Gerlach H, Hidalgo JL, Hollenberg SM, Jones AE, KarnadDR KRM, Koh Y, Lisboa TC, Machado FR, Marini JJ, Marshall JC, Mazuski JE, LA MI, AS ML, Mehta S, Moreno RP, Myburgh J, Navalesi P, Nishida O, Osborn TM, Perner A, Plunkett CM, Ranieri M, Schorr CA, Seckel MA, Seymour CW, Shieh L, Shukri KA, Simpson SQ, Singer M, Thompson BT, Townsend SR, Van der Poll T, Vincent JL, Wiersinga WJ, Zimmerman JL, Dellinger RP (2017) Surviving SepsisCampaign: international guidelines for Management of Sepsis and Septic Shock:2016. Intensive Care Med 43(3):304–377. https://doi.org/10.1007/s00134-017-4683-6

Sauer CM, Dong J, Celi LA, Ramazzotti D (2019) Improved survival of Cancer patients admitted to the intensive care unit between 2002 and 2011 at a U.S. teaching hospital. Cancer Res Treat 51(3):973–981. https://doi.org/10.4143/crt.2018.360

Scheich S, Weber S, Reinheimer C, Wichelhaus TA, Hogardt M, Kempf VAJ, Kessel J, Serve H, Steffen B (2018) Bloodstream infections with gram-negative organisms and the impact of multidrug resistance in patients with hematological malignancies. Ann Hematol 97(11):2225–2234. https://doi.org/10.1007/s00277-018-3423-5

Schnell D, Azoulay E, Benoit D, Clouzeau B, Demaret P, Ducassou S, Frange P, Lafaurie M, Legrand M, Meert AP, Mokart D, Naudin J, Pene F, Rabbat A, Raffoux E, Ribaud P, Richard JC, Vincent F, Zahar JR, Darmon M (2016) Management of neutropenic patients in the intensive care unit (NEWBORNS EXCLUDED) recommendations from an expert panel from the French Intensive Care Society (SRLF) with the French Group for Pediatric Intensive Care Emergencies (GFRUP), the French Society of Anesthesia and Intensive Care (SFAR), the French Society of Hematology (SFH), the French Society for Hospital Hygiene (SF2H), and the French infectious diseases society (SPILF). Ann Intensive Care 6(1):90. https://doi.org/10.1186/s13613-016-0189-6

Schuitemaker, L. M., Marcella C.A. Müller, Nuray Kusadasi, A.E.C. Dieers, M.G.E.C. Hilkens, N.M.A. Blijlevens and David J. van Westerloo. "Guideline summary: intensive care admission, treatment and discharge of critically ill haemato-oncological patients." (2017)

Shrime MG, Ferket BS, Scott DJ, Lee J, Barragan-Bradford D, Pollard T, Arabi YM, Al-Dorzi HM, Baron RM, Hunink MG, Celi LA, Lai PS (2016) Time-limited trials of intensive Care for Critically ill Patients with Cancer: how long is long enough? JAMA Oncol 2(1):76–83. https://doi.org/10.1001/jamaoncol.2015.3336

de Vries VA, Müller MCA, SesmuArbous M, Biemond BJ, Blijlevens NMA, Kusadasi N, Choi GCW, Vlaar APJ, van Westerloo DJ, Kluin-Nelemans HC, van den Bergh WM, HEMA-ICU Study Group (2018) Time trend analysis of long term outcome of patients with haematological malignancies admitted at Dutch intensive care units. Br J Haematol 181(1):68–76. https://doi.org/10.1111/bjh.15140

Wise MP, Barnes RA, Baudouin SV, Howell D, Lyttelton M, Marks DI, Morris EC (2015) Parry-Jones N; British Committee for Standards in Haematology. Guidelines on the management and admission to intensive care of critically ill adult patients with haematological malignancy in the UK. Br J Haematol 171(2):179–188. https://doi.org/10.1111/bjh.13594

Gram-Positive Infections

11

Alessandro Busca, Silvia Corcione, and Francesco Giuseppe De Rosa

11.1 Epidemiology and Risk Factors

Despite remarkable improvements achieved in the management of patients with malignant hematologic disorders, infectious complications persist as a leading cause of morbidity and mortality, particularly during the neutropenic phase subsequent to chemotherapy treatment.

Bloodstream infection (BSI) affects 11% to 40% of neutropenic patients with an associated mortality ranging from 5% up to 60% in cases of multi-drug resistant (MDR) BSI (Gudiol et al. 2011; Gaytan-Martinez et al. 2000; Cl et al. 2012). The epidemiology of BSI has been changing during the years: during the 1990s, Gram-positive BSI emerged as a leading cause of BSI following the increased use of intravascular devices and the extensive use of prophylaxis with fluoroquinolones (FQ). Subsequently, this trend was followed by a gradual rise of Gram-negative bacteria and more recently MDR Gram-negative extended spectrum β-lactamase (ESBL) or carbapenem-resistant enterobacteriaceae are becoming a critical issue in the daily clinical practice (Mikulska et al. 2009; Cattaneo et al. 2008; Tumbarello et al. 2012). Despite the shift in the epidemiology of BSI in hematologic patients, Gram-positive bacteria are still the dominating cause of BSI in many studies. A recent review by the ECIL group showed a reduction of Gram-positive to Gram-negative ratio from 60%:40% to 55%:45% reported by the studies published between 2005 and 2011 (Mikulka et al. 2014). The most frequent Gram-positive pathogens were coagulase-negative staphylococci (CoNS) (24%) followed by enterococci (8%), viridans streptococci (6%), and *Staphylococcus aureus* (5%). Several risk factors have been associated with the emergence of Gram-positive BSI (Table 11.1). In this respect, a scoring system for predicting Gram-positive coccal infections in neutropenic patients has been developed, based on four risk factors, namely, the use of high-dose cytarabine, proton pump inhibitors, gut decontamination with colimycin without aminoglycosides, and the presence of chills at the onset of fever (Cordonnier et al. 2003).

11.2 Etiology

Staphylococci are the most frequent pathogen isolated in BSI (Balletto and Mikulska 2015). CoNS are responsible for approximately a quarter of BSI. *S. aureus*, even if more aggressive, is found in 5% of cases (Mikulska et al. 2014).

A. Busca (✉)
Stem Cell Transplant Center, AOU Citta' della Salute e della Scienza, Turin, Italy
e-mail: abusca@cittadellasalute.to.it

S. Corcione (✉) · F. G. De Rosa (✉)
Infectious Diseases 2, AOU Citta' della Salute e della Scienza, Turin, Italy

© Springer Nature Switzerland AG 2021
O. A. Cornely, M. Hoenig (eds.), *Infection Management in Hematology*, Hematologic Malignancies, https://doi.org/10.1007/978-3-030-57317-1_11

Table 11.1 Risk factors for Gram positive bloodstream infections

Risk factors for gram positive bloodstream infections
Central venous catheter.
Fluoroquinolone prophylaxis.
High-dose cytarabine.
Gut decontamination.
Toxic enterocolitis.
High-grade mucositis.
Use of proton pump inhibitors.
Disease or therapy-related changes of human gut microbiota.

Among CoNS, the prevalent pathogen is *S. epidermidis*, which dwells in skin and mucous membranes, followed by *S. hominis, S. saprophyticus, S. lugdunensis,* and *S. haemolyticus.* More frequent risk factors associated with CoNS infections are oral mucositis, central venous lines, previous use of cephalosporins, and fluoroquinolone prophylaxis. CoNS infection is easily derived from central venous catheter (CVC) local infections and surgical wounds (Bowden et al. 2010). Overall, they have low-grade virulence with poor propensity to invade, but they have the peculiar ability to generate a biofilm. Mortality is rare even if methicillin-resistant strains are rising (Becker et al. 2014).

S. aureus is more virulent than CoNS, in particular if methicillin resistance occurs, mortality can increase. Risk factor for methicillin-resistant Staphylococcus aureus (MRSA) is previous nasal colonization. Usually, *S. aureus* infections are attributed to CVC sites. Graft-versus-host disease (GvHD) can be confused with staphylococcal-scalded skin syndrome. GvHD itself through lengthening the hospitalization can promote *S. aureus* infections.

Enterococci are Gram-positive facultative anaerobes. They are commensals of the gastrointestinal tract and can affect 10–12% of hematopoietic stem cell transplant (HSCT) recipients (Cappellano et al. 2007). *Enterococcus faecalis* is the main strain encountered even if in some centers *E. faecium* is replacing it. For both strains, vancomycin resistance is causing mortality rate increases (DiazGranados and Jernigan 2005). Co-morbidities, enteric mucositis, and previous antibiotic use are

risk factors for enterococcal infection. Generally, they occur during the late post-transplant period and are often catheter related.

Viridans streptococci cause approximately 5% of BSI. Main strain is *S. mitis,* followed by *S. sanguis,* and *S. viridans.* They are facultative anaerobic, Gram-positive cocci. They usually are part of the flora of the oral cavity, upper respiratory tract, gastrointestine (GI), and female genital tract. BSI infections appear mostly in neutropenic patients. Main risk factors are oral mucositis, antibiotic prophylaxis with fluoroquinolones, and β-lactam exposure. Viridans streptococci can cause not only BSI but also acute respiratory syndrome (ARDS) (Freifeld and Razonable 2014a) resulting with high mortality. This frequently leads to a higher use of vancomycin in empiric therapy, causing a high pharmacological pressure and risk of selection of more resistant pathogens, with no clear advantage (Freifeld and Razonable 2014b).

Streptococcal infections can also lead to streptococcal toxic shock-like syndrome due to pyrogenic exotoxins A, B, and C produced by group A beta-hemolytic streptococci (*S. pyogenes*). Patients present with fever, rash, desquamation, hypotension, and multi-organ-system dysfunction. In HSCT recipients, *S. pneumoniae* can be responsible for invasive infections like bacteremia and meningitis and obviously respiratory infection. Of note, these diseases may occur even months or years following the transplantation, more rarely they can also happen in the neutropenic period. Main risk factors are GvHD and immunoglobulin deficiency, usually in subclasses IgG2 and IgG4 (Sheridan et al. 1990).

Clostridium difficile is one of the most frequent causes of diarrhea in hematologic patients and HSCT recipients; however, it rarely causes the potentially fatal complication of pseudomembranous colitis. It can affect up to 24.7% HSCT recipients within 1 year after transplant (Bruminhent et al. 2014). Risk factors are not entirely clear as hematologic patients may present all characteristics of frailty that predispose to *C. difficile* infections, including immunocompromise, broad-spectrum antibiotics, damaged intestinal mucosa, and prolonged hospital stay.

11.3 Resistance Mechanisms

Resistance mechanisms are usually transmitted by mobile genetic elements (MGEs) like plasmids, transposons, bacteriophages, pathogenicity islands, and cassette chromosomes (for staphylococci). Plasmids and staphylococcal cassette chromosomes have been particularly convenient for conferring resistance to β-lactam antibiotics and vancomycin.

Others mechanisms include biofilm production (*S. aureus* and *S. epidermidis*). CoNS and *S. aureus* can also be ingested by human host cells, non-professional phagocytes, to escape patient immune defense and antibiotic exposure (Becker et al. 2014). Nowadays, nosocomial CoNS are frequently methicillin resistant and this has to be considered in the therapeutic choice. Glycopeptides and daptomycin resistance imply bacterial cell wall alterations, oxazolidinone, tetracycline, and glycylcycline derivatives cause ribosomal changes.

S. aureus vancomycin-resistant strains are increasing. Vancomycin intermediate-resistant *S. aureus* [VISA, minimum inhibitory concentration (MIC) 4–8 μg/mL], has a polygenic involvement and is poorly understood, probably genes conditioning cell envelop biosynthesis are involved. VISA are more frequent than *S. aureus* with complete resistance to vancomycin (MIC ≥16 μg/mL) and influence treatment failure and worse clinical outcome (McGuinness et al. 2017).

Viridans streptococci resistance to the macrolide class is associated with the frequent use of these drugs (Ardanuy et al. 2005). Most strains are susceptible to penicillin; if resistance is present, it is usually caused by penicillin-binding protein (PBP). Quinolone resistance is often found in patients who received antibiotic prophylaxis. Pneumococci also are frequently resistant to macrolides; moreover, penicillin-resistant strains show resistance to other classes of antimicrobials, too, in particular fluoroquinolones, through alteration in topoisomerase IV and DNA gyrase and drug efflux mechanisms (Akova 2016).

Enterococci are intrinsically resistant to many antimicrobials and easily develop mutations. *E. faecium* is resistant to aminopenicillins in 90% of nosocomial strains. Moreover, the increase of *E. faecium* in particular in hematological cancer patients is a major problem for vancomycin-resistant infections. Enterococci are usually sensitive to linezolid, daptomycin, and tigecycline, these are the remaining options as enterococci are often resistant to aminoglycosides and quinolones too (Bender et al. 2018). The mechanisms involved in daptomycin resistance temper with membrane homeostasis, including structural alterations to the cell envelope and reduction in cell membrane fluidity.

C. difficile resistance to metronidazole and vancomycin are still sporadic, even if observed MIC is rising. Mechanisms are still not clear (Spigaglia et al. 2011; Baines and Wilcox 2015). Usually, recrudescences are caused by how badly antibiotic therapy affected gut microflora, IgG antitoxin response, and *C. difficile* spores concentration remaining in the colon. Some hypervirulent *C. difficile* strains are associated with recurrence; the more frequent is PCR-ribotype (RT) 027, which can carry a multidrug resistance (MDR) phenotype.

Specific resistance mechanisms are listed in Table 11.2.

11.4 Empiric Treatment

Therapeutic options are conditioned by resistance frequencies, which can change along the setting, and patient's characteristics, frailties, comorbidities, previous antibiotic use, and presence of venous lines. In this respect, it is worthwhile recalling that local epidemiology of bacterial isolates and resistance patterns are crucially important in determining the first-choice empirical therapy.

When fever occurs in neutropenic patients, it is mandatory to start an antibiotic treatment including an agent for Gram-negative bacteria, considering local frequencies of MDR bacteria, in particular ESBL; regarding Gram-positive BSI, the risk for MRSA has to be considered. As already mentioned, patients with central venous lines, history of MRSA colonization, cutaneous infections, pneumonia, or shock have a greater

Table 11.2 Resistance mechanisms of Gram-positive pathogens

Bacteria	Drugs	Mechanism of resistance
CoNS and *S. aureus* (Becker et al. 2014)	Penicillin	Penicillinases staphylococcal β-lactamase: Hydrolysis of the β-lactam ring
	Penicillins, most cephalosporins, and carbapenems (except cephalosporins with MRSA activity, such as ceftobiprole and ceftaroline)	Additional penicillin-binding protein (PBP), PBP2a: Cell-wall biosynthesis can continue
	Glycopeptides	Cell wall alterations
	Daptomycin	Cell membrane phenotypic changes occur in addition to other perturbations of the cell membrane Increased cell wall teichoic acid production, progressive cell wall thickening
	Oxazolidinones	Ribosomal alterations
	Tetracyclines and glycylcyclines	Ribosomal protection through dissociation of tetracyclines from their ribosomal binding sites Drug efflux
	Fusidic acid	Altered ribosomal translocase
	Fosfomycin	Development of covalent bond between fosfomycin and a sulfhydryl group in glutathione
Viridans streptococci and *S. pneumoniae* (Ardanuy et al. 2005; Chancey et al. 2012)	Penicillins	Penicillin-binding protein (PBP)
	Macrolides	Ribosomal alterations Drug efflux
	Tetracycline	Ribosomal alterations
	Glycopeptide	Bacterial cell wall synthesis
	Fluoroquinolones	Alteration in topoisomerase IV and DNA gyrase Active FQ efflux
Enterococci (Bender et al. 2018; Gagetti et al. 2018)	Ampicillin	Cell wall alterations
	Vancomycin	Cell wall alterations
	Oxazolidinone	Ribosomal alterations
	Tigecycline	Ribosomal alterations and efflux pumps
	Daptomycin	Structural alterations to the cell envelope Reduction in cell membrane fluidity

possibility of MRSA infection; based on these considerations vancomycin, teicoplanin, or daptomycin, if lungs are not involved, can be a good choice. In localized infections where blood stream is not involved, for example, pneumonia or soft tissue infection, linezolid, sulfamethoxazole/trimethoprim, new cephalosporins with MRSA activity, or tigecycline may be considered as a good alternative (Olson et al. 2002). In case of *S. aureus* BSI, endocarditis should be excluded and blood cultures should be repeated until negative result.

De-escalation is recommended once a susceptible strain is isolated, choosing the drug with lower genetic barrier; beta-lactams, fluoroquinolones, tetracycline derivatives, and clindamycin are possible choices. For VISA or VRA strains, linezolid, daptomycin, or telavancin can be considered.

In catheter-related CoNS blood stream infection, device removal may be sufficient, and in case of prolonged fever, a short course of antibiotic (5–7 days) is suggested. When a catheter cannot be removed, antibiotics should be continued up to 14 days and an antibiotic lock approach should be added (Mermel et al. 2009).

Therapy for viridans streptococci should follow local resistance prevalence to methicillin. As these infections are usually not aggressive, a first step therapy with a beta-lactam should be considered in order to preserve glycopeptide susceptibility, evaluating risk factors like central venous lines, which should be removed as soon as possible in case of positive blood cultures, or other patient conditions. In case of the presence of additional risk factors, vancomycin should be considered (Bowden et al. 2010), and in case of drug-sensitive strains any cephalosporin, amoxicillin, or carbapenems are suitable.

For enterococcal infections, considering the increasing diffusion, *E. faecium* prevalence, and subsequent resistance, vancomycin has to be considered as first choice for hematologic patients until the pattern of susceptibility is available.

Alternatives can be daptomycin, tigecycline, or linezolid. Tigecycline and linezolid are preferably not used in blood stream infections because of their great volume of distribution, while daptomycin should be avoided if lungs are involved. It is still not clear whether empiric treatment of VRE strains is associated with a true advantage in clinical outcomes (Kamboj et al. 2018). For sensitive strains, ampicillin, oxacillin, piperacillin/tazobactam, or carbapenems may be considered as alternative therapies (Cunha and Cunha 2017).

C. difficile guidelines have been modified recently. Main recommendation remains to discontinue therapy with the inciting antibiotic(s) as soon as possible; as for drug choice either vancomycin (125 mg QID p.o. for 10 days) or fidaxomicin are recommended, and thus preferred over metronidazole (400 mg TID for 10 days) for an initial episode of *Clostridium difficile* infection (CDI). Metronidazole can be considered for an initial episode of non-severe CDI, if at all, and prolonged courses should be avoided due to risk of cumulative neurotoxicity (McDonald et al. 2018). Fidaxomicin is also recommended for recurrent episodes. It is a macrocyclic narrow spectrum, bactericidal antimicrobial agent, poorly absorbed after oral administration.

Another new possibility is bezlotoxumab, a human monoclonal antibody approved to reduce the recurrence of this bacterial infection as it binds to *C. difficile* toxin B. Bezlotoxumab is not an antibacterial drug so it is not indicated for the treatment of CDI but to reduce recurrences (Baines and Wilcox 2015). In patients with underlying congestive heart failure, special attention should be raised, as an unexplained increased risk of heart failure was noted (Lee et al. 2017).

References

Akova M (2016) Epidemiology of antimicrobial resistance in bloodstream infections. Virulence 7(3):252–266

Ardanuy C, Tubau F, Liñares J, Domínguez MA, Pallarés R, Martín R (2005) Distribution of subclasses mefA and mefE of the mefA gene among clinical isolates of macrolide-resistant (M-phenotype) Streptococcus pneumoniae, Viridans group streptococci, and Streptococcus pyogenes. Antimicrob Agents Chemother 49(2):827–829

Baines SD, Wilcox MH (2015) Antimicrobial Resistance and Reduced Susceptibility in Clostridium difficile: Potential Consequences for Induction, Treatment, and Recurrence of C. difficile Infection. Antibiotics (Basel) 4(3):267–298

Balletto E, Mikulska M (2015) Bacterial Infections in Hematopoietic Stem Cell Transplant Recipients. Mediterr J Hematol Infect Dis 7(1):e2015045. Published 2015 Jul 1. https://doi.org/10.4084/MJHID.2015.045

Becker K, Heilmann C, Peters G (2014) Coagulase-negative staphylococci. Clin Microbiol Rev 27(4):870–926

Bender JK, Cattoir V, Hegstad K, Sadowy E, Coque TM, Westh H et al (2018) Update on prevalence and mechanisms of resistance to linezolid, tigecycline and daptomycin in enterococci in Europe: towards a common nomenclature. Drug Resist Updat 40:25–39

Bowden RA, Ljungman P, Snydman DR (2010) Transplant infections, 3rd edn. Wolters Kluwer Health/Lippincott Williams & Wilkins, Philadelphia

Bruminhent J, Wang Z-X, Hu C, Wagner J, Sunday R, Bobik B et al (2014) Clostridium difficile colonization and disease in patients undergoing hematopoietic stem cell transplantation. Biol Blood Marrow Transplant 20(9):1329–1334

Cappellano P, Viscoli C, Bruzzi P, Van Lint MT, Pereira CAP, Bacigalupo A (2007) Epidemiology and risk factors for bloodstream infections after allogeneic hematopoietic stem cell transplantation. New Microbiol 30(2):89–99

Cattaneo C, Quaresmini G, Cesari S et al (2008) Recent changes in bacterial epidemiology and the emergence of fluoroquinolone-resistant Escherichia coli among patients with hematological malignancies: results of a prospective study on 823 patients at a single institution. J Antimicrob Chemother 61:721–728

Chancey ST, Zähner D, Stephens DS (2012) Acquired inducible antimicrobial resistance in gram-positive bacteria. Future Microbiol 7:959–978

Cl G, Bodro M, Simonetti A et al (2012) Changing aetiology, clinical features, antimicrobial resistance, and outcomes of bloodstream infection in neutropenic cancer patients. Clin Microbiol Infect 19:474–479

Cordonnier C, Buzyn A, Leverger G et al (2003) Epidemiology and risk factors for gram-positive coccal infections in neutropenia: toward a more targeted antibiotic strategy. Clin Infect Dis 36:149–158

Cheston B Cunha - Burke A Cunha . Antibiotic Essentials 2017 - Jaypee Brothers Medical Publishers, New Delhi

DiazGranados CA, Jernigan JA (2005) Impact of vancomycin resistance on mortality among patients with neutropenia and enterococcal bloodstream infection. J Infect Dis 191(4):588–595

Freifeld AG, Razonable RR (2014a) Viridans group streptococci in febrile neutropenic cancer patients: what should we fear? Clin Infect Dis 59(2):231–233

Freifeld AG, Razonable RR (2014b) Editorial commentary: Viridans group streptococci in febrile neutropenic Cancer patients: what should we fear? Clin Infect Dis 59(2):231–233

Gagetti P, Bonofiglio L, García Gabarrot G, Kaufman S, Mollerach M, Vigliarolo L et al (2018) Resistance to β-lactams in enterococci. Rev Argent Microbiol

Gaytan-Martinez JL, Mateos-Garcia E, Sanchez-Cortes E et al (2000) Microbiological findings in febrile neutropenia. Arch Med Res 31:388–392

Gudiol C, Tubau F, Calatayud L et al (2011) Bacteremia due to multidrug-resistant gram-negative bacilli in cancer patients: risk factors, antibiotic therapy and outcomes. J Antimicrob Chemother 66:657–663

Kamboj M, Cohen N, Huang Y-T, Kerpelev M, Jakubowski A, Sepkowitz KA et al (2018) Impact of empiric treatment for vancomycin-resistant Enterococcus (VRE) in colonized patients early after allogeneic hematopoietic stem cell transplantation. Biol Blood Marrow Transplant 15

Lee Y, Lim WI, Bloom CI, Moore S, Chung E, Marzella N (2017) Bezlotoxumab (Zinplava) for Clostridium Difficile infection. P T 42(12):735–738

McDonald LC, Gerding DN, Johnson S, Bakken JS, Carroll KC, Coffin SE et al (2018) Clinical practice guidelines for Clostridium difficile infection in adults and children: 2017 update by the Infectious Diseases Society of America (IDSA) and Society for Healthcare Epidemiology of America (SHEA). Clin Infect Dis 66(7):e1–e48

McGuinness WA, Malachowa N, DeLeo FR (2017) Vancomycin resistance in Staphylococcus aureus. Yale J Biol Med 90(2):269–281

Mermel LA, Allon M, Bouza E, Craven DE, Flynn P, O'Grady NP et al (2009) Clinical practice guidelines for the diagnosis and Management of Intravascular Catheter-Related Infection: 2009 update by the Infectious Diseases Society of America. Clin Infect Dis 49(1):1–45

Mikulka M, Viscoli C, Orasch C et al (2014) Aetiology and resistance in bacteraemias among adult and paediatric haematology and cancer patients. J Infect 68:321–331

Mikulska M, De Bono V, Raiola AM et al (2009) Blood stream infections in allogeneic hematopoietic stem cell transplant recipients: reemergence of gram-negative rods and increasing antibiotic resistance. Biol Blood Marrow Transplant 15:47–53

Mikulska M, Viscoli C, Orasch C, Livermore DM, Averbuch D, Cordonnier C et al (2014) Aetiology and resistance in bacteraemias among adult and paediatric haematology and cancer patients. J Infect 68(4):321–31.1

Olson ME, Ceri H, Morck DW, Buret AG, Read RR (2002) Biofilm bacteria: formation and comparative susceptibility to antibiotics. Can J Vet Res 66(2):86–92

Sheridan JF, Tutschka PJ, Sedmak DD, Copelan EA (1990) Immunoglobulin G subclass deficiency and pneumococcal infection after allogeneic bone marrow transplantation. Blood 75(7):1583–1586

Spigaglia P, Barbanti F, Mastrantonio P, Ackermann G, Balmelli C, Barbut F et al (2011) Multidrug resistance in European Clostridium difficile clinical isolates. J Antimicrob Chemother 66(10):2227–2234

Tumbarello M, Viale P, Viscoli C et al (2012) Predictors of mortality in bloodstream infections caused by Klebsiella pneumoniae carbapenemase-producing K. pneumoniae: importance of combination therapy. Clin Infect Dis 55:943–950

Matteo Bassetti, Elda Righi, and Murat Akova

12.1 Epidemiology of Gram-Negative Bacterial Infections in Haematology Patients

During the last 50 years, two major shifts could be noticed in the epidemiology of bacteria causative for infections and particularly bloodstream infections in febrile neutropenic cancer patients. Until the mid-1980s, gram-negative bacteria, particularly *Escherichia coli* and *Pseudomonas aeruginosa*, were the main infectious agents in these patients. Then, presumably due to the increased use of high-intensity chemotherapeutic regimens leading to a higher incidence of severe mucositis, the frequent use of fluoroquinolone (FQ) prophylaxis and indwelling long-term vascular catheters, gram-positive bacteria, particularly coagulase-negative staphylococci and viridans streptococci, became the dominant infecting agents.

M. Bassetti (✉)
Infectious Diseases Clinic, Policlinico San Martino Hospital – IRCCS, Genoa, Italy

Department of Health Sciences, University of Genoa, Genoa, Italy

E. Righi (✉)
Infectious Diseases, Department of Diagnostics and Public Health, University of Verona, Verona, Italy

M. Akova (✉)
Department of Infectious Diseases and Clinical Microbiology, Hacettepe University School of Medicine, Ankara, Turkey

Since the turn of the twenty-first century, gram-negative bacteria have re-emerged in many haematology centres throughout the world (Gustinetti and Mikulska 2016). However, the main difference between gram-negative bacteria in 2000s and those in 1970s and 1980s is the significant antimicrobial resistance in the former, which causes a severe compromise in patients with acute leukaemia (AL) and other haematological malignancies and in those undergoing haematopoietic stem cell transplantation (HSCT) (Akova 2016). Currently, enteric gram negatives (particularly *E. coli* and *Klebsiella pneumoniae*) and non-fermentative bacteria (*P. aeruginosa*, *Acinetobacter baumannii* and *Stenotrophomonas maltophilia*) are primarily responsible for gram-negative bloodstream infections (BSIs) in febrile neutropenic cancer patients (Alp and Akova 2013; Kara et al. 2015). Since multidrug resistance (MDR) is a common problem among these pathogens, empirical therapy in febrile neutropenic cancer patients may need to be devised accordingly. However, most of the current guidelines do not recommend empirical regimens for these highly resistant bacteria. This may delay antibiotic therapy (Freifeld et al. 2010; Averbuch et al. 2013). Current standard microbiological techniques do not allow identification of both bacteria and antimicrobial resistance earlier than within 36–48 h, thus delaying appropriate antibiotic therapy (Kirn and Weinstein 2013).

© Springer Nature Switzerland AG 2021
O. A. Cornely, M. Hoenig (eds.), *Infection Management in Hematology*, Hematologic Malignancies, https://doi.org/10.1007/978-3-030-57317-1_12

12.1.1 Mechanisms of Emerging Antimicrobial Resistance in Gram-Negative Bacteria

The main resistance mechanism of MDR in gram-negative bacilli is the production of various beta-lactamase enzymes including extended-spectrum beta-lactamases (ESBLs) and carbapenemases (Alp and Akova 2017). The latter enzymes are encoded by multicopy plasmids in these bacteria. These plasmids often also carry resistance determinants for other antibiotics, thus leading to multi- or extended-drug resistance (MDR, XDR phenotypes) (Magiorakos et al. 2012). Other mechanisms contributing to resistant phenotypes are porin mutations, efflux pumps and target modifications. Usually, two or more of these mechanisms can be found simultaneously in the same strain (Eichenberger and Thaden 2019).

12.1.2 Carbapenem and Extended-Spectrum Cephalosporin-Resistant Enterobacteriaceae

Extended-spectrum beta-lactamases, especially the CTX-M type, confer resistance against broad-spectrum cephalosporins and penicillins, particularly in *E. coli*, but also in other members of Enterobacteriaceae. ESBL-encoding plasmids may also encode resistance to aminoglycosides, tetracyclines, sulphonamides and trimethoprim. These plasmids frequently encode an inhibitor-resistant beta-lactamase, namely OXA-1, which provides resistance to beta-lactamase inhibitors including amoxicillin/clavulanate and piperacillin/tazobactam (Livermore 2012). One of the new beta-lactamase inhibitor combinations, namely ceftolozane/tazobactam, may overcome this resistance, since ceftolozane is resistant to hydrolysis by OXA-1 (Zhanel et al. 2014). *Escherichia coli* sequence type ST131 with CTX-M-15 ESBL production is emerging worldwide and has a high epidemic potential.

Carbapenem resistance (CR) may occur due to the production of various carbapenemases, expression of efflux pumps, porin mutations, or combination of these mechanisms (Eichenberger and Thaden 2019). Three different types of carbapenemases are usually accounted for CR in most of the carbapenem-resistant Enterobacteriaceae (CRE): *Klebsiella pneumoniae* carbapenemase (KPC), an Ambler Class A enzyme (Ambler 1980), is highly prevalent in the United States, Western Europe and South East Asia. The KPC gene is located on a plasmid that can be transferred between species. KPC can hydrolyse and thereby inactivate almost all penicillins, cephalosporins and aztreonam along with carbapenems, but most of the new beta-lactam/beta-lactamase inhibitor combinations can inhibit KPC. The most common Class D beta-lactamases in Enterobacteriaceae are OXA-48-like enzymes (Mairi et al. 2018). These enzymes are weak carbapenemases; thus, the bacteria usually remain susceptible to broad-spectrum cephalosporins. However, Enterobacteriaceae harbouring these enzymes often additionally carry an ESBL gene that provides resistance to cephalosporins. OXA-48-producing *K. pneumoniae* was first described in Turkey in 2001 and has been spread to Europe, North Africa, the Middle East and India. These enzymes are rarely encountered in the United States and South East Asia. Metallo-beta-lactamases (MBLs) are Class B carbapenemases and can hydrolyse all beta-lactams except aztreonam. Unfortunately, none of the new beta-lactamase inhibitors is active against the new classes of carbapenemases. Two new agents, namely aztreonam/avibactam and cefiderocol, which are currently being evaluated in Phase 3 trials, show a strong in vitro activity and may be useful against MBL-producing Enterobacteriaceae (Theuretzbacher et al. 2019). New Delhi metallo (NDM-type) enzymes are the most prevalent enzymes in this group and are endemic in the Indian subcontinent. They have also been found in the European continent, but are less frequent in Americas (Eichenberger and Thaden 2019). Verona integron-encoded metallo-beta-lactamase (VIM) is another metalloenzyme that has chemical characteristics similar to those of NDM enzymes. VIM is frequently reported in non-enteric gram-negative bacteria. Enterobacteriaceae with VIM production are usually found in Southern European countries (Matsumura et al. 2017).

When compared with *K. pneumoniae*, the production of carbapenemases and CR are lower in *E. coli* (Poirel et al. 2018). Like ESBL-producing strains, carbapenem-resistant strains of Enterobacteriaceae frequently acquire resistance to other classes of antibiotics, including aminoglycosides, FQs, tetracyclines and trimethoprim–sulfamethoxazole (TMP-SMX) by various mechanisms.

Although polymyxins have usually been active against these XDR pathogens, the emergence of colistin resistance has become widespread in certain locations (Jeannot et al. 2017). Resistance to polymyxins typically results from chromosomally determined lipopolysaccharide modifications; however, a plasmid-mediated resistance has also been described. The latter type of resistance was recently reported in *E. coli* from faecal samples collected from three patients with acute leukaemia (Lalaoui et al. 2019).

Extensively drug-resistant (XDR) *Pseudomonas aeruginosa*: Loss of porins and presence of efflux pumps (such as MexA-MexB-OprM) can cause intrinsic resistance to several antibiotics, including rifampin plus TMP-SMX, tetracycline and most beta-lactam antibiotics, including carbapenems, in *P. aeruginosa* (Eichenberger and Thaden 2019). The porin protein OprD allows carbapenem uptake through the outer membrane. Loss of this protein confers resistance to imipenem and reduced susceptibility to meropenem. When OprD loss is combined with upregulated MexA-MexB-OprM, *P. aeruginosa* gains an XDR phenotype that is resistant to almost all beta-lactams, quinolones and tetracyclines.

P. aeruginosa intrinsically possesses Class C chromosomal beta-lactamases (AmpC). Mutations can lead to hyperproduction (derepressed state) of these enzymes which results in resistance to all broad-spectrum cephalosporins, penicillins and aztreonam. Additional acquisition of plasmid-mediated broad-spectrum beta-lactamases (such as PER-1, VEB-1, GES-1 and some OXA-type enzymes) enhances resistance to all beta-lactams except carbapenems. The latter

can be hydrolysed by acquired MBLs including VIM, IMP, SMP and GIM.

Aminoglycoside-modifying enzymes are also encoded on transferable plasmids and confer resistance to aminoglycosides. Mutations in FQ targets such as *parC* and gyrA can lead and augment quinolone resistance in addition to that conferred by efflux pumps. Several clones exert an XDR phenotype, and the globally most frequent clone is ST235, which may have 39 different beta-lactamases from Class A (PER-1, GES), Class B (VIM) and Class D (OXA type) enzymes (Eichenberger and Thaden 2019).

Extensively drug-resistant (XDR) *Acinetobacter baumannii*: This microorganism has similar mechanisms of antibiotic resistance as described for *P. aeruginosa*. CR is the hallmark of an XDR phenotype. EARS-Net surveillance by ECDC reported prevalence of CR in *A. baumannii* in the EU at 49% (European Centre for Disease Prevention and Control 2019). This figure may be up to >90% in South East Asia and South America. A hyperexpressed adeABC efflux pump combined with OXA-type carbapenemases (OXA-23, 40 and 58-like enzymes) leads to high-level CR (Akova 2016).

12.1.3 Current Epidemiological Figures and Emerging Threat of Resistant Gram-Negative Bacilli

Since the turn of the twenty-first century, gram-negative bacteria with various antibiotic resistance patterns have become the dominating life-threatening microorganisms in patients with haematological malignancies. A multicentre survey by the European Conference on Infections in Acute Leukaemia (ECIL-4) from 39 centres in 18 countries from Europe and Near East in 2011 revealed a reduction of the gram-positive to gram-negative ratio when compared with previously published literature (55%:45% vs. 60%:40%, respectively) (Mikulska et al. 2014). The rate of Enterobacteriaceae has increased (30% vs. 24%, respectively), whereas the rates of *P. aeruginosa* has declined (5% vs. 14%). One particular finding in this survey is that, although overall resistance rates were lower than those already published, South-Eastern European countries have a significantly higher frequency of resistance compared to those in North-Western Europe. The north to the south shift in Europe in antimicrobial resistance has been significant over the years, and recently, a complex scheme of contributing factors has been described that goes beyond antimicrobial usage (Collignon et al. 2018).

Similar observations were reported in a recent European Society for Blood and Marrow Transplantation (EBMT) survey with HSCT recipients (Averbuch et al. 2017). Sixty-five HSCT centres from Europe, Asia and Australia reported data on 591 patients with 655 gram-negative BSI episodes caused by 704 pathogens. Enterobacteriaceae accounted for 73% of all episodes and non-fermentative bacteria for 24%. FQ resistance was present in 50.4% of all isolates, non-carbapenem beta-lactam resistance in 50.9%, CR in 18.5% and MDR in 35.2%. *Klebsiella pneumoniae* isolates had the highest rate of CR (25%), whereas this figure was low in non-Klebsiella Enterobacteriaceae (2.3% in *E. coli*, 7.3% in *Enterobacter* spp.). *Acinetobacter baumannii* was resistant to carbapenems in 63.6% of the isolates and *P. aeruginosa* in 37.9%. In centres where FQ prophylaxis was provided, higher rates of FQ resistance in gram negatives were observed (79% vs. 50%, p = 0.001). Patients with allogeneic HSCT (allo-HSCT) showed higher resistance rates, and similar to the previous report by Mikulska et al. (Mikulska et al. 2014), higher resistance rates were shown in South East vs. North East Europe.

A sevenfold increase in carbapenem-resistant *K. pneumoniae* isolates from BSIs among HSCT recipients was reported between 2010 and 2013 in 52 Italian centres (Girmenia et al. 2015). Another prospective Italian study with 2743 HSCT patients reported a cumulative incidence for gram-negative BSIs of 17.3% and 9% in the pre-engraftment period of allo- and auto-HSCT (Girmenia et al. 2017). *Escherichia coli* was the most frequent pathogen, followed by *K. pneu-*

moniae and *P. aeruginosa* in both allo- and auto-HSCT.

A total of 2388 HSCT patients with neutropenia (61.6% with allo-HSCT) were analysed in a prospective, multicentre study in 20 HSCT centres from Germany, Austria and Switzerland between 2002 and 2014. The incidence of BSIs did not change over the study period (15.8%). Although gram-positive bacteria were predominating agents of BSIs (63.9%), the incidence of gram-negative BSIs increased in both allo-HSCT patients (1.4% in 2002 vs. 6.4% in 2014, p < 0.001) and auto-HSCT patients (3.6% in 2002 vs. 7.4% in 2014, p = 0.001). *Escherichia coli* was the leading pathogen (19.9% of all BSIs) for which the incidence increased threefold in allo-HSCT patients. Overall, 11% of Enterobacteriaceae from BSIs produced ESBL, and no significant increase in this pattern occurred during the study period.

A recent systematic review and meta-analysis of 22 studies between 1998 and 2014 with 5650 BSI patients with cancer reported a pooled prevalence of 11% of ESBL production among Enterobacteriaceae in patients with haematological malignancy (Alevizakos et al. 2017). Stratification according to geographic region indicated pooled prevalence figures of 7% in Europe (Turkey, Italy, Germany, Sweden and Spain), Eastern Mediterranean region (Saudi Arabia, Jordan) and South America (Brazil); 10% in Western Pacific region (China, Malaysia, South Korea, Hong Kong); and 30% in South East Asia (India). In addition, an annual increase of 7.1% in the production of ESBL in enteric gram negatives was observed.

Beyond multicentre analysis, single-centre data have shown greater variations both in epidemiology and in antibacterial resistance. Bodro et al. (Bodro et al. 2014) reported on 1148 bacteraemia episodes in adult cancer patients (58% with haematological malignancies) between 2006 and 2011. ESKAPE pathogens (*Enterococcus faecium, Staphylococcus aureus, K. pneumoniae,* and *P. aeruginosa* and *Enterobacter* spp.) caused bacteraemia in 392 episodes (34%). In 54 episodes (4.7%), resistant ESKAPE pathogens were isolated: 33.3% carbapenem- and quinolone-resistant *P. aeruginosa*, 22.2% stably derepressed and ESBL-producing *Enterobacter cloacae*, 13% ESBL-producing *K. pneumoniae* and 7.4% carbapenem-resistant *A. baumannii*.

Between 2005 and 2009, 3703 neutropenic episodes in 2098 patients with haematological malignancies were analysed in a large tertiary care centre in Turkey (Kara et al. 2015). The frequency of BSIs was 14.5%. Among them, gram-negative pathogens were the predominant bacteria (52.6%). *Escherichia coli* (17.3%), *Klebsiella* spp. (11%), *Acinetobacter* spp. (7.1%) and *P. aeruginosa* (6.7%) were the most frequently isolated bacteria. Extended-spectrum beta-lactamase production was 45% in *E. coli* and 23% in *Klebsiella* spp. and did not change much during the study period. Overall FQ resistance was 33.3% in gram-negative bacteria, ceftazidime resistance was 28% in *P. aeruginosa*, and MDR pattern was found 87% in *A. baumannii*. Meropenem resistance was observed in 11.5% of all gram-negative bacteria in high-risk haematology patients (i.e. acute leukaemia and HSCT recipients), 10% in *K. pneumoniae*, 20% in *P. aeruginosa* and 35.3% in *Acinetobacter* spp. No CR was in found in *E. coli*. A follow-up surveillance in 153 patients with 254 BSI isolates revealed ESBL production in 41.9% of *E. coli* and 42.6% of *K. pneumoniae* and CR was present in 5.1% of *E. coli* and in 44.2% of *K. pneumoniae* (a > fourfold increase over the previous period) and in all *A. baumannii* isolates (Ayaz et al. 2018).

A total of 2083 patients with haematological malignancy were retrospectively evaluated in a Taiwanese hospital between 2008 and 2013 (Chen et al. 2017). Lymphoma was the most common underlying disease (38.1%), closely followed by acute myeloid leukaemia (30.9%). Gram-negative bacteria were the leading cause (53.7%) of bacteraemia among 1310 non-duplicate isolates in neutropenic patients. The isolates included *E. coli* (13.8%), *K. pneumoniae* (9.5%), *A. calcoaceticus–baumannii* (ACB) complex (5.7%) and *P. aeruginosa* (4.0%). MDR was detected in 21.8% of the ACB complex isolates. Comparing the distribution of resistant bacteria in three different periods (1995–2011, 2002–2006 and 2008–2013), the investigators detected significant increases in rates of cefotaxime-resistant *E. coli*, and CR rates in *E. coli*, *P. aeruginosa* and ACB complex isolates.

Varying incidences up to 32% of polymicrobial BSIs have been reported for all episodes of BSIs (Rolston et al. 2007). However, more recent series noted an incidence of around 10% with a dominance of resistant gram-negative bacteria as the causative agents (Royo-Cebrecos et al. 2017).

Analysis of the so-called blood microbiome by high-throughput sequencing (HTS) method in neutropenic cancer patients can lead to the identification of non-culturable microorganisms (Gyarmati et al. 2015; Gyarmati et al. 2016; Horiba et al. 2018). In a study with 130 blood samples in 33 patients, 98% of the identified reads by HTS were known human pathogens and 65% of them belonged to the normal human gut microbiota, confirming that a translocation from the gut has a critical role in the pathogenesis of BSIs in neutropenic patients (Gyarmati et al. 2015; Song and Peter 2019). While only bacteria belonging to *Firmicutes* phylum were isolated with blood cultures, 5 phyla and 30 genera mostly belonging to anaerobic and facultative genera were identified with HTS. Although the importance of this finding is yet to be determined in larger series, one point deserves to be mentioned: The *Shewanella* genus (formerly classified as *Pseudomonas*) was detected in over 80% of the samples analysed by HTS. The authors suggested that its relevance might have been underestimated since these bacteria are not routinely diagnosed. Although preliminary, these findings may explain why most neutropenic patients with fever of unknown origin (i.e. those with negative blood cultures) respond to initial empirical antibacterial therapy.

12.1.4 Risk Factors for Gram-Negative Infections and Related Mortality

Several risk factors have been described for severe, antibiotic-resistant gram-negative bacterial sepsis and the related mortality in neutropenic, haemato-

Table 12.1 Factors facilitating gram-negative bacterial sepsis in HSCT recipients

Age of the recipient
Severity of immunosuppression and neutropenia
Comorbidities and organ dysfunctions
Type of HSCT transplantation (Allo- vs. auto-transplantation)
Degree of stem cell match (full matched, mismatched, haploidentical)
Mucosal injury
Central venous catheter
Previous exposure to antimicrobials (such as fluoroquinolone prophylaxis)
Change in host microbiota
Previous colonisation by resistant gram negatives
Presence of acute or chronic graft versus host disease (GVHD)

logical cancer patients. In HSCT transplant patients, a complex interplay between various host and graft factors may predispose patients to have serious gram-negative infections. Table 12.1 summarises the most important predisposing factors to gram-negative bacteraemia and related mortality in haematological cancer patients.

The relationship between severity and longevity of neutropenia and gram-negative bacteraemia has long been known (Gustinetti and Mikulska 2016; Akova 2016). Previous antibiotic exposure may lead to gram-negative colonisation. Then, these bacteria can translocate from the gut through the chemotherapy-disrupted mucosa, leading to bacteraemia (Song and Peter 2019). However, a recent literature review of FQ prophylaxis in neutropenic patients and a large surveillance study identified conflicting results on colonisation or infection with MDR strains after prophylaxis (Mikulska et al. 2018a; Kern et al. 2018).

In a multicentre, prospective observational study with 2226 admissions in 18 haematological institutions in Italy revealed that 144 patients (6.5%) were colonised with MDR gram negatives at admission (Cattaneo et al. 2018). ESBL-producing bacteria were found in 44% of the colonised patients and CRE was found in 59%. Overall, 25.7% of the colonised patients developed at least one episode of BSI. In 62.2% of the BSIs, previously colonised bacteria were the

responsible agents. Overall survival at 3 months was significantly lower in CRE-colonised patients (83.6%) as compared with ESBL colonisers (96.8%). In another multicentre trial, a total of 278 episodes of *K. pneumoniae* BSI was analysed between 2010 and 2014 (Trecarichi et al. 2016). CR was present in 57.9% of the isolates. Overall 21-day mortality was 36.3%. Factors related to mortality were septic shock, acute respiratory failure, inadequate antimicrobial therapy and CR (Trecarichi et al. 2016). In a retrospective survey involving 52 centres in Italy, carbapenem-resistant *K. pneumoniae* (CRKp) colonisation before or after transplant was followed by infection in 25.8% and 39.2% of auto- and allo-HSCT recipients, respectively (Girmenia et al. 2015). The infection-related mortality rates were 16% and 64.4% in respective recipients. Multivariate analyses revealed that CRKp infection before transplantation and subsequent CRKp-targeted first-line antibiotic therapy were significantly related with mortality due to infection after allo-HSCT. A global prevalence study and systematic review also indicated that CR in gram negatives infecting neutropenic patients is correlated with mortality and previous exposure to carbapenems (Righi et al. 2017).

MDR *P. aeruginosa* was identified in 7% of 589 episodes of BSIs in 357 acute leukaemia cases. The related factors for MDR phenotype were found to be prior anti-pseudomonal cephalosporin and current beta-lactam use, shock and pulmonary source of infection. Inappropriate treatment of BSIs caused by this pathogen was significantly associated with mortality in patients (Garcia-Vidal et al. 2018).

The type of HSCT may affect the frequency and severity of gram-negative BSIs. Due to the higher intensity of immunosuppression, allo-HSCT recipients are more prone to severe infections and increased mortality than auto-HSCT recipients. In a single-centre study in China, 1847 patients undergoing haploidentical or human leukocyte antigen (HLA)-identical sibling HSCTs between 2013 and 2016 were analysed (Yan et al. 2018). Haploidentical transplant recipients had more and earlier BSIs than HLA-identical transplant recipients. A multivariate analysis revealed that diagnosis of myelodysplastic syndrome, interval from diagnosis to HSCT >190 days, carbapenem therapy and grade 3–4 mucositis were related with the occurrence of BSI, mostly by *E. coli* and *K. pneumoniae* as gram-negative pathogens. BSI was an independent risk factor for an increased all-cause mortality in haploidentical recipients at 3 months.

12.2 Emerging Issues in the Diagnosis of Gram-Negative Infections

Blood cultures are still considered the gold standard for diagnosing BSIs (Kirn and Weinstein 2013). However, only 10–30% of blood cultures are positive in febrile neutropenic patients (Gyarmati et al. 2015). With modern automated systems, time-to-culture positivity could be less than 24 h for most of the MDR pathogens (Puerta-Alcalde et al. 2019), but antibiotic susceptibility test results may take another 7–24 h even with the most advanced automatisation (Marschal 2017). When one considers the consequences of inappropriate empirical antimicrobial therapy in neutropenic cancer patients, this lag time is too long. Thus, the current interest in developing point-of-care tests for bedside identification of the causative microorganisms and their resistance mechanisms is very high. Multiplex polymerase chain reaction (PCR) methodology can identify multiple bacterial species simultaneously, and several commercial tests are available (Lebovitz and Burbelo 2013). However, with these tests, only a limited of number of bacteria can be identified. Species identification with matrix-assisted laser desorption ionisation–time of flight (MALDI-TOF) mass spectrometry and molecular techniques have been used in combination to shorten the time to diagnosis, aiming for earlier appropriate antimicrobial therapy (Egli et al. 2015; de Souza et al. 2018). Combining MALDI-TOF identification with real-time antimicrobial stewardship intervention has been shown to shorten the time to appropriate antibiotic therapy (Beganovic et al. 2017). The 16S metagenomics sequencing library can be used to detect bacteria

simultaneously in blood samples. It is based on PCR amplification of the 16S ribosomal RNA gene and subsequent sequencing of the amplicons. This gene is highly conserved in prokaryotes but not present in humans (Rutanga et al. 2018). By combining these methods, not only bacterial pathogens can be identified but also information about their antimicrobial resistance mechanisms can be obtained. In a few small-scale trials, several uncultured bacteria could be identified in blood samples from neutropenic patients. However, these techniques still require ample time for positive results and are no point-of-care tests. Nonetheless, identifying several bacterial phyla in a patient with neutropenia without fever may help to predict future bacteraemia episodes and may lead to a tailored empirical antimicrobial therapy. An extensive review on the diagnosis of BSIs from positive blood cultures and directly from blood samples was recently published (Peker et al. 2018).

12.3 Current Approaches for Empirical Therapy of Gram-Negative Bacteria: Escalation and De-Escalation Therapy

The choice of effective antimicrobial therapy among haematological patients is hampered by an increased number of gram-negative bacteria (GNB) that re-emerged as the most common pathogen isolated from blood cultures along with high resistance rates to broad-spectrum antibiotics (Montassier et al., 2013; Gudiol et al., 2013; Rolston, 2005). Most commonly isolated GNBs include Enterobacteriaceae such as *Escherichia coli* and *Klebsiella pneumoniae*, *Pseudomonas aeruginosa* and, less frequently, *Acinetobacter* spp. (Klastersky et al., 2007). In areas where antimicrobial resistance in GNB is common, the correct choice of empirical therapy is particularly challenging, especially among patients with severe infections that require prompt treatment. MDR pathogens responsible for life-threatening infections among haematological patients include extended-spectrum beta-lactamase (ESBL)-producing Enterobacteriaceae and carbapenem-resistant bacteria (e.g. *A. baumannii, K. pneumoniae* and *P. aeruginosa*) (Satlin et al., 2013). Among neutropenic patients, infections caused by carbapenem-resistant bacteria have been associated with increased mortality (Righi et al., 2017). Various risk factors have been associated with the development of MDR GNB infection, including advanced underlying disease with severe clinical presentation, prolonged hospital stay, colonisation or previous infections with resistant bacteria, exposure to broad-spectrum antibiotics and urinary catheter placement (Sahin et al., 2009; Gudiol et al., 2011; Gudiol et al., 2010; Kang et al., 2012). The use of inadequate antimicrobial regimens due to the presence of MDR bacteria is a frequent cause of delayed initiation of appropriate treatment and represents one of the main causes for adverse outcomes in patients with severe infections, especially among those with profound immunosuppression (Cosgrove, 2006; Ramphal, 2004). The correct approach to severe infections in haematological patients is based on the assessment of various factors, including patient's characteristics (e.g. age, duration of aplasia, liver and/or kidney impairment, history of previous infections or colonisation due to MDR GNB), infection characteristics (e.g. type of infection and disease severity), as well as the site's local epidemiology and resistance patterns. Prompt initiation of appropriate empiric therapy is paramount in haematological patients, and should be followed by clinical reassessment after the availability of susceptibility tests (Bassetti & Righi, 2013). Finally, the choice of a correct targeted therapy should take the patient's comorbidities, type and site of the infection, and pathogen resistances into account (Averbuch et al., 2013).

According to these factors, an 'escalation' or a 'de-escalation' approach can be selected to treat severe infections in haematological patients (Table 12.2). Escalation therapy usually includes coverage against non-resistant Enterobacteriaceae and *P. aeruginosa*, using monotherapy with a beta-lactam (e.g. ceftazidime, cefepime or piper-

Table 12.2 Escalation and de-escalation approaches in the treatment of infections among patients with haematological malignancies

Escalation approach	
Indication	Antimicrobial therapy
• Sites where infections due to MDR bacteria are rare, and strict surveillance system is in place. • Uncomplicated clinical presentation. • No known colonisation with MDR bacteria. • No previous infection with MDR bacteria.	• Anti-pseudomonal cephalosporin (e.g. cefepime, ceftazidime). • Piperacillin/tazobactam.
De-escalation approach	
• ESBL prevalence is high or MDR pathogens are regularly seen. • Known colonisation or previous infection with ESBL-producing or other resistant GNB. • Previous exposure (<30 days) to broad-spectrum antibiotics. • Seriously ill patients (e.g. septic shock, pneumonia).	• Carbapenem monotherapy. • Anti-pseudomonal beta-lactam + aminoglycoside or fluoroquinolone. • Colistin + beta-lactam. • Early coverage of MDR gram-positive bacteria.

MDR, multidrug-resistant; *ESBL*, extended-spectrum beta-lactamase; *GNB*, gram-negative bacteria

acillin/tazobactam). This approach reduces the use of carbapenems and combination treatment, thus limiting toxicities and selection pressure, and can be modified in case of clinical deterioration or isolation of a resistant pathogen. In case of compromised patients with severe presentation or risk for infections caused by MDR GNB (e.g. high local prevalence of ESBL-producing bacteria, previous history of colonisation or infection due to MDR GNB, or other risk factors for resistance), a strategy using a narrow-spectrum antibiotic may lead to inadequate early treatment and potential negative outcomes. In these cases, a de-escalation therapy using broad-spectrum regimens (e.g. a carbapenem or combination therapy with an aminoglycoside plus a beta-lactam, or colistin with a beta-lactam) that are active against highly resistant pathogens is recommended. De-escalation therapy should always be followed by clinical reassessment after 48–72 h of treatment to optimise antimicrobial therapy according to the results of susceptibility tests.

In conclusion, MDR GNB threat should be taken into consideration when choosing an empirical treatment for haematological patients, according to clinical parameters and the local epidemiology. Prompt patient evaluation, risk assessment and treatment with broad-spectrum antibiotics are required when MDR GNB involvement is suspected. Reassessment after 48–72 h from the beginning of an empiric treatment is mandatory to optimise a targeted therapy, in case of documented multiple resistances, and to avoid an unnecessary use of broad-spectrum antibiotics. Implementation and review of infection control policies are mandatory if MDR pathogens are regularly seen at the onset of febrile neutropenia.

12.4   New Antimicrobial Options for the Treatment of MDR Gram-Negative Infections

The emergence of MDR GNB strains, including MDR *P. aeruginosa* and extended-spectrum beta-lactamases (ESBLs)-producing Enterobacteriaceae, has dramatically narrowed the choices for targeted treatment and increased the risk of empirical inadequate therapy (Kanj & Kanafani, 2011). Furthermore, the increased use of broad-spectrum antimicrobials led to the emergence of isolates that were resistant to the majority of available molecules, including carbapenems and colistin (Gupta et al., 2011; Munoz-Price et al., 2013; Liu et al., 2016).

In the past decades, the increase in MDR GNB has not been counterbalanced by the availability of new compounds (Hersh et al., 2012). Fortunately, new molecules with in vitro activity against carbapenem-resistant GNB have just recently been developed. The new molecules include a combination of beta-lactam antibiotics with beta-lactamase inhibitors (BLBLIs), novel beta-lactam antibiotics and drugs that do not belong to the beta-lactam class. Novel BLBLIs include avibactam, relebactam and vaborbactam

that show the ability to inhibit Class A carbapenemases-producing bacteria such as *Klebsiella pneumoniae* carbapenemase-producing *K. pneumoniae* (KPC-Kp) (Toussaint & Gallagher, 2015). New FDA-approved BLBLIs with activity against carbapenem-resistant Enterobacteriaceae (CRE) include ceftazidime/avibactam and meropenem/vaborbactam.

Among other novel beta-lactam antibiotics, ceftolozane has been approved in combination with tazobactam and showed high efficacy against MDR *P. aeruginosa* (Munita et al., 2017). Other non-beta-lactam antibiotics recently approved by the FDA include plazomicin, a novel aminoglycoside and eravacycline (Rodríguez-Avial et al., 2015; Bassetti & Righi, 2014a).

Novel compounds such as cefiderocol (S-649266), a novel siderophore cephalosporin and the association of aztreonam with avibactam are currently under investigation and may provide new tools against other carbapenemases (Falagas et al., 2017; Davido et al. 2017).

The new molecules show promising results when compared to a combination of old molecules such as carbapenems, colistin, tigecycline and aminoglycosides (Shields et al., 2016; Van Duin et al., 2018; Shields et al., 2017; Ayaz et al. 2018). Here, we discuss the characteristics and efficacy of newly FDA-approved compounds with activity against carbapenem-resistant GNB.

Ceftazidime/avibactam has shown activity against CRE and carbapenem-resistant *P. aeruginosa* (Chen et al. 2017). Avibactam is a non-beta-lactam, beta-lactamase inhibitor that inhibits the activity of Ambler Class A (ESBL and KPC), Class C (AmpC) and some Class D (OXA-48) enzymes, but it is not active against metallo-beta-lactamases such as NDM, VIM and IMP (Keepers et al., 2015). Based on the results of Phase 3 trials, ceftazidime/avibactam is approved for use in complicated urinary tract infections (cUTI), complicated intra-abdominal infections (cIAI) and hospital-acquired pneumonia (HAP), including ventilator-associated pneumonia (VAP).

The emergence of resistance has been reported during treatment with ceftazidime/avibactam (Shields et al., 2016), and its use has later been reported in association with other antimicrobials

(Van Duin et al., 2018; Shields et al., 2017; Royo-Cebrecos et al. 2017). Promising results were shown by real-world studies comparing ceftazidime/avibactam with a combination of older antibiotics, such as a carbapenem plus an aminoglycoside or colistin, in the treatment of KPC-producing strains (Shields et al., 2017). Compared to colistin, ceftazidime/avibactam showed lower 30-day adjusted all-cause hospital mortality (9% vs. 32%, respectively, p = 0.001) (Van Duin et al., 2018). In Phase 3 clinical trials, adverse events were similar between ceftazidime/avibactam and comparators, and no safety concerns have emerged for ceftazidime/avibactam from recent studies (Mazuski et al., 2016; Gyarmati et al. 2016; Torres et al., 2017).

Among haematological patients, the experience with ceftazidime/avibactam remains limited. A study including 30 patients showed similar mortality but a higher 14-day clinical cure for those treated with ceftazidime/avibactam (n = 8) compared with other treatments (85.7% vs. 34.8%, respectively, p = 0.031) (Castón et al., 2017).

This novel antibiotic may be an effective alternative for treating haematological patients with CRE, although more data are needed to confirm its efficacy in this patient population.

Meropenem/vaborbactam is a novel Class A and Class C BLBLI and displays a high affinity for serine beta-lactamases (Hackel et al., 2017). In a study including 991 isolates of KPC-producing Enterobacteriaceae, vaborbactam was able to reduce meropenem MIC50 and MIC90 from 32 to 0.06 μg/mL and 1 μg/mL, respectively (Hackel et al., 2017; Sun et al., 2017). Overall, meropenem/vaborbactam has demonstrated high in vitro activity against KPC-producing Enterobacteriaceae (Hackel et al., 2017) but has no activity on Class D and Class B carbapenemases and against CR non-fermenting GNB (Lomovskaya et al., 2017). Meropenem/vaborbactam received FDA approval in August 2017 for the treatment of cUTI based on the results of the TANGO1 trial, showing its superiority versus piperacillin/tazobactam in the treatment of cUTI and acute pyelonephritis (Kaye et al., 2018). Meropenem/vaborbactam was well tolerated

with headache, diarrhoea and infusion site phlebitis being the most frequently reported adverse events (Kaye et al., 2018).

In a Phase 3 trial encompassing 72 patients with BSI, cUTI, HAP/VAP, or cIAI due to carbapenem-resistant Enterobacteriaceae, meropenem/vaborbactam was associated with increased clinical cure and lower all-cause mortality. The comparator was best available therapy including ceftazidime/avibactam monotherapy or combination treatment with a carbapenem or an aminoglycoside, polymyxin B/colistin or tigecycline (27% vs. 68%, p = 0.008 and 5% vs. 33%, p = 0.03, respectively) (Ayaz et al. 2018).

Although data in immunocompromised patients are lacking, meropenem/vaborbactam may represent a promising option for the treatment of CRE infections in various patient populations.

Ceftolozane/tazobactam is a BLBLI combination characterised by high activity against *P. aeruginosa*, including strains with resistance caused by derepressed AmpC or upregulated efflux pumps (Livermore et al., 2009), but excluding carbapenemases such as KPC and MBL-producing strains (Takeda et al., 2007). The combination with tazobactam enhances the activity against ESBL-producing Enterobacteriaceae (Armstrong et al., 2015). Ceftolozane/tazobactam is currently approved for the treatment of cIAI, in combination with metronidazole, and for cUTI based on the results of clinical trials (Huntington et al., 2016; Solomkin et al., 2015). Post-marketing studies have explored the efficacy of ceftolozane/tazobactam for the treatment of MDR *P. aeruginosa*, including respiratory infections (Munita et al., 2017; Marschal 2017).

A multicentre, retrospective study including 35 patients with infections due to carbapenem-resistant *P. aeruginosa* treated with ceftolozane/tazobactam showed successful outcome in 74% of the patients (Munita et al., 2017). Another recent study encompassing 101 patients (78% with carbapenem-resistant *P. aeruginosa*) showed overall clinical success rates of 83.2% (Bassetti et al., 2018).

Preliminary studies have shown the efficacy and favourable profiles of ceftolozane/tazobactam among patients with haematological malignancies (Fernández-Cruz et al., 2018; de Souza et al. 2018). In a single-centre study including 19 patients (>60% neutropenic), similar cure rates at day 14 of treatment and lower 30-day mortality were reported among patients treated with ceftolozane/tazobactam compared with those receiving alternative therapies for MDR *P. aeruginosa* infections (Fernández-Cruz et al., 2018).

This compound appears promising due to the increased rates of MDR *P. aeruginosa* among neutropenic patients, including areas where resistances to broad-spectrum antibiotics are relatively low (Righi et al., 2017).

Plazomicin is a novel aminoglycoside characterised by higher activity against KPC-producing bacteria compared to other aminoglycosides (Galani et al., 2012). Plazomicin demonstrated in vitro activity against aminoglycoside-resistant Enterobacteriaceae, ESBL-producing bacteria and CRE (Walkty et al., 2014). A study including 17 patients with BSI or HAP/VAP due to CRE showed lower mortality among those treated with plazomicin compared to colistin, when the antimicrobials were used in combination with meropenem or tigecycline, while creatinine levels were higher among patients treated with colistin compared to plazomicin (38% vs. 8%, respectively) (McKinnell et al., 2017). Plazomicin has recently been approved for the treatment of cUTI. A recent FDA briefing document, however, did not note substantial evidence for recommending plazomicin use in BSI (FDA Briefing Document 2018).

Eravacycline is a novel fluorocycline similar to tigecycline with efficacy against MDR Enterobacteriaceae including ESBL, KPC and OXA-producing strains and *A. baumannii* (Zhanel et al. 2018). Eravacycline has recently received FDA approval for the treatment of cIAI based on the results of a randomised, double-blind, multicentre study showing intravenous eravacycline non-inferiority compared to ertapenem (Solomkin et al. 2017).

In conclusion, novel FDA-approved compounds appear promising for the treatment of MDR GNB. More data, however, are awaited to confirm the superiority of novel strategies in the treatment of MDR GNB and the benefits for haematological patients in real-world practice.

12.5   Prevention Strategies: Antimicrobial stewardship, Infection Control Strategies and Targeted Decolonisation

Haematological patients may show prolonged intestinal colonisation with MDR GNB that poses them at high risk of developing resistant infections, especially during periods of chemotherapy-induced neutropenia and following HSCT (Birgand et al. 2013; Girmenia et al. 2015a; Zuckerman et al. 2011). A survey including tertiary hospitals showed the highest KPC-Kp colonisation rates and KPC-Kp attributable mortality in haematology compared to ICU, internal medicine and surgery wards (Bartoletti et al. 2013). Rates of infections among carriers in haematology, transplant surgery, ICU and medicine were 38.9%, 18.8%, 18.5% and 16%, respectively (Giannella et al. 2014).

In patients undergoing HSCT in areas with significant MDR GNB spread, monitoring of resistant bacteria such as KPC-Kp colonisation is suggested to implement infection control and to potentially guide empirical therapy in neutropenic febrile patients (Girmenia et al. 2015b).

Various studies have analysed the impact of decolonisation strategies in haematological patients but show variable results (Zuckerman et al. 2011; Tascini et al. 2014; Saidel-Odes et al. 2012; Lübbert et al. 2013; Oren et al. 2013; Lambelet et al. 2017). Oral gentamicin and oral colistin used in patients with CRE colonisation accomplish decontamination rates ranging from 37% to 71% (Zuckerman et al. 2011; Tascini et al. 2014; Saidel-Odes et al. 2012; Lübbert et al. 2013; Oren et al. 2013; Lambelet et al. 2017), but the persistence of resistant strains in up to 40% of patients.

Tascini et al. performed a prospective study encompassing 50 consecutive patients with gut colonisation due to gentamicin-susceptible KPC-Kp who received oral gentamicin and 6 months of post-treatment follow-up (Tascini et al. 2014). Less effective decolonisation occurred among patients with ongoing infections receiving antimicrobial treatment (44% vs. 96%, P < 0.001). Although a lower number of KPC-Kp infections was detected among patients receiving oral gentamicin compared to those who did not (15% vs. 73%, P < 0.001), mortality rates were similar among groups, and 25% persistent carriers presented gentamicin-resistant KPC-Kp colonisation after treatment.

A multidisciplinary consensus statement suggests to consider decontamination in carriers undergoing HSCT (Girmenia et al. 2015b) but highlighted that there is poor evidence to support a recommendation due to the limited experience in haematological populations and the need for further data regarding the risk of resistance selection. Specifically, the selection of colistin resistance could be detrimental since this compound is still often used as a backbone for the treatment of CRE infections (Bassetti and Righi 2014b). Furthermore, the timing to define definitive decolonisation is difficult to establish. A recent randomised trial showed a transient effect of oral colistin administration (2 MU q6h) on MDR/XDR GNB intestinal colonisation (in the 47% of cases due to *K. pneumoniae*) in 62 patients with haematological malignancies (Stoma et al. 2018). Efficacy of colistin treatment was demonstrated among patients receiving colistin versus no treatment (61.3% vs. 32.3%, respectively; p = 0.02) after 14 days, while no statistical difference was seen on day 21 post-treatment among both groups. Lower BSIs were reported in the decolonisation arm in the first 30 days after the intervention (3.2% vs. 12.9%), but the results were not confirmed at the 90-day follow-up. In conclusion, there is currently not enough evidence to recommend a decolonisation with oral antibiotics among haematological patients who are CRE carriers, and the decision should be taken on an individual patient basis.

Haematological patients are particularly exposed to antibiotics for the prevention or treatment of infection due to the frequent episodes of neutropenia caused by multiple courses of immunosuppressive treatments. Collateral damage

from the use of broad-spectrum antibiotics (e.g. cephalosporins or quinolones) includes the selection of multiple resistances to different antibiotic classes as well as an increased risk of developing candidemia and *Clostridioides difficile* infection (Das et al. 2011; Gifford and Kirkland 2006). A recent critical appraisal of the European Conference on Infections in Leukaemia (ECIL) guidelines for patients with prolonged neutropenia systematically revised the evidence of FQ prophylaxis impact on BSIs, showing a decreased incidence of BSIs but no impact on overall mortality rates (Mikulska et al. 2018b). Due to FQ toxicity and resistance, it is suggested to weigh the benefits of their use as prophylaxis in patients with severe neutropenia according to the changes in local ecology (Mikulska et al. 2018b).

Due to the frequent exposure to prolonged broad-spectrum antibiotics, haematological patients would largely benefit from antimicrobial stewardship (AMS) programmes which have the objective to limit, when possible, the unnecessary use of antibiotics (Gyssens et al. 2013). AMS programmes in haematology aim to improve outcomes, guarantee cost-effective therapy and reduce adverse effects of antimicrobial use, including collateral damage such as antimicrobial resistance. Elements of therapy optimisation include de-escalation of broad empirical regimens, once the susceptibility test is available, and dose optimisation, especially in severe infections and among critically ill patients (Kaki et al. 2011). Specifically, antibiotic regimens should be individualised according to pharmacokinetic/pharmacodynamic (PK/PD) principles, considering that, similarly to ICU patients, high-risk haematological patients often have large volumes of distribution and may require higher doses and/or extended infusion of antimicrobials (e.g. beta-lactams) to obtain target concentrations (Abbott and Roberts 2012; Lortholary et al. 2008).

Infection control measures are strictly correlated with AMS programmes and share the objective of limiting the number of infections caused by MDR bacteria. Infection control measures in haematology are well established and include patient's isolation and cohorting, strict hand hygiene measures enforcing antisepsis with alcohol-based hand-rubs, standard barrier precautions, use of single rooms and high-efficiency particulate air (HEPA) filtration for HSCT recipients (Freifeld et al. 2011; Pittet et al. 2000).

To ensure the optimisation of the different aspects involved in AMS programmes, a multidisciplinary approach is necessary, involving microbiologists, hospital pharmacy, haematologists and infectious diseases specialists. Shared protocols, mutual training, frequent clinical rounds with discussion of patient management, antimicrobial drug use and infection control are recommended to ensure a successful collaboration among different specialists. Gyssens et al. have recently summarised the principles of AMS for haematological cancer patients (Gyssens et al. 2013), emphasising the importance of regular reviews of local surveillance data, including rates of antibiotic consumption and resistance, to increase the optimisation of empirical therapy and to develop local protocols and algorithms. The performance of surveillance cultures to document colonisation with MDR pathogens is also important, although their relevance should be supported by data documenting the outcome of patients with BSI caused by different pathogens that may be

detected as colonisers. Furthermore, the development of local management algorithms should take into consideration patients' risk stratification (e.g. Multinational Association for Supportive Care in Cancer—MASSC risk index score) as well as the individualised risk assessment for infections due to MDR pathogens. A prompt availability of microbiological results should be guaranteed, and implementation of rapid techniques for identification of susceptibility profiles should be favoured to optimise treatment. When possible, de-escalation or treatment discontinuation should be considered. Tailored de-escalation and discontinuation have proven to be safe in selected high-risk haematological patients (Slobbe et al. 2009; Cornelissen et al. 1995; la Martire et al. 2018), also during pre-engraftment neutropenia (Gustinetti et al. 2018). AMS main interventions and expected benefits are summarised in Table 12.3.

In conclusion, the optimisation of AMS programmes in haematology is crucial in the era of growing microbial resistance. AMS implementation is justified by the global resistance crisis, the limited number of novel antibiotics available against MDR GNB, and high rates of mortality caused by infections due to resistant pathogens in

Table 12.3 Aims and related interventions associated to potential AMS programmes in haematology

Aims	Interventions
• Optimisation of therapy duration. • Reduction of antibiotic resistances.	• Interactive bedside education on antimicrobial drug use. • Reporting of positive clinical cultures. • Implementation of rapid techniques for bacterial identification. • De-escalation to narrow-spectrum antibiotics. • Discontinuation of therapy in stable patients. • Limitation of prophylaxis to selected high-risk patients. • Reassessment of empirical therapy after 48–72 h of treatment.
• Optimisation of antimicrobial dosing. • Reduction of antimicrobial toxicity.	• Use of high doses, beta-lactam extended infusion. • Therapeutic drug monitoring. • Risk stratification for type of infection and disease severity.
• Optimisation of management protocols. • Optimisation of empirical therapy.	• Multidisciplinary approach, protocol sharing. • Performance of surveillance cultures. • Monitoring of BSI outcomes. • Periodic update of local epidemiology data (at least twice yearly). • Surveillance of most common GNB resistance. • Monitor antimicrobial consumption (DDDs). • Perform patients' risk factor analysis for resistant infections.

BSI, bloodstream infections; *GNB*, gram-negative bacteria; *DDDs*, defined daily doses haematological patients. Infection control measures are paramount and complementary to AMS programmes to prevent the spread of resistant pathogens.

References

Abbott IJ, Roberts JA (2012) Infusional beta-lactam antibiotics in febrile neutropenia: has the time come? Curr Opin Infect Dis 25(6):619–625

Akova M (2016) Epidemiology of antimicrobial resistance in bloodstream infections. Virulence 7:252–266

Alevizakos M, Gaitanidis A, Andreatos N, Arunachalam K, Flokas ME, Mylonakis E (2017) Bloodstream infections due to extended-spectrum β-lactamase-producing Enterobacteriaceae among patients with malignancy: a systematic review and meta-analysis. Int J Antimicrob Agents 50:657–663

Alp S, Akova M (2013) Management of febrile neutropenia in the era of bacterial resistance. Ther Adv Infect Dis 1:37–43

Alp S, Akova M (2017) Antibacterial resistance in patients with hematopoietic stem cell transplantation. Mediterr J Hematol Infect Dis. 9:e2017002

Ambler RP (1980) The structure of beta-lactamases. Philos Trans R Soc Lond Ser B Biol Sci 289:321–331

Armstrong ES, Farrell DJ, Palchak M et al (2015) In vitro activity of Ceftolozane-Tazobactam against anaerobic organisms identified during the ASPECT-cIAI study. Antimicrob Agents Chemother 60:666–668

Averbuch D, Orasch C, Cordonnier C et al (2013) ECIL4, a joint venture of EBMT, EORTC, ICHS, ESGICH/ESCMID and ELN. European guidelines for empirical antibacterial therapy for febrile neutropenic patients in the era of growing resistance: summary of the 2011 4th European conference on infections in Leukaemia. Haematologica 98:1826–1835

Averbuch D, Tridello G, Hoek J et al (2017) Antimicrobial resistance in gram-negative rods causing bacteremia in hematopoietic stem cell transplant recipients: intercontinental prospective study of the infectious diseases working Party of the European Bone Marrow Transplantation Group. Clin Infect Dis 65:1819–1828

Ayaz CM, Sancak B, Ceylan S, Akova M. Distribution of gram negative bacteria isolated from blood cultures of febrile neutropenic patients and their antimicrobial susceptibilities: seven years of experience. 20th symposium on infections in the immunocompromised host. Abstract no. 27. June 17-19, 2018. Athens, Greece

Bartoletti M, Girometti N, Lewis RE, Tumietto F, Cristini F, Ambretti S, Tedeschi S, Ciliberti MF, Di Lauria N, Finzi G, Viale P. Prospective, Cross-Sectional Observational Study of Hospitalized Patients Colonized with Carbapenemase-Resistant Klebsiella pneumoniae (CR-KP). Presented at 23th European Congress of Clinical Microbiology and Infectious Diseases (ECCMID), Berlin, Germany; 2013

Bassetti M, Righi E (2013) Multidrug-resistant bacteria: what is the threat? Hematology Am Soc Hematol Educ Program 2013:428–432

Bassetti M, Righi E (2014a) Eravacycline for the treatment of intra-abdominal infections. Expert Opin Investig Drugs 23:1575–1584

Bassetti M, Righi E (2014b) SDD and colistin resistance: end of a dream? Intensive Care Med 40(7):1066–1067

Bassetti M, Castaldo N, Cattelan A, Mussini C, Righi E, Tascini C, Menichetti F, Mastroianni CM, Tumbarello M, Grossi P, Artioli S, Carrannante N, Cipriani L, Coletto D, Russo A, Digaetano M, Losito R, Peghin M, Capone A, Nicolè S, Vena A (2018) Ceftolozane/tazobactam for the treatment of serious P. aeruginosa infections: a multicentre nationwide clinical experience. Int J Antimicrob Agents. pii: S0924–8579(18)30326–1

Beganovic M, Costello M, Wieczorkiewicz SM (2017) Effect of matrix assisted laser desorption ionization–time of flight mass spectrometry (MALDI-TOF MS) alone versus MALDI-TOF MS combined with real-time antimicrobial stewardship interventions on time to optimal antimicrobial therapy inpatients with positive blood cultures. J Clin Microbiol 55:1437–1445

Birgand G, Armand-Lefevre L, Lolom I, Ruppe E, Andremont A, Lucet JC (2013) Duration of colonization by extended-spectrum ß-lactamase-producing Enterobacteriaceae after hospital discharge. Am J Infect Control 41(5):443–447

Bodro M, Gudiol C, Garcia-Vidal C et al (2014) Epidemiology, antibiotic therapy and outcomes of bacteraemia caused by drug-resistant ESKAPE pathogens in cancer patients. Support Care Cancer 22:603–610

Castón JJ, Lacort-Peralta I, Martín-Dávila P, Loeches B, Tabares S, Temkin L, Torre-Cisneros J, Paño-Pardo JR (2017) Clinical efficacy of ceftazidime/avibactam versus other active agents for the treatment of bacteraemia due to carbapenemase-producing Enterobacteriaceae in hematologic patients. Int J Infect Dis 59:118–123

Cattaneo C, Di Blasi R, Skert C et al (2018) Bloodstream infections in haematological cancer patients colonized by multidrug-resistant bacteria. Ann Hematol 97:1717–1726

Chen CY, Tien FM, Sheng WH et al (2017) Clinical and microbiological characteristics of bloodstream infections among patients with haematological malignancies with and without neutropenia at a medical Centre in northern Taiwan, 2008-2013. Int J Antimicrob Agents 49:272–281

Collignon P, Beggs JJ, Walsh TR, Gandra S, Laxminarayan R (2018) Anthropological and socioeconomic factors contributing to global antimicrobial resistance: a univariate and multivariable analysis. Lancet Planet Health 2:e398–e405

Cornelissen JJ, Rozenberg-Arska M, Dekker AW (1995) Discontinuation of intravenous antibiotic therapy during persistent neutropenia in patients receiving prophylaxis with oral ciprofloxacin. Clin Infect Dis 21(5):1300–1302

Cosgrove SE (2006) The relationship between antimicrobial resistance and patient outcomes: mortality, length of hospital stay, and health care costs. Clin Infect Dis 42:S82–S89

Das I, Nightingale P, Patel M, Jumaa P (2011) Epidemiology, clinical characteristics, and outcome of candidemia: experience in a tertiary referral center in the UK. Int J Infect Dis 15(11):e759–e763

Davido B, Fellous L, Lawrence C et al (2017) Ceftazidime-Avibactam and Aztreonam, an Interesting Strategy To Overcome β-Lactam Resistance Conferred by Metallo-β-Lactamases in Enterobacteriaceae and Pseudomonas aeruginosa. Antimicrob Agents Chemother:61(9)

Egli A, Osthoff M, Goldenberger D et al (2015) Matrix-assisted laser desorption/ionization time-of-flight mass spectrometry(MALDI-TOF) directly from positive blood culture flasks allows rapid identification of bloodstream infections in immunosuppressed hosts. Transpl Infect Dis 17:481–487

Eichenberger EM, Thaden JT (2019) Epidemiology and mechanisms of resistance of extensively drug resistant gram-negative bacteria. Antibiotics 8:37

European Centre for Disease Prevention and Control (2019). Surveillance of Antimicrobial Resistance in Europe 2017. European Center for Disease Prevention: Sona, Sweden. https://ecdc.europa.eu/en/publications-data/surveillance-antimicrobial-resistance-europe-2017. Accessed 11 May 2019

Falagas ME, Skalidis T, Vardakas KZ, Legakis NJ (2017) Activity of cefiderocol (S-649266) against carbapenem-resistant gram-negative bacteria collected from inpatients in Greek hospitals. J Antimicrob Chemother 72:1704–1708

FDA Briefing Document. Plazomicin sulfate Injection Meeting of the Antimicrobial Drugs Advisory Committee (AMDAC); 2018 [cited 2018 Jun 10]. https://www.fda.gov

Fernández-Cruz A, Alba N, Semiglia-Chong MA, Padilla B, Rodríguez-Macías G, Kwon M, Cercenado E, Chamorro-de-Vega E, Machado M, Pérez-Lago L, de Viedma DG, Díez Martín JL, Muñoz P (2018) Real-life experience with ceftolozane/tazobactam in patients with hematologic malignancy and Pseudomonas aeruginosa infection: a case-control study. Antimicrob Agents Chemother. pii: AAC.02340–18

Freifeld AG, Eric J, Bow EJ, Kent A et al (2010) Clinical practice guideline for the use of antimicrobial agents in neutropenic patients with Cancer: 2010 update by the Infectious Diseases Society of America. Clin Infect Dis 62:e56–e93

Freifeld AG, Bow EJ, Sepkowitz KA, Boeckh MJ, Ito JI, Mullen CA et al (2011) Clinical practice guideline for the use of antimicrobial agents in neutropenic patients with cancer: 2010 update by the Infectious Diseases Society of America. Clin Infect Dis 52(4):e56–e93

Galani I, Souli M, Daikos GL, Chrysouli Z et al (2012) Activity of plazomicin (ACHN-490) against MDR clinical isolates of Klebsiella pneumoniae, Escherichia coli, and Enterobacter spp. from Athens, Greece. J Chemother 24:191–194

Garcia-Vidal C, Cardozo-Espinola C, Puerta-Alcalde P et al (2018) Risk factors for mortality in patients with acute leukaemia and bloodstream infections in the era of multiresistance. PLoS One 13(6):e0199531

Giannella M, Trecarichi EM, De Rosa FG, Del Bono V, Bassetti M, Lewis RE, Losito AR, Corcione S, Saffioti C, Bartoletti M, Maiuro G, Cardellino CS, Tedeschi S, Cauda R, Viscoli C, Viale P, Tumbarello M (2014) Risk factors for carbapenem-resistant Klebsiella pneumoniae bloodstream infection among rectal carriers: a prospective observational multicentre study. Clin Microbiol Infect 20(12):1357–1362

Gifford AH, Kirkland KB (2006) Risk factors for Clostridium difficile-associated diarrhoea on an adult hematology-oncology ward. Eur J Clin Microbiol Infect Dis 25(12):751–755

Girmenia C, Rossolini GM, Piciocchi A et al (2015) Gruppo Italiano Trapianto Midollo Osseo (GITMO); Gruppo Italiano Trapianto Midollo Osseo GITMO. Infections by carbapenem-resistant Klebsiella pneumoniae in SCT recipients: a nationwide retrospective survey from Italy. Bone Marrow Transplant 50:282–288

Girmenia C, Rossolini GM, Piciocchi A et al (2015a) Infections by carbapenem-resistant Klebsiella pneumoniae in stem cell transplant recipients: a nationwide retrospective survey from Italy. Bone Marrow Transplant 50(2):282–288

Girmenia C, Viscoli C, Piciocchi A et al (2015b) Management of carbapenem resistant Klebsiella pneumoniae infections in stem cell transplant recipients: an Italian multidisciplinary consensus statement. Haematologica 100(9):e373–e376

Girmenia C, Bertaina A, Piciocchi A, Gruppo Italiano Trapianto di Midollo Osseo (GITMO) and Associazione Microbiologi Clinici Italiani (AMCLI) et al (2017) Incidence, risk factors and outcome of pre-engraftment gram-negative bacteraemia after allogeneic and autologous hematopoietic stem cell transplantation: an Italian prospective multicentre survey. Clin Infect Dis 65:1884–1896

Gudiol C, Calatayud L, Garcia-Vidal C et al (2010) Bacteraemia due to extended-spectrum beta-lactamase-producing Escherichia coli (ESBL-EC) in cancer patients: clinical features, risk factors, molecular epidemiology and outcome. J Antimicrob Chemother 65(2):333–341

Gudiol C, Tubau F, Calatayud L, Garcia-Vidal C, Cisnal M, Sánchez-Ortega I, Duarte R, Calvo M (2011) Carratalà J Bacteraemia due to multidrug-resistant gram-negative bacilli in cancer patients: risk factors, antibiotic therapy and outcomes. J Antimicrob Chemother 66(3):657–663

Gudiol C, Bodro M, Simonetti A et al (2013) Changing aetiology, clinical features, antimicrobial resistance, and outcomes of bloodstream infection in neutropenic cancer patients. Clin Microbiol Infect 19(5):474–479

Gupta N, Limbago BM, Patel JB, Kallen AJ (2011) Carbapenem resistant Enterobacteriaceae: epidemiology and prevention. Clin Infect Dis 53:60–67

Gustinetti G, Mikulska M (2016) Bloodstream infections in neutropenic cancer patients: A practical update. Virulence 7:280–297

Gustinetti G, Raiola AM, Varaldo R, Galaverna F, Gualandi F, Del Bono V, Bacigalupo A, Angelucci E, Viscoli C, Mikulska M (2018) De-Escalation and Discontinuation of Empirical Antibiotic Treatment in a Cohort of Allogeneic Hematopoietic Stem Cell Transplantation Recipients during the Pre-Engraftment Period. Biol Blood Marrow Transplant 24(8):1721–1726

Gyarmati P, Kjellander C, Aust C, Kalin M, Öhrmalm L, Giske CG (2015) Bacterial landscape of bloodstream infections in neutropenic patients via high throughput sequencing. PLoS One 10(8):e0135756

Gyarmati P, Kjellander C, Aust C, Song Y, Öhrmalm L, Giske CG (2016) Metagenomic analysis of bloodstream infections in patients with acute leukaemia and therapy-induced neutropenia. Sci Rep 6:23532

Gyssens IC, Kern WV, Livermore DM (2013) ECIL-4, a joint venture of EBMT, EORTC, ICHS and ESGICH of ESCMID. The role of antibiotic stewardship in limiting antibacterial resistance among hematology patients. Haematologica 98(12):1821–1825

Hackel MA, Lomovskaya O, Dudley MN, Karlowsky JA, Sahm DF (2017) In Vitro Activity of Meropenem-Vaborbactam against Clinical Isolates of KPC-Positive Enterobacteriaceae. Antimicrob Agents Chemother 62. pii: e01904–17

Hersh AL, Newland JG, Beekmann SE et al (2012) Unmet medical need in infectious diseases. Clin Infect Dis 54:1677–1678

Horiba K, Kawada JI, Okuno Y et al (2018) Comprehensive detection of pathogens in immunocompromised children with bloodstream infections by next-generation sequencing. Sci Rep 8:3784

Huntington J, Sakoulas G, Umeh O et al (2016) Efficacy of ceftolozane/tazobactam versus levofloxacin in the treatment of complicated urinary tract infections (cUTI) caused by levofloxacin-resistant pathogens: results from the cUTI trial. J Antimicrob Chemother 71:2014–2021

Jeannot K, Bolard A, Pleisat P (2017) Resistance to polymyxins in gram-negative organisms. Int J Antimicrob Agents 49:526–535

Kaki R, Elligsen M, Walker S, Simor A, Palmay L, Daneman N (2011) Impact of antimicrobial stewardship in critical care: a systematic review. J Antimicrob Chemother 66(6):1223–1230

Kang CI, Chung DR, Ko KS et al (2012) Risk factors for infection and treatment outcome of extended-spectrum beta-lactamase producing Escherichia coli and Klebsiella pneumoniae bacteraemia in patients with hematologic malignancy. Ann Hematol 91(1):115–121

Kanj SS, Kanafani ZA (2011) Current concepts in antimicrobial therapy against resistant gram-negative organisms: extended spectrum beta-lactamase-producing Enterobacteriaceae, carbapenem-resistant Enterobacteriaceae, and multidrug-resistant Pseudomonas aeruginosa. Mayo Clin Proc 86:250–259

Kara O, Zarakolu P, Ascioglu S et al (2015) Epidemiology and emerging resistance in bacterial bloodstream infections in patients with hematologic malignancies. Infect Dis (Lond) 47:686–693

Kaye KS, Bhowmick T, Metallidis S, Bleasdale SC, Sagan OS, Stus V, Vazquez J, Zaitsev V, Bidair M, Chorvat E, Dragoescu PO, Fedosiuk E, Horcajada JP, Murta C, Sarychev Y, Stoev V, Morgan E, Fusaro K, Griffith D, Lomovskaya O, Alexander EL, Loutit J, Dudley MN, Giamarellos-Bourboulis EJ (2018) Effect of Meropenem-Vaborbactam vs Piperacillin-Tazobactam on Clinical Cure or Improvement and Microbial Eradication in Complicated Urinary Tract Infection: The TANGO I Randomized Clinical Trial. JAMA 319(8):788–799

Keepers TR, Gomez M, Biek D, Critchley I, Krause KM (2015) Effect of In Vitro Testing Parameters on Ceftazidime-Avibactam Minimum Inhibitory Concentrations. Int Sch Res Notices 2015:489547. Published 2015 May 19. https://doi.org/10.1155/2015/489547

Kern WV, Weber S, Dettenkofer M, Hospital Infection Surveillance System for Patients with Haematologic/Oncologic Malignancies Study Group (ONKO-KISS) et al (2018) Impact of fluoroquinolone prophylaxis during neutropenia on bloodstream infection: data from a surveillance program in 8755 patients receiving high-dose chemotherapy for haematologic malignancies between 2009 and 2014. J Infect 77:68–74

Kirn TJ, Weinstein MP (2013) Update on blood cultures: how to obtain, process, report, and interpret. Clin Microbiol Infect 19:513–520

Klastersky J, Ameye L, Maertens J et al (2007) Bacteraemia in febrile neutropenic cancer patients. Int J Antimicrob Agents 30(Suppl 1):S51–S59

Lalaoui R, Djukovic A, Bakour S, Sanz J et al (2019) Detection of plasmid-mediated colistin resistance, mcr-1 gene, in Escherichia coli isolated from high-risk patients with acute leukaemia in Spain. J Infect Chemother. pii: S1341-321X(19)30072–8

Lambelet P, Tascini C, Fortunato S, Stefanelli A, Simonetti F, Vettori C, Leonildi A, Menichetti F (2017 Jul) Oral gentamicin therapy for Carbapenem-resistant Klebsiella pneumoniae gut colonization in hematologic patients: a single center experienc. New Microbiol 40(3):161–164

Lebovitz EE, Burbelo PD (2013) Commercial multiplex technologies for the microbiological diagnosis of sepsis. Mol Diagn Ther 17:221–231

Liu YY, Wang Y, Walsh TR, Yi LX, Zhang R, Spencer J, Doi Y, Tian G, Dong B, Huang X, Yu LF, Gu D, Ren H, Chen X, Lv L, He D, Zhou H, Liang Z, Liu JH, Shen J (2016) Emergence of plasmid mediated colistin resistance mechanism MCR1 in animals and human beings in China: a microbiological and molecular biological study. Lancet Infect Dis 16(2):161–168

Livermore DM (2012) Current epidemiology and growing resistance of gram-negative pathogens. Korean J Intern Med 27:128–142

Livermore DM, Mushtaq S, Ge Y et al (2009) Activity of cephalosporin CXA-101 (FR264205) against Pseudomonas aeruginosa and Burkholderia cepacia group strains and isolates. Int J Antimicrob Agents 34:402–406

Lomovskaya O, Sun D, Rubio-Aparicio D et al (2017) Vaborbactam: Spectrum of Beta-Lactamase Inhibition and Impact of Resistance Mechanisms on Activity in Enterobacteriaceae. Antimicrob Agents Chemother 61. pii: e01443–17

Lortholary O, Lefort A, Tod M, Chomat AM, Darras-Joly C, Cordonnier C (2008) Pharmacodynamics and pharmacokinetics of antibacterial drugs in the management of febrile neutropenia. Lancet Infect Dis 8(10):612–620

Lübbert C, Faucheux S, Becker-Rux D et al (2013) Rapid emergence of secondary resistance to gentamicin and colistin following selective digestive decontamination in patients with KPC-2-producing Klebsiella pneumoniae: a single-Centre experience. Int J Antimicrob Agents 42(6):565–570

Magiorakos AP, Srinivasan A, Carey RB et al (2012) Multidrug-resistant, extensively drug-resistant and pandrug-resistant bacteria: an international expert proposal for interim standard definitions for acquired resistance. Clin Microbiol Infect 18:268–281

Mairi A, Pantel A, Sotto A, Lavigne JP, Touati A (2018) OXA-48-like carbapenemases producing Enterobacteriaceae in different niches. Eur J Clin Microbiol Infect Dis 37:587–604

Marschal M (2017) Evaluation of the accelerate pheno system for fast identification and antimicrobial susceptibility testing from positive blood cultures in bloodstream infections caused by gram-negative pathogens. J Clin Microbiol 55:2116–2126

la Martire G, Robin C, Oubaya N, Lepeule R, Beckerich F, Leclerc M, Barhoumi W, Toma A, Pautas C, Maury S, Akrout W, Cordonnier-Jourdin C, Fihman V, Venditti M, Cordonnier C (2018) De-escalation and discontinuation strategies in high-risk neutropenic patients: an interrupted time series analyses of antimicrobial consumption and impact on outcome. Eur J Clin Microbiol Infect Dis 37(10):1931–1940

Matsumura Y, Peirano G, Devinney R et al (2017) Genomic epidemiology of global VIM-producing Enterobacteriaceae. J Antimicrob Chemother 72:2249–2258

Mazuski JE, Gasink LB, Armstrong J et al (2016) Efficacy and safety of ceftazidime-avibactam plus metronidazole versus Meropenem in the treatment of complicated intra-abdominal infection: results from a randomized, controlled, double-blind, phase 3 program. Clin Infect Dis 62(11):1380–1389

McKinnell JA, Connolly LE, Pushkin R et al (2017) Improved outcomes with Plazomicin (PLZ) compared with Colistin (CST) in patients with bloodstream infections (BSI) caused by Carbapenem-resistant Enterobacteriaceae (CRE): results from the CARE study. Open Forum Infect Dis 4:S531

Mikulska M, Viscoli C, Orasch C et al (2014) On behalf of the fourth European conference on infections in Leukaemia group (ECIL-4), a joint venture of EBMT, EORTC, ICHS, ELN and ESGICH/ESCMID. Aetiology and resistance in bacteraemias

among adult and paediatric haematology and cancer patients. J Infect 68:321–331

Mikulska M, Averbuch D, Tissot F et al (2018a) European conference on infections in Leukaemia (ECIL). Fluoroquinolone prophylaxis in haematological cancer patients with neutropenia: ECIL critical appraisal of previous guidelines. J Infect 76:20–37

Mikulska M, Averbuch D, Tissot F, Cordonnier C, Akova M, Calandra T, Ceppi M, Bruzzi P, Viscoli C (2018b) Fluoroquinolone prophylaxis in haematological cancer patients with neutropenia: ECIL critical appraisal of previous guidelines. J Infect 76(1):20–37

Montassier E, Batard E, Gastinne T et al (2013) Recent changes in bacteraemia in patients with cancer: a systematic review of epidemiology and antibiotic resistance. Eur J Clin Microbiol Infect Dis 32(7):841–850

Munita JM, Aitken SL, Miller WR et al (2017) Multicenter evaluation of Ceftolozane/Tazobactam for serious infections caused by Carbapenem-resistant Pseudomonas aeruginosa. Clin Infect Dis 65(1):158–161

Munoz-Price LS, Poirel L, Bonomo RA, Schwaber MJ, Daikos GL, Cormican M, Cornaglia G, Garau J, Gniadkowski M, Hayden MK, Kumarasamy K, Livermore DM, Maya JJ, Nordmann P, Patel JB, Paterson DL, Pitout J, Villegas MV, Wang H, Woodford N, Quinn JP (2013) Clinical epidemiology of the global expansion of Klebsiella pneumoniae carbapenemases. Lancet Infect Dis 13:785–796

Oren I, Sprecher H, Finkelstein R et al (2013) Eradication of carbapenem resistant Enterobacteriaceae gastrointestinal colonization with nonabsorbable oral antibiotic treatment: A prospective controlled trial. Am J Infect Control 41(12):1167–1172

Peker N, Couto N, Sinha B, Rossen JW (2018) Diagnosis of bloodstream infections from positive blood cultures and directly from blood samples: recent developments in molecular approaches. Clin Microbiol Infect 24:944–955

Pittet D, Hugonnet S, Harbarth S, Mourouga P, Sauvan V, Touveneau S et al (2000) Effectiveness of a hospital-wide programme to improve compliance with hand hygiene. Infection Control Programme Lancet 356(9238):1307–1312

Poirel L, Madec JY, Lupo A et al (2018) Antimicrobial resistance in Escherichia coli. Microbiol Spectr:6(4). https://doi.org/10.1128/microbiolspec.ARBA-0026-2017

Puerta-Alcalde P, Cardozo C, Suárez-Lledó M et al (2019) Current time-to-positivity of blood cultures in febrile neutropenia: a tool to be used in stewardship de-escalation strategies. Clin Microbiol Infect 25:447–453

Ramphal R (2004) Changes in the etiology of bacteraemia in febrile neutropenic patients and the susceptibilities of the currently isolated pathogens. Clin Infect Dis 39:S25–S31

Righi E, Peri AM, Harris PNA et al (2017) Global prevalence of carbapenem resistance in neutropenic patients and association with mortality and carbapenem use:

systematic review and meta-analysis. J Antimicrob Chemother 72:668–677

Rodríguez-Avial I, Pena I, Picazo JJ, Rodríguez-Avial C, Culebras E (2015) In vitro activity of the next-generation aminoglycoside plazomicin alone and in combination with colistin, meropenem, fosfomycin or tigecycline against carbapenemase-producing Enterobacteriaceae strains. Int J Antimicrob Agents 46:616–621

Rolston KV (2005) Challenges in the treatment of infections caused by gram-positive and gram-negative bacteria in patients with cancer and neutropenia. Clin Infect Dis 40:S246–S252

Rolston KV, Bodey GP, Safdar A (2007) Polymicrobial infection in patients with cancer: an underappreciated and underreported entity. Clin Infect Dis 45:228–233

Royo-Cebrecos C, Gudiol C, Ardanuy C, Pomares H, Calvo M, Jordi CJ (2017) A fresh look at polymicrobial bloodstream infection in cancer patients. PLoS One 12(10):e0185768

Rutanga JP, Puyvelde SV, Heroes A-S, Muvunyi CM, Jacobs J, Deborggraeve S (2018) 16S metagenomics for diagnosis of bloodstream infections: opportunities and pitfalls. Expert Rev Mol Diagn 18:749–759

Sahin E, Ersoz G, Goksu M, et al. Risk factors for hospital infections with multidrug-resistant bacteria in patients with cancer (abstract P1450). Presented at the 19th European Congress of Clinical Microbiology and Infectious Diseases, Helsinki, Finland, May 16–19, 2009

Saidel-Odes L, Polachek H, Peled N et al (2012) A randomized, double-blind, placebo-controlled trial of selective digestive decontamination using oral gentamicin and oral polymyxin E for eradication of carbapenem-resistant Klebsiella pneumoniae carriage. Infect Control Hosp Epidemiol 33(1):14–19

Satlin MJ, Calfee DP, Chen L et al (2013) Emergence of carbapenem-resistant Enterobacteriaceae as causes of bloodstream infections in patients with hematologic malignancies. Leuk Lymphoma 54(4):799–806

Shields RK, Potoski BA, Haidar G et al (2016) Clinical outcomes, drug toxicity, and emergence of ceftazidime-avibactam resistance among patients treated for Carbapenem-resistant Enterobacteriaceae infections. Clin Infect Dis 15(63):1615–1618

Shields RK, Nguyen MH, Chen L et al (2017) Ceftazidime-avibactam is superior to other treatment regimens against Carbapenem-resistant Klebsiella pneumoniae bacteremia. Antimicrob Agents Chemother 61:8

Slobbe L, Waal L, Jongman LR, Lugtenburg PJ, Rijnders BJ (2009) Three-day treatment with imipenem for unexplained fever during prolonged neutropaenia in haematology patients receiving fluoroquinolone and fluconazole prophylaxis: a prospective observational safety study. Eur J Cancer 45(16):2810–2817

Solomkin J, Hershberger E, Miller B, Popejoy M, Friedland I, Steenbergen J, Yoon M, Collins S, Yuan G, Barie PS, Eckmann C (2015) Ceftolozane/Tazobactam plus metronidazole for complicated intra-abdominal infections in an era of multidrug resistance: results from a randomized, double-blind, phase 3 trial (ASPECT-cIAI). Clin Infect Dis 60(10):1462–1471

Solomkin J, Evans D, Slepavicius A et al (2017) Assessing the efficacy and safety of Eravacycline vs Ertapenem in complicated intra-abdominal infections in the investigating gram-negative infections treated with Eravacycline (IGNITE 1) trial: a randomized clinical trial. JAMA Surg 152:224–232

Song Y, Peter GP (2019) Bacterial translocation in acute lymphocytic leukaemia. PLoS One 14:e0214526

de Souza ILA, Quiles MG, Boettger BC, Pignatari ACC, Cappellano P (2018) Tailoring antimicrobials in febrile neutropenia: using faster diagnostic and communication tools to improve treatment in the era of extensively resistant pathogens. Braz J Infect Dis 22:239–242

Stoma I, Karpov I, Iskrov I et al (2018) Decolonization of intestinal carriage of MDR/XDR gram-negative Bacteria with Oral Colistin in patients with Haematological malignancies: results of a randomized controlled trial. Mediterr J Hematol Infect Dis 10(1):e2018030

Sun D, Rubio-Aparicio D, Nelson K et al (2017) Meropenem-Vaborbactam resistance selection, resistance prevention, and molecular mechanisms in mutants of KPC-producing Klebsiella pneumoniae. Antimicrob Agents Chemother 61(12):e01694–e01e17

Takeda S, Nakai T, Wakai Y et al (2007) In vitro and in vivo activities of a new cephalosporin, FR264205, against Pseudomonas aeruginosa. Antimicrob Agents Chemother 51:826–830

Tascini C, Sbrana F, Flammini S et al (2014) Oral gentamicin gut decontamination for prevention of KPC-producing Klebsiella pneumoniae infections: the relevance of concomitant systemic antibiotic therapy. Antimicrob Agents Chemother 58(4):1972–1976

Theuretzbacher U, Gottwalt S, Beyer P et al (2019) Analysis of the clinical antibacterial and antituberculosis pipeline. Lancet Infect Dis 19:e40–e50

Torres A, Zhong N, Pachl J et al (2017) Ceftazidime-avibactam versus meropenem in nosocomial pneumonia, including ventilator-associated pneumonia (REPROVE): a randomised, double-blind, phase 3 non-inferiority trial. Lancet Infect Dis 10:747–748

Toussaint KA, Gallagher JC (2015) β-Lactam/β--lactamase inhibitor combinations: from then to now. Ann Pharmacother 49:86–98

Trecarichi EM, Pagano L, Martino B et al (2016) Bloodstream infections caused by Klebsiella pneumoniae in onco-hematological patients: clinical impact of carbapenem resistance in a multicentre prospective survey. Am J Hematol 91:1076–1081

Van Duin D, Lok JJ, Earley M et al (2018) Antibacterial resistance leadership group. Colistin versus ceftazidime-avibactam in the treatment of infections due to Carbapenem-resistant Enterobacteriaceae. Clin Infect Dis 66:163–171

Walkty A, Adam H, Baxter M et al (2014) In vitro activity of plazomicin against 5,015 gram-negative and gram-positive clinical isolates obtained from patients in Canadian hospitals as part of the CANWARD study, 2011–2012. Antimicrob Agents Chemother 58(5):2554–2563

Yan C-H, Mo X-D, Sun Y-Q et al (2018) Incidence, risk factors, microbiology and outcomes of pre-engraftment bloodstream infection after haploidentical hematopoietic stem cell transplantation and comparison with HLA-identical sibling transplantation. Clin Infect Dis 67(S2):S162–S173

Zhanel GG, Chung P, Adam H et al (2014) Ceftolozane/tazobactam: a novel cephalosporin/beta-lactamase inhibitor combination with activity against multidrug-resistant gram-negative bacilli. Drugs 74:31–51

Zhanel GG, Baxter MR, Adam HJ et al (2018) In vitro activity of eravacycline against 2213 gram-negative and 2424 gram-positive bacterial pathogens isolated in Canadian hospital laboratories: CANWARD surveillance study 2014-2015. Diagn Microbiol Infect Dis 91:55–62

Zuckerman T, Benyamini N, Sprecher H et al (2011) SCT in patients with carbapenem resistant Klebsiella pneumoniae: a single center experience with oral gentamicin for the eradication of carrier state. Bone Marrow Transplant 46(9):1226–1230

Herpes Viruses

13

Rosanne Sprute, Philipp Koehler,
and Oliver A. Cornely

13.1 Introduction

The family of herpes viridae comprises more than 200 members that infect a variety of eukaryotic organisms (Roizman and Baines 1991; Bharucha et al. 2019). Herpes viruses are extremely widespread on a global scale. In humans, ten herpes viruses have been identified as disease-causing with a wide variety of clinical manifestations. Human herpes viruses (HHV) are a family of nine deoxyribonucleic acid (DNA) viruses with no other reservoir known than humans: herpes simplex virus (HSV) 1 and 2, varicella zoster virus (VZV), Epstein–Barr virus (EBV), cytomegalovirus (CMV), human herpes virus 6 type A and type B, human herpes virus 7 and Kaposi sarcoma-associated herpes virus (KSHV). Simian herpes virus B is found in non-human primates and is mainly transmitted by macaque monkeys. It is a very rare cause of human infections (Bharucha et al. 2019).

All herpes viruses share common characteristics. They have an architecturally similar virion with a double-stranded DNA genome. They all establish latency—the property to maintain their genome after primary infection in host cells over the host's lifespan—and they may reactivate upon external stimuli or during periods of immunosuppression. Due to this, infections are currently incurable. The reactivation can be entirely asymptomatic or may lead to disease manifestations, particularly in immunocompromised individuals.

Based on their distinct biological characteristics, herpes viruses can be differentiated in three subclasses: Alpha herpes viruses are neurotropic viruses that establish latency primarily but not exclusively in sensory ganglia. They have a relatively short reproductive cycle. Beta herpes viridae persist predominantly in glandular, kidney and lymphoid tissue. They frequently cause massive cell enlargement (cytomegalia) and have a long reproductive cycle with slow infection in culture. Gamma viruses have a tropism for lymphocytes and have oncogenic potential (Table 13.1) (Roizman and Baines 1991).

This chapter discusses epidemiology, signs and symptoms, diagnostic procedures and therapy for the human herpes viruses. For prophylactic implications, please see chapter 'Antiviral Prophylaxis' and chapter 'Vaccine-Preventable Disease'.

R. Sprute (✉) · P. Koehler (✉) · O. A. Cornely (✉)
Department I for Internal Medicine, Excellence
Center for Medical Mycology (ECMM), University
of Cologne, Cologne, Germany

Cologne Excellence Cluster on Cellular Stress
Responses in Aging-Associated Diseases (CECAD),
University of Cologne, Cologne, Germany
e-mail: rosanne.sprute@uk-koeln.de; philipp.
koehler@uk-koeln.de; oliver.cornely@uk-koeln.de

© Springer Nature Switzerland AG 2021
O. A. Cornely, M. Hoenigl (eds.), *Infection Management in Hematology*, Hematologic
Malignancies, https://doi.org/10.1007/978-3-030-57317-1_13

Table 13.1 Human-pathogenic members of the herpes viridae family

Subtype		Features	Common clinical presentation	Presentation in population at risk/immunocompromised hosts
HHV-1 and HHV-2	Herpes simplex virus 1 and herpes simplex virus 2 (HSV-1, HSV-2)	Alpha herpes viruses	Primary infection: Stomatitis Reactivation: Herpes labialis, genital lesions	Encephalitis, esophagitis, hepatitis, pneumonia, ocular infections, stomatitis
HHV-3	Varicella-zoster virus (VZV)	Alpha herpes virus	Primary infection: Chickenpox Reactivation: Herpes zoster (shingles)	Cutaneous dissemination of herpes zoster, haemorrhagic lesions Hepatic and gastrointestinal involvement, meningoencephalitis, pneumonia
HHV-4	Epstein–Barr virus (EBV)	Gamma herpes virus	Infectious mononucleosis, chronic active EBV infection	Oral hairy leucoplakia Burkitt lymphoma, Hodgkin lymphoma, nasopharyngeal carcinoma, T cell lymphoma Lymphoproliferative disorders: Haemophagocytic lymphohistiocytosis, lymphomatoid granulomatosis and posttransplant lymphoproliferative disorders
HHV-5	Human cytomegalovirus (CMV), human beta herpes virus 5	Beta herpes virus	Infectious mononucleosis	Colitis, encephalitis, esophagitis, hepatitis, pneumonia, retinitis, bone marrow failure
HHV-6A and HHV-6B		Beta herpes virus	Roseola infantum	Encephalitis, hepatitis, pneumonitis, graft failure
HHV-7		Beta herpes virus	Roseola infantum	
HHV-8	Kaposi sarcoma-associated herpes virus (KSHV)	Gamma herpes virus	Kaposi sarcoma, lympho-proliferative disorders	Kaposi sarcoma, Kaposi sarcoma-associated herpesvirus inflammatory cytokine syndrome, lymphoproliferative disorders
	Herpes virus simiae B	Alpha herpes virus	Encephalitis, meningitis, myelitis, vesicular rash	

13.2 Herpes Simplex Virus 1 and 2 Infections in Haematology Patients

HSV-1 and HSV-2 infections are frequently diagnosed and seroprevalence is high, especially in low- and middle-income countries (Looker et al. 2015; Looker et al. 2020). In high-income countries, the overall seroprevalence is declining. Data from the United States show a decrease of the prevalence of both HSV-1 and HSV-2 from 2000 to 2016 (from 59.4% to 48.1%, and from 18.0% to 12.1%, respectively) in individuals between 14 and 49 years of age (McQuillan et al.

2018). Possible reasons are improvements in living and hygiene conditions (Xu et al. 2006).

For the most part primary infection is unapparent. HSV-1 transmission usually occurs during early childhood through oral contact with secretions or mucous membranes, while primary HSV-2 infection is associated with the advent of sexual activity.

HSV establishes latency in the neuronal cells of sensory nerve ganglia. Symptomatic HSV-1 reactivations usually manifest as recurrent orolabial and facial lesions, but HSV-1 is also found in increasing proportions as the cause of genital herpes (Bernstein et al. 2013; Roberts et al. 2003). In immunocompromised individuals, both primary infection and reactivation may cause severe disease.

HSV infections in patients with haematological malignancy are triggered by lack of host control of the virus and mainly manifest as a localized efflorescence of the oral and pharyngeal mucosa (Wade 2006; Baden et al. 2016). The loss of mucosal integrity during haematological treatment increases the risk of infectious complications, and reactivation of HSV-1 is the most common viral cause for stomatitis in patients with cancer. HSV reactivation typically manifests with vesicular lesions and may also cause ulcerations of the oral mucosa (Baden et al. 2016). Of note, the characteristic vesicular lesions may not always be present, mimicking other pathogens. For diagnosis, a swab of the lesions should be examined via polymerase chain reaction (PCR) or viral culture (Baden et al. 2016; Styczynski et al. 2009).

In patients with dysphagia, odynophagia or retrosternal burning, clinicians should consider HSV oesophagitis. Confirmation of the diagnosis by endoscopy should be considered, and in unclear cases, a confirmatory biopsy is the gold standard for diagnosing invasive oesophageal infections.

HSV infections among haematological patients are associated with prolonged viral shedding, as well as dissemination of infection to visceral sites. Both HSV-1 and HSV-2 may cause serious end-organ infections such as encephalitis, hepatitis, pneumonia, and ocular infections.

HSV encephalitis, the most common sporadic encephalitis in the western world, is caused by HSV-1 in the majority of cases and often affects the temporal lobe and limbic system. The clinical presentation is characterized by acute focal neurologic symptoms, headache, seizures, impaired consciousness, often accompanied by the rapid onset of fever. Rapid diagnosis and treatment are essential to lower morbidity and mortality of this devastating disease.

Diagnosing HSV is generally based on virologic confirmation through DNA detection via PCR or virus culture.

In immunocompromised patients, acyclovir is efficacious in terms of viral shedding, decrease and resolution of pain, and healing (Wade 2006; Styczynski et al. 2009). Intravenous acyclovir

remains the standard treatment for severe mucocutaneous or visceral HSV infections (Table 13.2). Resistance to acyclovir remains infrequent. In case of acyclovir-resistant HSV strains, foscarnet may be used as alternative treatment (Baden et al. 2016; Styczynski et al. 2009). For double- or multidrug-resistant strains, cidofovir was shown to be efficacious (Styczynski et al. 2009). Oral acyclovir or valacyclovir may be considered alternatives for less serious manifestations of HSV disease (Styczynski et al. 2009).

13.3 Varicella Zoster Infections in Haematology Patients

VZV causes two clinically distinct diseases. Chickenpox (varicella) results from a primary infection with VZV and are highly contagious with a manifestation rate of >85% (Wharton 1996). Transmission occurs via aerosolized droplets from nasopharyngeal secretions or by direct contact with vesicle fluid from skin lesions. Reactivation results in a distinct clinical disease—herpes zoster (shingles).

Chickenpox is characterized by prodromal symptoms such as fever, fatigue and anorexia, followed by a generalized vesicular rash. The primary infection usually has a mild disease course in children, but occasionally causes VZV-associated complications such as bacterial or fungal superinfections or serious neurologic complications, for example, encephalitis. In adults and particularly in immunocompromised individuals, the primary infection can be very severe with high fevers and visceral dissemination such as encephalitis, hepatitis and pneumonia (Styczynski et al. 2009).

During primary VZV infection, the virus establishes latency primarily in the trigeminal and dorsal root ganglia. The occurrence of viral reactivation is influenced by age-associated immune senescence, disease-related immunocompromise or iatrogenic immunosuppression. Approximately 30% of persons in the United States are estimated to experience herpes zoster during their lifetime (Harpaz et al. 2008). The rash starts as erythematous papules, typically in a

Table 13.2 Antiviral agents

Agent	Indication	Common dosages (in adults)	Renal impairment	Side effects
Acyclovir	HSV-1 and 2, VZV	Primary infection: HSV: 3 × 400 mg/d or 5 × 200 mg/d p.o. for 5–10d VZV: 5 × 800 mg p.o. for 7d Reactivation: HSV hepatitis, herpes zoster, VZV pneumonia: 3 × 10 mg/kg i.v. for 7–14d	Dose adjustment	Elevated liver enzymes, gastrointestinal complaints, nephrotoxicity, neurological complications, seizures
Brivudine	VZV	1 × 125 mg p.o. for 7d	No dose adjustment	Cave: Fatal interactions with 5-fluoropyrimidines, hepatitis
Cidofovir	CMV	Retinitis: Initial 5 mg/kg i.v. weekly for 2 weeks, maintenance 5 mg/kg i.v. every two weeks	Contraindicated in patients with GFR <55 mL/min	Alopecia, gastrointestinal complaints, nephrotoxicity, neutropenia, skin rash
Famciclovir	VZV	Herpes zoster: 3 × 500 mg p.o. for 10d	Dose adjustment	Headache, gastrointestinal complaints
Foscarnet	HSV 1 and 2, CMV	HSV: 3 × 40 mg/kg i.v. for 2–3 weeks CMV: Initial 3 × 60 mg/kg i.v. for 2–3 weeks, maintenance 1 × 90–120 mg/kg i.v. for 1 week	Dose adjustment	Anaemia, hypocalcaemia hypokalaemia, hypomagnesaemia, gastrointestinal complaints, genital ulcers, neutropenia, nephrotoxicity, paraesthesia
Ganciclovir	CMV	Initial 2 × 5 mg/kg i.v. for 14d, maintenance 1 × 5 mg/kg i.v. until PCR results negative for 14d	Dose adjustment	Depression, dyspnoea, gastrointestinal complaints, pancytopenia, nephrotoxicity, retinal detachment, urinary tract infection
Valacyclovir	HSV 1 and 2, VZV	HSV: 2 × 1000 mg/d p.o. for 5d–10d Herpes zoster: 3 × 1000 mg/d p.o. for 7d	Dose adjustment	Dyspnoea, elevated liver enzymes, gastrointestinal complaints, skin rash
Valganciclovir	CMV	Initial 2 × 900 mg p.o. for 21d, maintenance 1 × 900 mg/d p.o. until PCR results negative for 14d	Dose adjustment	Depression, dyspnoea, gastrointestinal complaints, pancytopenia, nephrotoxicity, retinal detachment, urinary tract infection

single thoracic or lumbar dermatome or several contiguous dermatomes, and is often accompanied by severe pain caused by acute neuritis. The majority of VZV infections in adult patients with haematological malignancy are reactivations and 80% present with localized disease (Wade 2006).

However, immunocompromised hosts are at risk for repetitive episodes of herpes zoster and severe VZV-related complications. Herpes zoster may generalize with cutaneous dissemination,

present with atypical, for example, haemorrhagic lesions, or have visceral involvement (meningoencephalitis, hepatic and gastrointestinal involvement, pneumonia), which may occur occasionally in the absence of skin manifestations. Visceral dissemination in immunocompromised hosts has been associated with high mortality (Wade 2006).

Additionally, syndromes including trigeminal zoster (herpes zoster ophthalmicus), Ramsey

Hunt syndrome (herpes zoster oticus) or soft tissue infections with bacterial or fungal superinfections may complicate the disease course and raise morbidity. Post-herpetic neuralgia is a painful long-term complication (Wade 2006).

PCR for VZV DNA is very sensitive (95%) and specific (100%) and can be used to detect viral genomes in vesicle fluids, cerebrospinal fluids, tissues, bronchoalveolar lavages, or EDTA blood (Sauerbrei et al. 1999; Sauerbrei 2016). It is more rapid compared to conventional culture techniques and therefore preferred. Direct immunofluorescent-antibody staining is an alternative that provides results fast, but with a lower sensitivity than PCR. Candidates for haematopoietic stem cell transplantation (HSCT) should be tested for VZV IgG antibodies to determine their risk for reactivation or de novo infection (Ullmann et al. 2016).

Antiviral treatment for HSV or varicella-zoster virus infection is only indicated if there is clinical or laboratory evidence of active viral disease (Freifeld et al. 2011). Antiviral treatment is highly efficacious at preventing dissemination and visceral involvement. Acyclovir, valacyclovir, famciclovir and brivudine were shown to be efficacious in reduction of complications (Wade 2006; Styczynski et al. 2009). Rapid initiation of intravenous acyclovir therapy is particularly critical in severely immunocompromised patient, for example, acute leukaemia and HSCT patients. In stable cutaneous disease, the tablet applications of acyclovir, valacyclovir, famciclovir or brivudine are therapeutic options. Of note, brivudine is contraindicated in patients receiving 5-fluoropyrimidines due to potentially fatal interactions (Table 13.2) (Styczynski et al. 2009).

13.4 Epstein-Barr-Virus Infections in Haematology Patients

EBV is highly prevalent worldwide with approximately 90–95% of adults being seropositive (Fugl and Andersen 2019). The virus is transmitted by oropharyngeal secretion, mainly during childhood or adolescence. After oral transmission, EBV has a tropism specific to epithelial cells and B lymphocytes. The incubation period lasts several weeks and leads to an activation of cytotoxic T lymphocytes and natural killer cells. This activation in turn causes a cell-mediated immune response, occasionally leading to the clinical presentation of infectious mononucleosis (Fugl and Andersen 2019).

Infections with EBV account for 90% of infectious mononucleosis cases. Infections in children usually cause no symptoms, while in adolescents and adults, the primary infection may cause pharyngitis with tonsillar exudation, fatigue, fever, swollen lymph nodes, hepatomegaly and splenomegaly. The majority of infections are self-limiting, but acute complications such as airway obstruction, acute liver failure and splenic rupture can occur (Fugl and Andersen 2019).

Laboratory diagnostics include a complete blood count and peripheral smear revealing lymphocytosis with atypical lymphocytes and a blood test for heterophile antibodies. In heterophile antibody-negative patients with a strong clinical suspicion, an EBV viral capsid antigen IgG and IgM antibody test is of diagnostic value offering higher sensitivity and specificity (Fugl and Andersen 2019).

Delayed complications are chronic active EBV infection and the mucocutaneous manifestation of oral hairy leucoplakia. Furthermore, EBV has oncogenic potential and is associated with the development of malignancies and lymphoproliferative disorders, including Burkitt lymphoma, Hodgkin lymphoma, nasopharyngeal carcinoma, T cell lymphoma and haemophagocytic lymphohistiocytosis, lymphomatoid granulomatosis and posttransplant lymphoproliferative disorders (PTLD) (Styczynski et al. 2009).

In contrast to other herpes viruses, EBV reactivations usually do not cause end-organ manifestations and are of minor importance for patients with haematological malignancies undergoing conventional chemotherapy (Styczynski et al. 2009). The main complication, particularly in allogenic HSCT with unrelated or mismatched donor, is PTLD. EBV-related PTLD results from the uncontrolled neoplastic proliferation of lymphoid or plasmacytic cells and is one of the most severe complications associated with transplantation and confers a high mortality risk (Styczynski et al. 2016).

High-risk HSCT patients should be closely monitored by quantitative PCR of EBV-DNA. Screening should start within the first month after allo-HSCT and should continue for at least 4 months after HSCT, with a frequency of at least once a week (Fugl and Andersen 2019; Styczynski et al. 2016).

The diagnostic of EBV-PTLD is based on consistent signs and symptoms such as fever and lymphadenopathy and the detection of EBV from the involved tissue. Diagnosis of disease is preferably based on biopsy and histological examination. Peripheral EBV viral load and PET-CT may support diagnosis in extranodular disease (Fugl and Andersen 2019).

Rapid initiation of treatment is vital due to the risk of rapidly progressive multi-organ failure. For the first-line treatment of PTLD, anti-CD20 therapy with rituximab is the choice. Rituximab is usually administered once per week while monitoring EBV viral load. If feasible, a reduction of immunosuppression should be taken into account. As second-line therapy, chemotherapy or a cellular immunotherapy with in vitro–generated donor EBV cytotoxic T cells are alternative treatment modalities. Antiviral agents are not active in PTLD (Fugl and Andersen 2019; Styczynski et al. 2016).

13.5 Cytomegalovirus Infections in Haematology Patients

In high-income countries, CMV infection is prevalent in approximately 60% of the adults. The virus transmission can occur via multiple routes but is mainly acquired by contact with saliva of individuals with viral shedding. CMV establishes latency in epithelial cells and monocytes/macrophages. The primary infection is asymptomatic in most cases or may present as a mononucleosis-like syndrome (Clark et al. 2003). Serious infections or reactivations in immunocompetent hosts are rare.

In immunocompromised individuals, CMV causes a variety of diseases. In the absence of effective antiviral prophylaxis, the incidence of CMV disease among patients with haematological malignancy ranges from 5% to 75% (Wade 2006). Patients after allogenic HSCT and after treatment with cytarabine, fludarabine, alemtuzumab or idelalisib are particularly at high risk. Cytomegalovirus causes multi-organ disease both early (<100 days) and late (>100 days) after HSCT and remains one of the most important pathogens for transplant-associated complications (Ljungman et al. 2019). Manifestations include febrile syndromes without organ-specific focus, encephalitis, esophagitis, gastrointestinal manifestations (mainly colitis), hepatitis, pneumonia and retinitis. CMV has further been associated with graft-versus-host disease and delayed granulocyte and platelet engraftment (Wade 2006; Clark et al. 2003). Early and late CMV disease have a varied presentation, with retinitis, encephalitis and bone marrow failure being more common in late than in early CMV disease (Wade 2006).

For the detection of acute CMV infection, antigenaemia assays or methods detecting CMV DNA or RNA are recommended from peripheral blood (Ljungman et al. 2008). Diagnosis of CMV disease (with organ involvement) is challenging, as many other pathogens may cause similar symptoms and coinfections are common. Diagnosis is based on signs and symptoms of organ infection and the detection of CMV by an appropriate method applied to the obtained specimen, such as culture, histopathology, CMV-specific immunostaining or in situ hybridization in a biopsy specimen. The exception is CMV retinitis, where typical findings by ophthalmologic examination are sufficient for diagnosis (Wade 2006; Ljungman et al. 2008). Symptoms of organ involvement accompanied by detection of CMV in blood are not sufficient for diagnosis of CMV disease. PCR detection of CMV DNA on biopsy material is also usually insufficient due to limitations in differentiating active disease from latency (Ljungman et al. 2008).

Treatment options for CMV disease are ganciclovir, valganciclovir, foscarnet and cidofovir (Table 13.2). Intravenous ganciclovir is the gold standard for first-line treatment of symptomatic

CMV infection (Ljungman et al. 2019; Marchesi et al. 2018). Treatment with foscarnet or cidofovir are alternatives for CMV infections caused by ganciclovir-resistant strains. Valganciclovir can be used instead of intravenous ganciclovir or foscarnet. The combination of antiviral therapy and intravenous immune globulin is established for treatment of CMV pneumonia (Wade 2006; Ljungman et al. 2019). For other manifestations of CMV disease, data do not support the addition of immune globulin (Wade 2006; Ljungman et al. 2019). Combination therapy may be used as second-line therapy (Ljungman et al. 2008).

Prophylaxis of infection or early preemptive intervention, for example, with letermovir, after routine surveillance by quantitative PCR (at least once per week for 100 days after transplant) remain the foundations of effective CMV infection management for seropositive patients (see chapter 'Antiviral Prophylaxis') (Wade 2006; Clark et al. 2003).

13.6 HHV-6 Infections in Haematology Patients

HHV-6A and HHV-6B have been recognized as distinct species during the past years (Ward et al. 2019). Both establish latency in T lymphocytes, monocytes-macrophages, epithelial cells and neuronal cells. Additionally, both HHV-6A and HHV-6B have the ability to persist by integration of their viral genome into host chromosomes, leading to germline inheritance of the chromosomally integrated DNA in about 1% of the population (Clark et al. 2003; Leong et al. 2007).

Primary infection with HHV-6B is causative of the febrile disease exanthema subitum (roseola infantum), a widespread disease during early childhood, while no disease has yet been causally linked to HHV-6A (Wade 2006; Ward et al. 2019). Accordingly, HHV-6B gives potential for reactivation and is associated with disease in the immunocompromised.

In patients with haematological malignancies not receiving HSCT, there is little evidence that HHV-6 causes disease (Ward et al. 2019). Following HSCT, HHV-6B was associated with a range of clinical syndromes, including encephalitis, hepatitis, pneumonitis, delayed platelet engraftment and early and late graft failure. Particularly, HHV-6B encephalitis is the most significant manifestation and an important cause of morbidity and mortality after allogeneic HSCT (Wade 2006; Ljungman et al. 2008; Ward et al. 2019). Symptoms are characterized by altered mental status, short-term memory loss and seizures (Ward et al. 2019; Ogata 2009).

Quantitative real-time PCR analysis on blood and cerebrospinal fluid is the method of choice to diagnose HHV-6B encephalitis. The PCR method should distinguish between HHV-6A and HHV-6B. In suspected end-organ disease other than failed engraftment or encephalitis, tissue from the affected organ should be tested for HHV-6 infection by culture, immunostaining or in situ hybridization instead of PCR detection of viral DNA (Ward et al. 2019). Aside from infection, high levels of HHV-6 DNA can also be detected in individuals with chromosomally integrated HHV-6, leading to diagnostic pitfalls. Chromosomal integration should be suspected if the level of viremia does not respond to initiation of antiviral therapy (Clark et al. 2003; Ljungman et al. 2008). Other likely infectious or noninfectious causes must be excluded.

Ganciclovir, foscarnet and cidofovir are inhibitors of HHV-6 replication in vitro. Ganciclovir and foscarnet, alone and/or in combination, have been used with assumed clinical response as treatment for HHV-6 infections. Cidofovir may be applied as second-line therapy, as drug-resistant isolates particularly against ganciclovir have been described (Clark et al. 2003; Ward et al. 2019).

13.7 HHV-7 Infections in Haematology Patients

HHV-7 is genetically closely related to HHV-6 and primary infection similarly is highly prevalent and causes roseola infantum in young children (Clark et al. 2003). However, in contrast to HHV-6, available data on the pathogenicity in patients with haematological malignancies and in

HSCT recipients are weak (Ljungman et al. 2008; Agut et al. 2017). Similar to HHV-6, reactivation of HHV-7 is described in HSCT patients, but no obvious correlation between HHV-7 infection and clinical endpoints including GvHD and engraftment was found (Clark et al. 2003). The diagnostic strategy would be similar for HHV-7 infections, even though diagnostic strategies are less well developed (Agut et al. 2017). Ganciclovir, foscarnet and cidofovir were shown to inhibit the replication of HHV-7 in vitro (Clark et al. 2003; Ljungman et al. 2008).

13.8 Kaposi Sarcoma-Associated Herpes Virus Infections in Haematology Patients

Prevalence of KSHV is worldwide variable with high seroprevalence in Africa, the Amazon basin and the Mediterranean area compared to North America or northern Europe. The mode of transmission is not completely understood. Primary infection may be transmitted sexually but also non-sexually in areas of high endemicity, probably via saliva, and via blood products and solid organ transplants. KSHV infects a variety of cells and has a broad cellular tropism (Ljungman et al. 2008).

KSHV was originally identified in biopsy samples of Kaposi sarcoma but has also been linked to some rare lymphoproliferative disorders such as primary effusion lymphoma, Kaposi sarcoma-associated herpesvirus inflammatory cytokine syndrome and multicentric Castleman's disease (MCD) with MCD-associated plasmablastic lymphoma, especially in individuals infected with human immunodeficiency virus (Ljungman et al. 2008; Quadrelli et al. 2011). Both, non-malignant associations and development of Kaposi sarcoma are described very rarely in HSCT patients (Ljungman et al. 2008; Cuzzola et al. 2003; Erer et al. 1997; Luppi et al. 2000).

Several serologic assays for the detection of serum anti-KSHV antibodies exist with moderate sensitivity and specificity, but a gold-standard serological test is lacking and existing tests are of limited clinical utility for the identification of previous infection. For detection of KSHV-DNA, different PCR techniques have been used, but no standard method is established, and clinical application again is limited (Ljungman et al. 2008; Riva et al. 2013).

The effect of antiviral agents on KSHV replication has not been extensively studied. In vitro testing and observational studies suggest a susceptibility to ganciclovir, foscarnet and cidofovir (Kedes and Ganem 1997). In a randomized trial with 26 patients, valganciclovir was shown to reduce both the frequency and quantity of KSHV viral shedding. Similar results could be found for valacyclovir and famciclovir (Cattamanchi et al. 2011). The clinical efficacy for KSHV-associated disease remains to be evaluated. In KSHV-associated CMD, antiviral treatment, particularly valganciclovir, is sporadically added to a combination regime (Lurain et al. 2018).

References

Agut H, Bonnafous P, Gautheret-Dejean A (2017) Update on infections with human herpesviruses 6A, 6B, and 7. Med Mal Infect 47:83–91

Baden LR, Swaminathan S, Angarone M et al (2016) Prevention and treatment of Cancer-related infections, version 2.2016, NCCN clinical practice guidelines in oncology. J Natl Compr Cancer Netw 14:882–913

Bernstein DI, Bellamy AR, Hook EW 3rd et al (2013) Epidemiology, clinical presentation, and antibody response to primary infection with herpes simplex virus type 1 and type 2 in young women. Clin Infect Dis 56:344–351

Bharucha T, Houlihan CF, Breuer J (2019) Herpesvirus infections of the central nervous system. Semin Neurol 39:369–382

Cattamanchi A, Saracino M, Selke S et al (2011) Treatment with valacyclovir, famciclovir, or antiretrovirals reduces human herpesvirus-8 replication in HIV-1 seropositive men. J Med Virol 83:1696–1703

Clark DA, Emery VC, Griffiths PD (2003) Cytomegalovirus, human herpesvirus-6, and human herpesvirus-7 in hematological patients. Semin Hematol 40:154–162

Cuzzola M, Irrera G, Iacopino O et al (2003) Bone marrow failure associated with herpesvirus 8 infection in a patient undergoing autologous peripheral blood stem cell transplantation. Clin Infect Dis 37:e102–e106

Erer B, Angelucci E, Muretto P et al (1997) Kaposi's sarcoma after allogeneic bone marrow transplantation. Bone Marrow Transplant 19:629–631

Freifeld AG, Bow EJ, Sepkowitz KA et al (2011) Clinical practice guideline for the use of antimicrobial agents in neutropenic patients with cancer: 2010 update by the infectious diseases society of america. Clin Infect Dis 52:e56–e93

Fugl A, Andersen CL (2019) Epstein-Barr virus and its association with disease - a review of relevance to general practice. BMC Fam Pract 20:62

Harpaz R, Ortega-Sanchez IR, Seward JF (2008) Prevention of herpes zoster: recommendations of the Advisory Committee on Immunization Practices (ACIP). MMWR Recomm Rep 57:1–30, quiz CE2–4

Kedes DH, Ganem D (1997) Sensitivity of Kaposi's sarcoma-associated herpesvirus replication to antiviral drugs. Implications for potential therapy. J Clin Invest 99:2082–2086

Leong HN, Tuke PW, Tedder RS et al (2007) The prevalence of chromosomally integrated human herpesvirus 6 genomes in the blood of UK blood donors. J Med Virol 79:45–51

Ljungman P, de la Camara R, Cordonnier C et al (2008) Management of CMV, HHV-6, HHV-7 and Kaposisarcoma herpesvirus (HHV-8) infections in patients with hematological malignancies and after SCT. Bone Marrow Transplant 42:227–240

Ljungman P, de la Camara R, Robin C et al (2019) Guidelines for the management of cytomegalovirus infection in patients with haematological malignancies and after stem cell transplantation from the 2017 European conference on infections in Leukaemia (ECIL 7). Lancet Infect Dis 19:e260–ee72

Looker KJ, Magaret AS, May MT et al (2015) Global and regional estimates of prevalent and incident herpes simplex virus type 1 infections in 2012. PLoS One 10:e0140765

Looker KJ, Johnston C, Welton NJ et al (2020) The global and regional burden of genital ulcer disease due to herpes simplex virus: a natural history modelling study. BMJ Glob Health 5:e001875

Luppi M, Barozzi P, Schulz TF et al (2000) Nonmalignant disease associated with human herpesvirus 8 reactivation in patients who have undergone autologous peripheral blood stem cell transplantation. Blood 96:2355–2357

Lurain K, Yarchoan R, Uldrick TS (2018) Treatment of Kaposi sarcoma herpesvirus-associated multicentric Castleman disease. Hematol Oncol Clin North Am 32:75–88

Marchesi F, Pimpinelli F, Ensoli F, Mengarelli A (2018) Cytomegalovirus infection in hematologic malignancy settings other than the allogeneic transplant. Hematol Oncol 36:381–391

McQuillan G, Kruszon-Moran D, Flagg EW, Paulose-Ram R (2018) Prevalence of herpes simplex virus type 1 and type 2 in persons aged 14-49: United States, 2015-2016. NCHS Data Brief:1–8

Ogata M (2009) Human herpesvirus 6 in hematological malignancies. J Clin Exp Hematop 49:57–67

Quadrelli C, Barozzi P, Riva G et al (2011) β-HHVs and HHV-8 in lymphoproliferative disorders. Mediterr J Hematol. Infect Dis 3:e2011043

Riva G, Barozzi P, Quadrelli C et al (2013) Human herpesvirus 8 (HHV8) infection and related diseases in Italian transplant cohorts. Am J Transplant 13:1619–1620

Roberts CM, Pfister JR, Spear SJ (2003) Increasing proportion of herpes simplex virus type 1 as a cause of genital herpes infection in college students. Sex Transm Dis 30:797–800

Roizman B, Baines J (1991) The diversity and unity of Herpesviridae. Comp Immunol Microbiol Infect Dis 14:63–79

Sauerbrei A (2016) Diagnosis, antiviral therapy, and prophylaxis of varicella-zoster virus infections. Eur J Clin Microbiol Infect Dis 35:723–734

Sauerbrei A, Eichhorn U, Schacke M, Wutzler P (1999) Laboratory diagnosis of herpes zoster. J Clin Virol 14:31–36

Styczynski J, Reusser P, Einsele H et al (2009) Management of HSV, VZV and EBV infections in patients with hematological malignancies and after SCT: guidelines from the second European conference on infections in leukemia. Bone Marrow Transplant 43:757–770

Styczynski J, van der Velden W, Fox CP et al (2016) Management of Epstein-Barr Virus infections and post-transplant lymphoproliferative disorders in patients after allogeneic hematopoietic stem cell transplantation: sixth European conference on infections in leukemia (ECIL-6) guidelines. Haematologica 101:803–811

Ullmann AJ, Schmidt-Hieber M, Bertz H et al (2016) Infectious diseases in allogeneic haematopoietic stem cell transplantation: prevention and prophylaxis strategy guidelines 2016. Ann Hematol 95:1435–1455

Wade JC (2006) Viral infections in patients with hematological malignancies. Hematology Am Soc Hematol Educ Program 2006:368–374

Ward KN, Hill JA, Hubacek P et al (2019) Guidelines from the 2017 European conference on infections in Leukaemia for management of HHV-6 infection in patients with hematologic malignancies and after hematopoietic stem cell transplantation. Haematologica 104:2155–2163

Wharton M (1996) The epidemiology of varicella-zoster virus infections. Infect Dis Clin N Am 10:571–581

Xu F, Sternberg MR, Kottiri BJ et al (2006) Trends in herpes simplex virus type 1 and type 2 seroprevalence in the United States. JAMA 296:964–973

Polyomavirus, Adenovirus, and Viral Respiratory Diseases

Simone Cesaro, Silvio Ragozzino and Nina Khanna

14.1 Human Polyomaviruses, BK Virus, and Hemorrhagic Cystitis: Epidemiology and Virological Characteristics

BK polyomavirus (BKPyV) belongs to the genus *Polyomavirus* of the family *Polyomaviridae* that comprises 13 different species with human host (Calvignac-Spencer et al. 2016). BKPyV virions are small non-enveloped particles of 40–45 nm in diameter, with an icosahedral symmetry, resistant to heat, and environment exposure (Hirsch and Steiger 2003). Structurally, BKPyV consists of a circular 5.1 kb double-stranded DNA genome within a capsid made of proteins Vp1 on the outside and Vp2 and Vp3 on the inside. The BKPyV genome is divided into three regions: the noncoding control region (NCCR); the early viral gene region (EVGR); the late viral gene region (LVGR). The NCCR is responsible for DNA replication and bidirectional viral gene

S. Cesaro (✉)
Pediatric Hematology Oncology, Mother and Child Department, Azienda Ospedaliera Universitaria Integrata Verona, Verona, Italy
e-mail: simone.cesaro@aovr.veneto.it

S. Ragozzino · N. Khanna (✉)
Division of Infectious Diseases and Hospital Epidemiology, University and University Hospital of Basel, Basel, Switzerland
e-mail: silvio.ragozzino@usb.ch; nina.khanna@usb.ch

expression; the EVGR encodes the regulatory nonstructural proteins called small tumor antigen (sTag), large tumor antigen (LTag), and spliced variants called truncated Tag; the LVGR contains the genes for the structural proteins Vp1, Vp2, Vp3, and a small accessory protein of unknown function called agnoprotein. The Vp1 capsid protein is the main target of BKPyV-specific antibodies while LTag is used as target for immunohistochemical diagnosis in tissue samples. BKPyV was isolated for the first time in a patient (B.K.) who underwent a kidney transplant and presented in the urine particular epithelial cells with nuclear viral inclusions called "decoy cells" (Gardner et al. 1971). Subsequently, BKPyV has been associated with hemorrhagic cystitis (HC) after hematopoietic stem cell transplantation (HSCT) (Apperley et al. 1987; Arthur et al. 1986), and nephropathy after kidney transplantation (Binet et al. 1999; Randhawa et al. 1999). Serologic studies showed that up to 90% of the adult population has been exposed to BKPyV during infancy and childhood (Egli et al. 2009). The infection can be asymptomatic or causes flu-like symptoms indistinguishable from other causes of viral community respiratory tract infections. The transmission is thought to be by direct person-to-person contact or by exposure to respiratory secretions. After primary infection, the virus remains latent in renal tubular epithelial and urothelial cells and asymptomatic viruria can be detected in 5–10%

© Springer Nature Switzerland AG 2021
O. A. Cornely, M. Hoenigl (eds.), *Infection Management in Hematology*, Hematologic Malignancies, https://doi.org/10.1007/978-3-030-57317-1_14

of healthy individuals (Hirsch and Steiger 2003; Egli et al. 2009). The urinary shedding increases to 60–80% in patients undergoing HSCT, as well as the BKPyV viruria load increases to less than 3 $\log_{10}$ to >7 $\log_{10}$ copies/mL (Cesaro et al. 2018a; Cesaro et al. 2015).

The incidence of BKPyV-HC is 8–25% and 7–54% in pediatric and adult patients, respectively, being higher in allogeneic than autologous HSCT and in haploidentical HSCT with post-transplant exposure to cyclophosphamide as prophylaxis of graft versus host reaction (GVHD) (Cesaro et al. 2018a). The occurrence of BKPyV-HC has a negative impact on duration and quality of hospitalization in the early post-transplant period while its effect on mortality and overall survival is still debated (Cesaro et al. 2015; Gilis et al. 2014).

The pathogenesis of posttransplant HC is multifactorial and the factors implicated are different according to the time of onset. The early-onset HC occurs during the conditioning regimen or by 48 hours from its end, and it is considered to be a consequence of the direct toxicity of drug catabolites or radiotherapy on the urothelial mucosa; its appearance can be facilitated by the presence of coagulopathy and thrombocytopenia. The late-onset HC is usually observed with the start of neutrophil engraftment (around the second week posttransplant) up to the first 2 months after transplant, and it is associated with infection by BKPyV (Apperley et al. 1987; Arthur et al. 1986; Cesaro et al. 2018a; Cesaro et al. 2015; Gaziev et al. 2010).

The current pathogenetic model of BKPyV-HC is based on the occurrence of the following events: (a) Urothelial toxicity due to the conditioning regimen with denudation of bladder mucosa. (b) High level of BKPyV replication due to the severe impairment of the immune system in the early weeks post-HSCT that increases further the damage of urothelial mucosa for the cytopathic effect of the virus. (c) Attraction and infiltration of the mucosa and submucosa by alloreactive inflammatory cells during the periengraftment period that determines the loss of urothelial lining, urinary bleeding, and macroscopic hematuria (Cesaro et al. 2018a).

14.1.1 Risk Factors

High-level of BKPyV viruria is found up to 50–80% of HSCT patients in the early months posttransplant, but its specificity is low because only less than 20–25% develop BKPyV-HC. The combination of BKPyV viremia >1 × 10^3 genomic copies/mL and viruria >7 × 10^6 genomic copies/mL resulted instead a more specific and sensitive predictive factors for late-onset BKPyV-HC in HSCT patients (Cesaro et al. 2015; Gaziev et al. 2010). Several other factors related to the type of transplant or transplant complications and recipient age are associated with a higher risk of BKPyV-HC: The use of cord blood (CB) and peripheral blood (PB) as stem cell source (Gilis et al. 2014; Rorije et al. 2014), unrelated donor transplant (Giraud et al. 2006), grade II–IV acute GvHD alone or combined with high BKPyV load in urine (Gaziev et al. 2010; Rorije et al. 2014; Bogdanovic et al. 2004; Hayden et al. 2015), myeloablative conditioning (MAC) containing anti-thymocyte globulin, cyclophosphamide or high-dose busulfan (Gaziev et al. 2010; Giraud et al. 2008; Peinemann et al. 2000), and in pediatric patients recipient age > 7 years (Laskin et al. 2013).

14.1.2 Definition, Clinical Findings, and Diagnostic Considerations

The severity of HC is defined by four grades: microscopic hematuria (grade 1); macroscopic hematuria (grade 2); macroscopic hematuria with clots (grade 3); and macroscopic hematuria with clots and impaired renal function secondary to urinary tract obstruction (grade 4) (Cesaro et al. 2018a). The diagnosis of BKPyV-HC is based on presence of signs of cystitis (dysuria, urinary frequency, lower abdominal pain), hematuria grade 2 or higher and the demonstration of BKPyV-viruria, with viral loads of >7 $\log_{10}$ genomic copies/mL. Plasma viral loads of >3–4 $\log_{10}$ copies/mL are seen in more than two thirds of allogeneic HSCT recipients with BKPyV-HC (Cesaro et al. 2015; Laskin et al. 2013; Cesaro et al. 2009;

Erard et al. 2005; Koskenvuo et al. 2013), and declining plasma loads have been found to correlate with clinical recovery. Ultrasound and computed tomography examinations can support the clinical diagnosis showing nonspecific signs of HC such as bladder wall thickness, mural edema, intraluminal clots, urethral obstruction, mucosal enhancement, and perivesical stranding (Schulze et al. 2008). BKPyV-HC generally resolves after 3–5 weeks, but it is associated with prolonged hospital care and significant patient pain or discomfort. Moreover, bleeding together with additional complications such as renal failure and delayed immune recovery may contribute to higher nonrelapse mortality and lower overall survival.

14.1.3 Prevention and Therapy

Apart from the early-onset HC that can be prevented by supportive measures such as hyperhydration, bladder irrigation, and in patients who receive cyclophosphamide in the conditioning regimen, the use of mesna (sodium mercaptoethanesulphonate), there are no effective measures to prevent BKPyV-HC. The use of fluoroquinolones that in vitro reduce BKPyV replication showed in retrospective studies modest or conflicting results (Cesaro et al. 2018a). Moreover, their use is associated with the increased risk of tendinitis and development of antibiotic resistance (Averbuch et al. 2017).

Considering BKPyV does not encode classic antiviral targets such as viral nucleoside kinases or DNA polymerase, the current antiviral drugs developed for herpesviruses are ineffective or suboptimal. Cidofovir (CDV), a nucleotide analogue that inhibits DNA replication for a broad range of viruses, is the antiviral more active against BKPyV. Its use has been reported by several authors in retrospective studies. Although there is no agreement on the optimal dose and the modality of administration of CDV, most authors used the dose of 3–5 mg/kg/weekly or every 2 weeks associated with probenecid to decrease nephrotoxicity. Overall, a complete clinical response was found in 74% of patients with a reduction ≥1 log of BKPyV load on urine and in blood in 38% and 84% of patients, respectively. Mild-to-moderate increase of creatinine level was found in 18% of the patients (Cesaro et al. 2018a). In a smaller number of patients treated with a low dose of cidofovir, 0.5–1.5 mg/kg/week, without probenecid, a complete clinical response was observed in 83% of patients with a reduction of BKPyV load in the urine and in blood in 62% and in 67% of patients, respectively. Mild-to-moderate renal toxicity was reported in 20% of patients (Cesaro et al. 2018a). There are anecdotal experiences where cidofovir at the dose of 5 mg/kg/week has been administered intravesically to avoid nephrotoxicity with 43% of complete clinical response and 50% of virological response (Cesaro et al. 2018a). Other drugs that have been associated with some efficacy against BKPyV-HC are leflunomide, an antimetabolite drug with immunomodulatory and antiviral activity, vidarabin, and oral levofloxacin. Brincidofovir, a lipid derivative of cidofovir, has shown in vitro the capacity to inhibit the replication of BKPyV in urothelial cell cultures but clinical data of efficacy and safety are awaited (Tylden et al. 2015). BKPyV-HC may benefit of nonspecific treatment aiming at speeding the reparation and regeneration of urothelial mucosa such as hyperbaric oxygen therapy (HOT) or the topical application of fibrin glue by cystoscopy (Zama et al. 2013; Tirindelli et al. 2014). Both procedures depend on local availability. Moreover, HOT also depends on patient tolerance because it can cause earache due to barotrauma and claustrophobia.

In absence of validated medical treatment for BKPyV-HC, the use of adoptive transfer of donor-derived virus-specific T cells (VSTs) is a possible option, especially in patients who undergo haploidentical HSCT with deep ex vivo T-cell depletion. This approach showed to be effective in infections caused by *Cytomegalovirus*, *Epstein-Barr* virus, and *Adenovirus*, although its use is limited by costs, complexity of production, time of preparation, and availability of a seropositive donor (Baugh et al. 2018). To overcome these obstacles, the preparation and banking of VST lines from third-party healthy donors has been proposed in order to treat timely HSCT recipients with drug-refractory infections. In a "proof of principle" phase II study, the use of pentavalent third-party-donor VSTs (directed against CMV, EBV, ADV, HHV-6, and BKPyV) in 16 HSCT patients with BKPyV disease (14 HC, 2 nephritis) obtained clinical benefit in all patients with a significant reduction of BKPyV viruria load by week 6 post infusion. Thirteen of 14 patients with BKPyV-HC had a complete resolution of macrohematuria, and in seven, increase of circulating BKPyV-VSTs was observed. In contrast, four of five patients with BKPyV-HC, who were screened for the study but not treated, had disease progression (Tzannou et al. 2017). The VST infusions were well tolerated, and none of the patients developed cytokine release syndrome. These results are encouraging and support further studies.

14.1.4 JC Polyomavirus

JC polyomavirus (JCPyV) was described in 1971, and its name derives from the initials of the patient in whom it was isolated for the first time (Padgett et al. 1971). JCPyV is member of the human polyomavirus family and shares with other polyomavirus, such as BKPyV, a common morphology, and structural organization. Seroprevalence studies showed that 40–80% of adult population has contracted JCPyV infection during infancy or adulthood. The infection is asymptomatic, and the route of transmission is supposed to be through fluids or secretions containing virus particles or also contaminated food or water. The contagion is followed by a viremia phase with the exposure of various target organs. JCPyV, as BKPyV, persists latently in the reno-urinary tract and intermittent low-level viruria has been described in healthy individuals who remain asymptomatic without any organ diseases (Dalianis and Hirsch 2013). In patients severely immunocompromised, such as patients affected by HIV/AIDS, patients with multiple sclerosis treated with natalizumab, or hematological patients, JCPyV has been associated with the

development of progressive multifocal leukoencephalopathy (PML) (Pavlovic et al. 2015). In hematological patients, PML has been reported in Hodgkin lymphoma, chronic lymphocytic leukemia, multiple myeloma, and autologous or allogeneic HSCT (Pelosini et al. 2008; Kharfan-Dabaja et al. 2007). The main risk factors are treatment with purine analogues, male sex, age > 55 years, CD4+ count $\leq 200 \times 10^9$/L, treatment with rituximab (Pelosini et al. 2008). The analysis of published data revealed that long-lasting lymphopenia, profound CD4+ and CD8+ deficiency, and reduced interferon-γ response are common findings described across different diseases and treatments associated with PML (Pavlovic et al. 2018). Mortality rates for PML ranges from 62% to 95% (Pelosini et al. 2008).

Retrospective studies on two allogeneic HSCT patients showed that JCPyV viremia preceded the neurological symptoms of PML by 105, and 126 days and that JCPyV viral load in blood strictly correlated with steroid dosage used for GvHD treatment. These observations suggest that the detection of persistent JCPyV viremia may predict the development of PML and that a faster withdrawal of immune suppression is allowed in patients with a good control of GvHD (Avivi et al. 2014). On the other hand, the lack of a clear correlation between the preemptive detection of JCPyV viremia and the development of PML underlines the role of other factors implicated such as neurotropism and virulence activity of a specific virus subtype (Pavlovic et al. 2018).

Currently, PML is still an untreatable disease with poor outcome and both prophylaxis and treatment represent unmet needs. In hematological patients, the main therapeutic measures aim at improving immune response to JCPyV by withdrawing steroids or other immunosuppressive drugs whilst anecdotal benefit has been reported with antivirals (brincidofovir, ganciclovir, and leflunomide), JCPyV cell entry inhibitors (chlorpromazine, citalopram, mirtazapine, risperidone), JCPyV vaccination, and administration of JCPyV or third-party BKPyV-specific cytotoxic T lymphocytes (Pavlovic et al. 2015; Balduzzi et al. 2011; Muftuoglu et al. 2018).

14.2 Adenovirus

14.2.1 Epidemiology and Virological Characteristics

The species of human adenovirus (HAdV) comprises seven subgroups, termed A–G, belonging to the family *Adenoviridae*, genus *Mastadenovirus*, with the species B divided in subspecies B1 and B2. Inside of each species, 51 HAdV were identified by serotyping but, from 2007, many other types were detected by genomic analysis (Lion 2014). The name comes from the initial isolation of HAdV from adenoids of subjects with acute febrile respiratory illness. HAdV species have a large (90–100 nm), icosahedral, non-enveloped structure containing a double-stranded DNA and can infect different mucosal sites. The most common site of entry is *Coxsackie Adenovirus* receptor (CAR) except for subgroup B that uses CD46 cell-surface antigen. The transmission occurs through airborne droplets, human direct contact or through secretions, biological fluids (vomitus, feces, saliva), contaminated water, medical instruments, airflow filters, hospital surfaces, and hands of personnel or caregivers. HAdV indeed is resistant to gastric and biliary secretions or low pH, and maintains its stability for weeks in dry environment. Moreover, the non-enveloped structure makes it resistant to many disinfectants and the inactivation requires the exposure to alcohol solutions for at least 2 min or to sodium hypochlorite solutions for 10 min. After infecting epithelial cells (incubation time of 2 days–2 weeks), the spectrum of clinical symptoms is variable and depends on the HAdV type. In the immunocompetent host, HAdV species cause usually mild-to-moderate, self-limiting diseases such as conjunctivitis, nephritis, upper respiratory tract infection, cystitis, gastroenteritis, and rarely they have been associated to severe form of pneumonia or myocarditis. HAdV species are responsible for 5–10% of febrile episodes during infancy and approximately 10% of pneumonia in infants and young children; moreover, 70–80% of children have serological evidence of a prior HAdV infec-

tion by the age of 5 years, and almost all children have contracted a HAdV infection by the age of 10 years. Following primary infection, HAdV remains latent in the lymphoid tissue of tonsils, adenoids, lung, and gastrointestinal tract. HAdV DNA encodes for a viral DNA polymerase that is important for the process of viral replication, but at the same time, it represents an important target for antiviral drugs. In the immunocompromised host, HAdV infection can be a primary infection by transmission from the donor graft, environment, health personnel, caregivers, or secondary to endogenous reactivation, this latter being the most frequent. In fact, HAdV infection in stem cell transplant recipient is not related to cold season (winter, early spring), and the patients who are HAdV seropositive have higher risk of post-transplant infection; moreover, the detection of HAdV on nasopharyngeal aspirate or feces before transplant or during the first weeks is a risk factor for HAdV viremia and disease (Kosulin et al. 2018; Lion et al. 2010). In the hematopoietic stem cell transplant (HSCT) setting, the incidence of multi-organ involvement or disseminated disease is as high as 6–42% in pediatric patients and 3–15% in adult patients (Lion 2014). In a survey conducted among European transplant centers over a 5-year period (2013–2017), the incidence of HAdV infection in recipients of allogeneic HSCT was 15% for pediatric patients (<18 years) and 4% for adult patients (Cesaro et al. 2018b). The incidence figures may vary according to the criterion or test used to define HAdV infection. In another retrospective study, HAdV infection in the first 6 months after HSCT was 32% for pediatric patients and 6% for adult patients if positivity in any sample (respiratory, urine, blood, feces) was considered, whereas it resulted 14% and 1.5%, respectively, if only HAdV viremia ≥ 1000 genomic copies/mL was taken into consideration (Sedlacek et al. 2018). The higher incidence of HAdV infection in the pediatric age is related to the persistent shedding of the virus for months or years also in healthy children, which makes the horizontal transmission of a primary infection or reinfection by different serotypes more frequent. Immune response to HAdV infection is both humoral, by generating protective neutralizing antibodies, and cellular, by induction of specific CD4+ and CD8+ T lymphocytes (Keib et al. 2019). The lack of specific cellular immunity in the first months after transplant is primarily responsible for increasing viral replication in a patient with HAdV latency following a previous exposure (Feuchtinger et al. 2008; Guerin-El Khourouj et al. 2011).

14.2.2 Risk Factors and Outcome

Severe HAdV infection is associated with high load viremia and disseminated disease, in particular pneumonia. The factors associated to post-transplant HAdV viremia are young age, detection of HAdV in stool or nasopharynx before or after the transplant, the use of mismatched or haploidentical donor, the use of a cord blood allograft, T-depletion of the graft by CD34+ cell selection or the use of serotherapy with anti-thymocyte globulin or alemtuzumab, the presence of graft-versus-host disease (GvHD) requiring steroids at the dose of >1 mg/kg of prednisone, and severe lymphopenia (<300 lymphocytes/μL) (Lee et al. 2017). On the basis of the type of transplant and graft, period after transplant, and therapy of GvHD, Lindemans et al. proposed a risk classification for HAdV infection: a high-risk group comprising HSCT recipients within the first month after a cord blood graft, recipients of *in vitro* T-cell-depleted (CD3 + cell <5 × 10^4/kg) graft, and/or patients receiving prednisone with a dose >1 mg/kg together with one or more lymphocyte-proliferation inhibitors (e.g., cyclosporine-A and mycophenolate mofetil); an intermediate risk group comprising recipients of cord blood or T-cell-depleted grafts between first month and fourth month after HSCT and/or patients with immunosuppressive therapy consisting of two lymphocyte proliferation inhibitors or one lymphocyte-proliferation inhibitor and prednisone >0.5 and <1 mg/kg for prophylaxis or treatment of acute GvHD; and a low-risk group comprising recipients of all other types of transplant other than cord blood or T-cell-depleted graft, or all transplants after 4 months, irrespective of the type of donor sources, receiving immunosuppressive therapy with one proliferation inhibitor and/or prednisone ≤0.5 mg/kg/d (Lindemans et al. 2010). This classification can help define the type of HAdV monitoring and the timing of intervention. Despite the severity of HAdV infection may vary from a self-limited infection with low viremia to a fatal disease, one of the most important factors influencing the outcome is the recovery of specific cellular immunity. The appearance or the increase of HAdV-specific T cells have been associated with the clearance of infection; therefore, the absence of T-cell recovery (CD3+ <25/μL) or the absence of T-cell response to HAdV viremia (CD3+ <300/μL within 2 weeks) is used as indicator of poor outcome of infection (Feuchtinger et al. 2007; Chakrabarti et al. 2002). HAdV viremia ≥1000 genomic copies/mL is an indicator of disseminated disease, and there is evidence that viral burden, peak of HAdV viremia, duration of HAdV viremia, and $\log_{10}$ reduction of HAdV viremia in response to treatment are independent risk factors for mortality (Mynarek et al. 2014; Zecca et al. 2019). Given the different incidence of HAdV infection, overall mortality is higher in pediatric than in adult patients but in high-risk patients with HAdV viremia ≥1000 genomic copies/mL, the figures are as high as 18–22% in both age groups (Zecca et al. 2019; Lee et al. 2016).

14.2.3 Diagnostic Considerations

The study of previous exposure by serology of the donor/recipient pair has no role in defining measures to prevent HAdV infection after transplant due to the wide diffusion of HAdV in the population, the cross-reactivity of available assays, and the lack of effective drugs for HAdV prophylaxis. It has been shown that the presence or the appearance of a specific T-cell response is associated with protection or rapid recovery from HAdV infection, but its use is limited to experimental studies or selected centers (Feuchtinger et al. 2007; Zandvliet et al. 2010). The diagnosis of HAdV infection in HSCT patients is based on the demonstration of viral replication. In the past, this required 1–3 weeks using cell culture method or 2–3 days using the shell vial method, but the turnaround time of both limited their use in clinical practice. A shorter turnaround time of 2–4 hours is possible by direct demonstration of HAdV antigen in clinical specimens of nasopharyngeal swabs or aspirate, bronchoalveolar fluid or tracheal aspirate, stool with agglutination assay, fluorescence-labeled monoclonal antibody, enzyme immuno assay. The most sensitive, specific, and rapid technique is the determination of HAdV DNA with PCR on routine clinical samples of blood, stool, respiratory secretions, urine, cerebrospinal fluid, and tissues (Matthes-Martin et al. 2012). In particular, the presence of a high HAdV load in the blood is a sign of disseminated disease. Therefore, the use of quantitative real-time PCR in blood is useful to initiate early treatment, monitor the response to the treatment, and to predict the outcome of infection. Although low-level of HAdV DNAemia can be found in the early phase of an asymptomatic allogeneic HSCT, especially in pediatric patients, the development of HAdV DNAemia ≥1000 copies/mL is a marker of severe disease and predict dissemination, whereas a HAdV DNAemia ≥10.000 copies/mL is usually associated with disseminated disease, organ involvement, and high mortality. HAdV DNAemia ≥1000 copies/mL has been found in 14% of pediatric HSCT and 2% of adult HSCT, representing 61% and 51% of those viremic within 6 months from transplant, respectively (Sedlacek et al. 2018). Moreover, the peak of viral load, the duration of viremia, and the log reduction of viral load in response to therapy are predictors of mortality in patients with HAdV DNAemia (Lion 2014; Mynarek et al. 2014; Zecca et al. 2019). Based on these findings, the recommendation is to perform an active surveillance of HAdV in patients at risk by at least weekly determination of DNAemia during the first 3–4 months after transplantation (Hiwarkar et al. 2018). In pediatric patients, it is also recommended an active surveillance by PCR of HAdV load on stool because peak levels >10^{5-6} copies/g

are significantly associated with the subsequent development of HAdV DNAemia in a median time of 8–11 days (Lion et al. 2010; Hum et al. 2018). Quick raising of HAdV stool is proposed as criterion to start a preemptive treatment earlier, before HAdV infection became invasive, especially in patients lacking T-cell recovery. Nasopharyngeal detection of HAdV before HSCT in pediatric patients has been associated with the development of posttransplant and HAdV viremia (de Pagter et al. 2009). This finding has to be considered together with the patient clinical situation to decide whether to proceed or postpone the transplant procedure. For screening purposes, the use of conserved regions of HAdV genome such as the hexon gene and the fiber gene is fundamental to perform a reliable assay with a good sensitivity toward the different (sero) types (Huang et al. 2008). Conversely, typing of HAdV species is limited to epidemiological studies or in case of investigation of nosocomial outbreaks and is not commonly used to decide the antiviral treatment except for the use of ribavirin. In this case, the traditional serological methods have been substituted by molecular techniques based on PCR amplification or genome analysis, which are more rapid and precise (Ebner et al. 2006).

14.2.4 Definitions and Clinical Symptoms

In the immunocompetent and immunocompromised subject, the different species of HAdV show a different cell and tissue tropism and cause different diseases (Table 14.1). Indeed, the

Table 14.1 Association between disease and species of human adenovirus

Disease	Adenovirus species
Cystitis, nephritis	B1, B2
Disseminated disease	A, B2, C, F
Gastroenteritis	F, G
Hepatitis	C
Keratoconjunctivitis	B1, C, D
Meningoencephalitis	B1, C
Respiratory tract disease	B1, B2, C, E

Table 14.2 Definitions of infection, replication, and disease for patients who underwent a hematopoietic stem cell transplantation

Virus infection	Evidence of virus infection by detecting a specific immune response, viral antigens, nucleic acids in the host
Asymptomatic virus replication	Evidence of viral replication based on increasing viral load, or detection of virus by cell culture or viral antigens in an asymptomatic patient
Probable virus disease	Evidence of viral replication in a symptomatic patient in absence of histological evidence of virus organ disease
Proven virus disease	Evidence of viral replication in a symptomatic patient with histological evidence of virus organ disease

viruses belonging to the same species have a high DNA homology and usually do not recombine with virus of other species. The terminology proposed by ECIL for the different stages of HAdV infection is shown in Table 14.2 and includes clinical, virological, and histopathological evidence of infection or disease (Matthes-Martin et al. 2012). Disseminated invasive HAdV disease is defined by the involvement of ≥2 organs (pneumonitis, encephalitis, enteritis, retinitis) in the presence of HAdV viremia in peripheral blood or other sites (bronchoalveolar lavage, cerebrospinal fluid, nasopharyngeal or respiratory secretion, urine) and in absence of other identifiable causes (Lion et al. 2010; Lion et al. 2003). HAdV-related death is defined by death occurring with a high-level of HAdV viremia, HAdV detected in multiple sites, and multiple organ involvement or failure. In the HSCT patients, HAdV disease develops typically within the first 100 days after transplant (Lion et al. 2003), and the most frequent symptoms are fever, enteritis, and hepatitis. HAdV is responsible for 5–6% respiratory tract infections in HSCT patients with fever, cough, and sore throat. The involvement of lower respiratory tract is frequent in patients with high viremia or disseminated HAdV disease with a high risk of respiratory failure and lethality of 40–70%. Gastrointestinal involvement is characterized by cramps, diar-

rhea, or hemorrhagic enterocolitis that is not easily distinguishable by severe gut GVHD. Asymptomatic shedding in the stools of HAdV is frequently observed in pediatric patients during the early phase of HSCT patients but viral loads $>1 \times 10^6$ copies/g identify patients at high risk for HAdV viremia and disseminated disease (Lion et al. 2010). Fulminant hepatitis in patients with disseminated disease has been reported, usually the association between HAdV infection and liver disease or the increase of transaminases is rarely observed in the post-HSCT course and its differentiation from severe liver GVHD may require biopsy. HAdV is a cause of hemorrhagic cystitis although less frequently than BKPyV. Bladder involvement determines dysuria, macroscopic hematuria, abdominal pain, and in the more severe cases, urinary obstruction; moreover, in the context of a disseminated disease, HAdV may affect the kidney and determines a tubulo-interstitial nephritis and renal failure. Meningoencephalitis with fever, headache, seizures, and disorder of consciousness is a rare complication of HAdV infection and affects mainly pediatric HSCT patients. Overall, mortality associated with HAdV infection is 6% for pediatric patients and <1% for adult patients but can reach up to 50% in patients with HAdV viremia and 60–80% in patients with disseminated disease (Lion 2014; Lion et al. 2010; La Rosa et al. 2001).

14.2.5 Treatment and Prevention

Prophylaxis for HAdV infection with the currently available virustatic drugs is not recommended (Matthes-Martin et al. 2012); moreover, there is no approved antiviral treatment for HAdV infection in immunocompromised patients. The mainstay is based on reduction or suspension of immunosuppression, if feasible, and on the off-label use of antiviral drugs such as cidofovir (CDV) and ribavirin. Ganciclovir is not effective because the lack of the thymidine kinase enzyme gene in HAdV prevents the first step of its phosphorylation into an active compound. Alike, foscarnet is not active against HAdV. In vitro studies showed that CDV is effective against all species of HAdV, whereas ribavirin is effective only against the species belonging to group C. Considering the limited data on its efficacy in vivo, the use of ribavirin is generally not recommended for the preemptive treatment or for therapy of HAdV disease, except for individual cases infected by C species. CDV is a monophosphate nucleotide analogue of cytosine that once phosphorylated intracellularly to diphosphate inhibits viral DNA polymerase and viral replication. The main drawback of CDV is the low bioavailability that determines a low intracellular concentration of the active phosphorylated metabolites, whereas more than 90% of the dose is excreted unchanged in urine. On the other hand, its excessive concentration on the renal tubular cells may cause tubular necrosis and renal insufficiency. Probenecid, an organic acid, is used to reduce the renal tubular cell uptake of CDV and increase its plasma levels because it competes with CDV for the same organic anion transporter at renal tubular cells. Hyperhydration represents another important measure to reduce renal concentration of CDV and its toxicity. CDV has been used for both preemptive and therapeutic purposes (Lion 2014; Lindemans et al. 2010). Usually the starting dose is 5 mg/kg/week for 2 weeks followed by 3–5 mg/kg biweekly, with probenecid. An alternative scheme is 1 mg/kg/day three times per week, with or without probenecid. The treatment is continued until lymphocyte recovery is achieved (lymphocyte >300 μL) or HAdV DNAemia becomes undetectable or stably below the threshold for treatment. In general, CDV has a limited efficacy in the treatment of overt HAdV disease, irrespective of the dose used, especially in patients lacking T-cell reconstitution, and mortality remains high. CDV showed to be more effective in the setting of preemptive treatment, in asymptomatic patients with high or increasing HAdV load to control viral replication and to prevent the progression to disseminated disease until immune recovery occurs (Lion 2014; Lindemans et al. 2010). Brincidofovir (CMX001) is a lipid derivative of CDV that is promising in terms of safety and efficacy compared to CDV. In fact, brincidofovir has a supe-

rior oral bioavailability that permits to achieve higher concentration in the infected cells, and not being a substrate of renal cell organic anion transporters, it is not concentrated in renal tubules. In a randomized, phase II study, brincidofovir, 2 mg/kg twice a week, showed a significant virological response, defined reduction of DNAemia load in 2 weeks and clearance of DNAemia in 4 weeks, in two thirds of patients (Grimley et al. 2017). Moreover, no nephrotoxicity or myelotoxicity was reported. The most frequent side effect was diarrhea that affected 38% of patients and may require drug interruption and the start of differential diagnosis procedures for other causes of gastrointestinal disease such as gut GVHD or different infections. A retrospective study comparing pre-emptive therapy with brincidofovir or CDV in pediatric HSCT patients that had a comparable immune-reconstitution and viral burden showed that brincidofovir was associated to higher virological response, 83% versus 9%; moreover, brincidofovir was effective also in 9 of 11 patients not responding to CDV. Importantly, the reduction of DNAemia was observed despite lymphopenia. Only 1 of 18 patients suspended brincidofovir for abdominal cramps and diarrhea, whereas no patient developed nephrotoxicity. Considering the efficacy and the good safety profile, brincidofovir may represent a step forward in the treatment of HAdV infection, but further clinical development is needed (Hiwarkar et al. 2017).

14.2.6 Immunotherapy

The key role of T-cell immunity in HAdV infection is demonstrated by the fact that severe lymphopenia and delayed T-cell reconstitution represent a risk factor for HAdV infection; that the clearance of HAdV infection is associated with appearance of HAdV-specific T cells; and that the survival of patients with HAdV viremia is better in patients who have the recovery of lymphocyte count and HAdV-specific T cells (Zandvliet et al. 2010; Matthes-Martin et al. 2012).

In a recent survey among EBMT centers, the transfer of HAdV-specific T cells is used in 20%

of centers for preemptive or therapeutic purposes (Cesaro et al. 2018b); despite that, this approach is still considered experimental and to be performed in the context of a clinical trial. The advantage of adoptive immunotherapy is that the specific T cells are reactive against all species of HAdV because the immunodominant target antigen is the hexon, a viral capsid component that contains several epitopes conserved among different species of HAdV. The number of specific T cells in a subject previously exposed to HAdV is low, so obtaining an adequate number of cells requires the selection of cells from the peripheral blood of a seropositive donor and in vitro expansion (under GMP conditions); after infusion, a further in vivo expansion occurs under viremia stimulation. Several approaches have been used based on the selection of T cells secreting interferon (IFN)-gamma after stimulation with HAdV antigen (Feuchtinger et al. 2007; Feucht et al. 2015) or the production of cytolytic T-cell lines obtained by antigen-presenting cells transduced with HAdV vectors (Leen et al. 2006). These methods have limitations due to the complexity of the manufacturing process, the costs, the availability of a seropositive donor, and the time of production; in particular, the time of manufacturing could interfere with the "on time" use of the specific HAdV cells as viremia occurs. To overcome these limitations, manufacturing processes using seropositive third-party donors to generate multi-pathogen-specific T cells directed against CMV, EBV, HAdV, HHV-6, and BKV (Bollard and Heslop 2016; Leen et al. 2013) have been assessed. A phase II study in 38 patients using third-party-derived pentavalent CTLs showed an overall efficacy of 92%, with CTLs persisting in circulation for up to 12 weeks after infusion (Tzannou et al. 2017). These studies show that adoptive transfer of HAdV-specific T cells from the stem cell donor or third-party donors is a promising approach for patients not responding to treatment with antivirals and lacking circulating HAdV-specific T cells or for patients with disseminated HAdV infection, although the clinical applicability still depends on the future broader availability and timely access to virus-specific T cells.

14.3 Community-Acquired Respiratory Viral Infections

14.3.1 Introduction

Community-acquired respiratory viruses include a variety of RNA viruses such as human orthomyxo-, paramyxo-, picorna-, and coronaviruses, and DNA viruses such as adeno-, boca-, and polyomaviruses (Englund et al. 1999; Whimbey et al. 1996). In patients with hematological malignancies (HM) and recipients of hematopoietic cell transplant (HCT), respiratory viruses have been recognized as a significant cause of morbidity and mortality (Chemaly et al. 2014). Clinical presentation of all respiratory virus infections in patients with HMs or after HCT does not differ from the illness described in the general population. However, immune compromised patients may have atypical presentation with shortness of breath as the only manifestation (Ison 2007). These possibilities highlight the importance of a high index of suspicion. Respiratory virus infections may present with upper respiratory tract infectious disease (RTID) or lower RTID. Upper RTID is defined as the detection of respiratory viruses in upper respiratory tract specimens together with symptoms and/or signs and other causes excluded. Definition of lower RTID is pathological sputum production, hypoxia, or pulmonary infiltrates together with viral identification in respiratory secretions, preferentially in samples taken from the sites of involvement (Hirsch et al. 2013).

Rapid and accurate diagnosis for all community-acquired respiratory viruses is crucial in this patient population to allow prompt introduction of infection control precautions, start of antiviral therapy—if available—and potential deferral of chemotherapy or transplantation.

Patients with HMs or after HCT are at increased risk for progression to lower RTID, respiratory failure, and fatal outcome. This is most probably due to the immunopathology of respiratory virus infection, which reflects a complex interplay involving direct effects by a given virus but also the response of resident respiratory

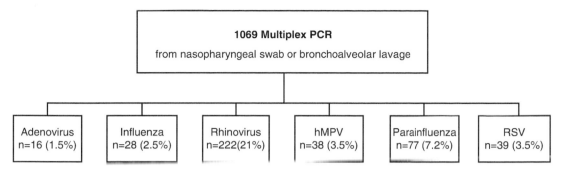

Fig. 14.1 Number of episodes of respiratory virus infections in HCT recipients at the University Hospital of Basel from 1/2010 until 12/2014

cells and recruited innate and adaptive immune cells to the lungs. Studies carried out over the last several decades suggest that the host response to respiratory virus infection dictates the type and extent of injury incurred (Newton et al. 2016).

Incidence of each virus can vary seasonally; however, rhinovirus (25–40%) has a higher incidence in HCT recipients than paramyxoviruses including respiratory syncytial virus (RSV) (2–17%), parainfluenza virus (PIV) (4–7%), or human metapneumovirus (hMPV) (3–9%) or influenza (1.3–2.6%), coronavirus (6.7–15.4%), and adenovirus (1–2%). At our institution, we have prospectively collected 1069 nasopharyngeal swabs and bronchoalveolar lavages in HCT recipients collected from January 2010 to December 2014 and found similar distribution as previously published (Martino et al. 2005) (Fig. 14.1). Mortality rates for HCT recipients range from 5% to 80% and seem to be overall higher for RSV (Whimbey et al. 1996; Hirsch et al. 2013; Martino et al. 2005; Chemaly et al. 2006; Nichols et al. 2001a; Peck et al. 2007; Avetisyan et al. 2009; Khanna et al. 2008; Ljungman 2001; Raboni et al. 2003).

14.3.2 Respiratory Syncytial Virus

14.3.2.1 Epidemiology

Respiratory syncytial virus (RSV) is a single-stranded RNA virus, member of the *Pneumoviridae* family. The virus is classified into two major antigenic groups, A and B, and infections by subtype A strains appear to be more severe (Walsh et al. 1997). Transmission occurs by contact with virus-containing secretions or fomites and subsequent inoculation of nasopharyngeal or ocular mucous membranes (Hall et al. 1981). The incubation period ranges between 2 and 8 days. RSV is worldwide in distribution, and it causes annual outbreaks: in temperate climates, these occur from late fall to spring, with a peak in January and February that usually precedes that of influenza season (Obando-Pacheco et al. 2018). RSV infections have a higher incidence among immunocompromised patients, especially those with hematologic malignancies submitted to HCT (Chatzis et al. 2018; Englund et al. 1988). The reported incidence in HCT recipients is about 2–17%, and such infections can be acquired through community outbreaks or by nosocomial transmission, generally through health care workers or infected visitors to inpatient units (Martino et al. 2005; Avetisyan et al. 2009; Khanna et al. 2008; Team RSVOI 2014; Shah et al. 2013). Male sex, allogeneic HCT, and pre-engraftment status are some of the factors that increase the risk for RSV acquisition in this population (Schiffer et al. 2009; Nichols et al. 2001b). It is well recognized that RSV infection among patients with HM significantly contribute to raise the burden of morbidity and mortality. These infections may lead to prolonged viral shedding, longer hospital stay, more severe disease with higher risk for progression to lower RTID and respiratory failure (Avetisyan et al. 2009; Khanna et al. 2008; Walsh et al. 2013). Mortality rate is reported up to 80% (Hertz et al. 1989; Harrington et al. 1992), although in more recent reviews, it ranges 10–30%, probably reflecting more sensitive diagnostics and earlier more aggressive treatment (Chatzis et al. 2018; Shah et al. 2013; Seo et al. 2013).

14.3.2.2   Clinical Presentation

RSV may produce a wide range of clinical manifestations, from self-limited upper RTID to severe pneumonia. Although symptoms are not specific, the presence of sinusitis and wheezing can be more suggestive of RSV infection than other pathogens (Hall et al. 2001). The clinical presentation depends upon age, health status, and degree of immunodeficiency. Patients with HM have a greater susceptibility to develop severe disease because of several factors: disruption of mucosal barrier integrity and IgA impairment, decrease in serum antibodies production, and deficient cytotoxic T-cell function increase the risk of infection in the lower airways and reduce the capacity for viral inactivation, resulting in an increase in disease severity and duration (Couch et al. 1997). A large proportion of HCT recipients (80–90%) experience initially upper RTID symptoms, such as cough, rhinorrhea, nasal congestion, sinusitis, otitis media, and subsequently, after an average time of 7 days, 30–40% of them develop a viral pneumonia (Boeckh 2008). The main risk factors for progression to lower RTID are lymphopenia, allogeneic HCT, early posttransplant period, graft-versus-host disease (Hirsch et al. 2013). Hematologic patients with RSV lower RTID usually present with dyspnea and hypoxemia together with new radiographic findings, which include bronchial wall thickening, peribronchial shadowing, air-trapping, multilobar patchy shadowing, or poorly defined nodularity (Gasparetto and Escuissato 2004). Without treatment, a great proportion of these patients develop respiratory failure, with need for ICU admission, mechanical ventilation, and high fatality rate (Chemaly et al. 2014; Shah et al. 2014). Progression to lower RTID, need for supplemental oxygen and higher degree of immunodeficiency are recognized as strong predictors of mortality among hematologic patients (Khanna et al. 2008; Seo et al. 2013). Moreover, RSV infection contributes to the development of respiratory superinfections by bacterial and fungal pathogens (Englund et al. 1988). As late complication, RSV lower RTID may also lead to bronchiolitis obliterans syndrome and to a decline in pulmonary function (Erard et al. 2006).

14.3.2.3   Diagnosis

Laboratory diagnosis has evolved considerably over recent decades. Adequate specimen collection from the site of infection (nasal washes, nasopharyngeal swabs, and bronchoalveolar lavages) and prompt transport to the laboratory are essential for the successful identification of the virus. Viral culture has been traditionally considered the gold standard for RSV detection, but it requires dedicated laboratory expertise and up to 7 days to become positive. Direct immunofluorescence antigen testing is a rapid and inexpensive method, but it has a low sensitivity (Ohm-Smith et al. 2004). Real-time polymerase chain reaction assays have a high sensitivity and specificity and represent currently the preferred method for diagnosing RSV infections. Multiplex PCR viral panels can efficiently test for multiple viruses at the same time and provide results in a short turnaround time (Layman et al. 2013).

14.3.2.4   Treatment

Deferral of chemotherapy or transplantation due to the high risk of fatal outcome needs to be considered (Hirsch et al. 2013). Early initiation of antiviral treatment is crucial to improve the prognosis of immunosuppressed patients with RSV infections. Treatment at the upper respiratory stage has demonstrated to reduce progression to lower RTID and thereby mortality (Chemaly et al. 2014). The therapeutic tools currently available for the treatment of RSV infections are ribavirin, intravenous immunoglobulins (IVIG), and palivizumab.

Ribavirin is a nucleoside analogue with activity against DNA and RNA viruses. Several studies have suggested that it is effective for the therapy of RSV infection in HCT recipients (Chemaly et al. 2006; Shah et al. 2013). Aerosolized ribavirin is the formulation most extensively studied: it allows to reach high concentration in the pulmonary parenchyma without systemic toxicity; the main disadvantages are the need for special air-flow, room conditions, and the potential teratogenicity for exposed caregivers and the high costs (Chemaly et al. 2014). In a randomized clinical trial, continuous (6 g over 18 hours daily) and intermittent (2 g over 3 hours every 8 hours daily) schedules of aerosolized ribavirin were equally effective in preventing progression to RSV lower RTID (Chemaly et al. 2012a). Systemic formulations (10–30 mg/kg body weight in three divided doses) have also been evaluated and have shown to be effective and well tolerated: intravenous ribavirin could be an alternative in patients with serious infections and/or pulmonary consolidation that prevents distribution of aerosolized medication (Molinos-Quintana et al. 2013); on the other hand, oral formulation is the least expensive form and does not require hospitalization (Khanna et al. 2008). Its bioavailability is around 50% but could be reduced in case of GVHD, thereby limiting its efficacy. In a recent retrospective study, effectiveness of oral and aerosolized ribavirin was compared in 46 patients with RSV infection (20 treated with oral ribavirin vs. 26 with aerosolized ribavirin). There were no differences in clinical outcomes between the two groups with regard to adverse events, progression from upper to lower RTID, escalation of care, or 30-day mortality (Trang et al. 2018).

Polyclonal immunoglobulins are an option for adjunctive therapy to ribavirin, especially in severe RSV infections. IVIG have demonstrated to prevent RSV replication in lung tissues and to induce anti-inflammatory effects that may be beneficial to reduce the airway damage caused by the inflammatory host immune response (Chemaly et al. 2014; Aschermann et al. 2010). RI-001 is a polyclonal IgG prepared from plasma donors with high-titer neutralizing anti-RSV antibody and has shown some promising results: its compassionate use in patients failing with standard of care therapy has shown to be effective and safe (Falsey et al. 2017). This strategy could offer advantages compared to standard IVIG.

Palivizumab is a monoclonal IgG that neutralizes RSV by binding the envelope protein F. It has been shown to reduce viral titers in pulmonary tissues and viral replication in animal models (Shah and Chemaly 2011). Furthermore, palivizumab has proven to have a prophylactic effect in infants at high risk for bronchiolitis, and it is currently registered for this indication (Tomblyn et al. 2009). Nevertheless, there is no strong evidence about its efficacy in adults and HCT recipients with RSV infections. Other limitations are represented by its high cost and the potential risk to select resistant mutants (Zhao and Sullender 2005).

There are no definite criteria for the management of RSV infection in with HM because of the lack of clinical randomized trials. Evidence is limited to few studies, mostly retrospective and from single centers. Despite the uncertainty regarding benefit, the European Conference on Infections in Leukemia (ECIL-4) recommends the treatment of RSV lower RTID and upper RTI at risk for progression to lower RTI with ribavirin and IVIG (0.5 g/kg bodyweight 1–3 times weekly) (Hirsch et al. 2013).

In view of the unmet clinical need of RSV and other paramyxovirus RTID after HCT and the undocumented efficacy of ribavirin and IVIG, the following key questions remain: who should be treated, and should all paramyxovirus RTID be treated with ribavirin and IVIG? Some studies have suggested classifications that can assist in the risk stratification (Table 14.3). Shah et al. (Shah et al. 2014) identified risk factors for poor outcome of RSV-RTIDs after allogeneic HCT and proposed a scoring index from 0 to 12 to classify patients with low (score 0–2), moderate (score 3–6), and high (7–12) for progression, in order to identify those who would benefit most from (inhaled ribavirin-based) antiviral therapy. At the University Hospital of Basel, we concluded from two retrospective studies that severe immunodeficient (SID) patients, particularly those fulfilling two or more SID criteria, are at high rsik for progression to LRTI and poor outcome (Khanna et al. 2008). The proposed criteria of Shah et al. are similar to ours but also introduced age $\geq$ 40 years, myeloablative conditioning regimen, and use of corticosteroids within the prior 30 days (Shah et al. 2014). Thus, there is a need to further validate such risk strata

Table 14.3 Risk stratification tools in hematologic patients with RSV infection

Immunodeficiency criteria [Khanna et al.] (Khanna et al. 2008)	Immunodeficiency scoring index ISI-RSV score [Shah et al.] (Shah et al. 2014)	
Moderate immunodeficiency	Neutrophil count	3
HSCT ≥6 months prior to diagnosis	<0.5 x 10⁹ cells/L	3
	Lymphocyte count	2
Immunosuppressive treatment	<0.2 x 10⁹ cells/L	1
	Age ≥ 40 y	1
T-cell depletion >3 months prior to diagnosis	Myeloablative conditioning regimen	1
	GVHD (acute or chronic)	12
Severe immunodeficiency	Corticosteroids	
Acute GVHD (grade ≥ 2)	<30 days prior to diagnosis	
HSCT <6 months prior to diagnosis	Allo-HCT <30 days prior to diagnosis or pre-engraftment	
Leukocyte count ≤2.0 x 10⁹ cells/L	Maximum overall score	
Lymphocyte count ≤0.1 x 10⁹ cells/L	Interpretation:	
T-cell depletion <3 months prior to diagnosis	0–2 low risk	
Pre-engraftment	3–6 moderate risk	
Immunoglobulin level < 6.5 g/L	7–12 high risk	
B cell depletion <3 months prior to diagnosis		
Patients with ≥2 severe immunodeficiency criteria have a significantly higher risk for mortality	ISI score predicts progression to LRTI and mortality. High-risk patients benefit the most from therapy at the URTI stage	

in prospective trials to balance treatment versus overtreatment and adverse events, particularly for HCT patients with low and moderate risk for poor outcome. Even more, their translation to other respiratory viruses needs to be investigated (Khanna et al. 2009; Spahr et al. 2018).

Regarding future perspectives in the therapy of RSV infections, there are currently several compounds being investigated in clinical trials, which can be divided into four different classes: immunoglobulins, nucleoside analogues, small interfering RNAs, and fusion inhibitors (Xing and Proesmans 2019). Among them, presatovir (GS-5806), a novel, orally bioavailable RSV

fusion inhibitor targeting the F protein, has been shown to be safe and to decrease the viral load, as well as the disease severity, in a challenge study of healthy adults (DeVincenzo et al. 2014).

14.3.2.5 Prevention

Given the high morbidity and mortality in this subset of patients, preventive measures remain the best approach to reduce the burden of RSV infection and to limit nosocomial transmission. Strict infection control precautions should be implemented, including respiratory isolation of infected patients, hand hygiene, wearing masks and gloves, and educational efforts targeting visitors and health care workers (Dykewicz, and National Center for Infectious Diseases CfDC, Prevention, Infectious Diseases Society of A, American Society for B, Marrow T 2001). These should be screened for signs and symptoms of respiratory illness and restricted from entering the unit if symptomatic. Passive immunoprophylaxis with monoclonal or polyclonal immunoglobulins may be considered in susceptible patients, especially in outbreak situations (Kassis et al. 2010). At present, there is no commercially available vaccine that can prevent RSV infection. Efforts are currently ongoing and focus on live attenuated and recombinant subunit vaccines.

14.3.3 Parainfluenza Virus

14.3.3.1 Epidemiology

Parainfluenza virus (PIV) is an enveloped, single-stranded RNA virus belonging to the *Paramyxoviridae* family. PIVs are divided into four types (PIV 1–4) based on their genetic and antigenic characteristics. Similar to in the general population, most clinical infections in HM patients and HCT recipients caused by PIV-3 followed by PIV-1 (Spahr et al. 2018; Fry et al. 2006). PIV infections occur year-round; peak seasonal activity has been reported biennially between late September and December for PIV-1 and during the spring and summer months for PIV-3 (Spahr et al. 2018; Fry et al. 2006; Ustun et al. 2012).

The incidence of parainfluenza infections in HCT recipients is 1–4%. Significantly higher rates can be found in asymptomatic HCT recipients (Chemaly et al. 2014; Peck et al. 2007; Chemaly et al. 2012b). PIV infections can occur early post-transplant, as well as also very late post-HCT, which possibly reflects the high risk of nosocomial transmission, as well as the circulation in the community (Peck et al. 2007; Spahr et al. 2018; Ustun et al. 2012).

14.3.3.2 Clinical Presentation

The clinical presentation of PIV infections in patients with HMs or after HCT does not differ from the illness described in the general population. Importantly, asymptomatic carriage in HCT recipients is frequent and reported in up to 18% (Peck et al. 2007). Upper RTID is the most common presentation in HCT recipients occurring in 56–87% (Spahr et al. 2018; Chartrand et al. 2012; Chemaly et al. 2012c). Clinical presentation of upper RTID may include any combination of symptoms like fever, rhinorrhea, nasal congestion, sinusitis, headache, cough, wheezing, and coryza (Wendt et al. 1992; Johny et al. 2002). Lower RTID is reported in 15–45% (Nichols et al. 2001a; Ljungman 2001; Spahr et al. 2018) with symptoms like dyspnea, hypoxemia, and new or changing pulmonary infiltrates on chest radiography.

Factors associated with progression to lower RTID in patients after HCT include lymphopenia ($<0.2 \times 10^9$ cells/L) and neutropenia ($<0.5 \times 10^9$ cells/L), the use of glucocorticoid treatment (≥ 1 mg/kg bodyweight) (Nichols et al. 2001a; Chemaly et al. 2012b; Seo et al. 2014). Mortality rates range between 4% and 46% (Spahr et al. 2018; Safdar et al. 2010). Risk factors for mortality include presence of lower RTID, receipt of transplants from a mismatched related donor and infection within 3 months after HCT and coinfections (Martino et al. 2005; Nichols et al. 2001a; Schiffer et al. 2009; Ustun et al. 2012; Chemaly et al. 2012b; Safdar et al. 2010; Srinivasan et al. 2011; Marcolini et al. 2003; Hodson et al. 2011).

PIV may activate immunological mechanisms in the lung and has been associated with risk of bronchiolitis obliterans syndrome (BOS) development. BOS belongs in HCT recipients to one of the most frequent late manifestation of noninfectious pulmonary complication (Yoshihara et al. 2007). The diagnosis is based on spirometry measurements, bronchiectasis, and computer tomography (Filipovich et al. 2005). Significant airflow decline was documented in 86% of HCT recipients who developed PIV attributable lower RTID during 100 days after HCT (Erard et al. 2006).

14.3.3.3 Diagnosis

Multiplex NAT by reverse-transcriptase polymerase chain reaction (RT–PCR) is today considered the reference test for diagnosis of PIV because of its sensitivity of 100% and specificity of 95–98%, as well as its rapid turnaround time (Fan and Henrickson 1996). Culture tests are slow and labor-intensive, making it poorly suited to guide the management of acutely ill patients. Antigen detection kits are commercially available. The sensitivity is poor with 28–84%, which limits their widespread use (Bowden et al. 2010).

14.3.3.4 Treatment

There is currently no licensed antiviral agent for the treatment of PIV. Thus, if possible, deferral of high intensity chemotherapy and allogeneic HCT is recommended (Hirsch et al. 2013).

The data on the use of ribavirin remain controversial. It had no effect on viral shedding, symptom duration, hospital stay, progression to lower RTID, or mortality following PIV infections (Nichols et al. 2001a; Boeckh 2008; Chemaly et al. 2012b). Interestingly, in a recent study, ribavirin showed some benefit associated with overall mortality but not with deaths due to respiratory failure or in patients with bronchoalveolar lavage confirmed PIV lower RTID (Seo et al. 2014). On the other hand, a study performed at our institution found that 16 of 19 patients with lower RTID had a beneficial outcome with IVIG alone. Therefore, the use of IVIG is usually recommended at the University Hospital of Basel (Spahr et al. 2018). The impact of IVIG on overall outcome following PIV infection still needs to be determined. Very few novel antiviral drugs have shown promising results for treating PIV infection in this patient population. DAS181 has shown efficacy against PIV in vitro and in vivo, and in three immunocompromised patients with respiratory infections, including two HCT recipients (Guzman-Suarez et al. 2012; Moscona et al. 2010; Chen et al. 2011). BCX2798 and BCX2855 have been found to have antiviral activity against PIV-3, significantly reducing pulmonary viral titers and mortality in rats when given intranasally within 24 hours of infection (Alymova et al. 2004).

14.3.4 Human Metapneumovirus

14.3.4.1 Epidemiology
Human metapneumovirus (HMPV) belongs to the *Pneumoviridae* family, and it is closely related to RSV. Incidence rates range from 3% to 9% (Martino et al. 2005; Debur et al. 2010; Williams et al. 2005; Oliveira et al. 2008) and did not differ in HM patients from that observed for HCT recipients (Shah et al. 2016). Peak seasonal activity for HMPV infections has been reported yearly between December and May in the Northern hemisphere (Spahr et al. 2018). The importance of HMPV in transplant recipients has not been studied as thoroughly as RSV. Progression from upper to lower RTID has been reported in 21–40% (Williams et al. 2005; Renaud and Campbell 2011) with fatality rates of up to 80% in HCT recipients.

14.3.4.2 Clinical Presentation
Disease manifestation of HMPV is indistinguishable from that of other respiratory viruses including rhinorrhea, sore throat, cough, and fever (Shah et al. 2016). Risk factors for HMPV lower RTID have not been studied in detail. One study examined 118 HCT recipients with HMPV infections and found significant association between steroid use at ≥1 mg/kg within 2 weeks prior to diagnosis, low lymphocyte count, and early onset of HMPV infection after HCT (before day 30 after HCT) and progression to lower RTID (Seo et al. 2016). Another study identified that high viral loads in bronchoalveo-lar lavage samples and viral RNA from serum samples of HCT recipients with pneumonia have been indicative of severe disease (Campbell et al. 2010).

14.3.4.3 Diagnosis
HMPV infection is commonly diagnosed by NAT, as it is faster and more sensitive than viral culture or antigen detection. Most laboratories currently use commercial multiplex NAT that includes many community-acquired respiratory viruses in parallel.

14.3.4.4 Treatment
No general recommendation for treatment can currently be made. Ribavirin is active in vitro and in vivo against HMPV (Wyde et al. 2003; Hamelin et al. 2006). Some centers consider treating HMPV lower RTID with ribavirin and/or IVIG despite the lack of supporting studies (Spahr et al. 2018; Renaud et al. 2013; Chu et al. 2014).

14.3.5 Influenza

14.3.5.1 Epidemiology
The influenza virus belongs to the orthomyxo-viridae family and is a segmented, single-stranded RNA virus. Classification of the virus into subtypes is based on its surface hemagglutinins and neuraminidases. Seasonal influenza activity can begin as early as October and continue into May in the Northern hemisphere. The seasonal prevalence of influenza infections in patients with HMs and recipients of HCT closely parallels the community-wide prevalence (Kmeid et al. 2016). The incidence of influenza infections in HCT recipients is 1.3–2.6%, and significantly higher rates may be seen during the peaks of influenza outbreaks in the community (Kmeid et al. 2016). Patients with HMs and HCT recipients have a higher risk of developing severe disease and higher rates of complications such as hospitalizations, prolonged shedding, emergence of resistance, and mortality compared to the general population (Khanna et al. 2009; Minnema et al. 2013; Nichols et al. 2004).

14.3.5.2 Clinical Presentation

Influenza is an acute, usually self-limited, febrile illness. In patients with HMs and HCT recipients up to 35% progress to lower RTID (Chemaly et al. 2006; Nichols et al. 2004).

Identified risk factors for progression to lower RTID or fatal outcome in patients after HCT include lymphopenia (0.1×10^9 cells/L and 0.2×10^9 cells/L) and neutropenia ($< 0.5 \times 10^9$ cells/L), older age and preexisting lung disease (Khanna et al. 2009; Kmeid et al. 2016; Protheroe et al. 2012; Ljungman et al. 2011; Choi et al. 2011). Influenza-related mortality and all-cause mortality ranges between 4–9.3% and 5–12.4% (Kmeid et al. 2016; Choi et al. 2011).

14.3.5.3 Diagnosis

Rapid and sensitive methods to diagnose influenza are important to initiate early treatment and to reduce the risk of nosocomial transmission. Reliable diagnosis depends on the quality of the collected respiratory sample. Samples should be collected at the site of infections, for upper RTID nasopharyngeal swabs, nasal washings, and for lower RTID preferably bronchoalveolar lavages. Respiratory specimens should be placed in virus transport media and investigated within 24 hours.

Multiplex NAT and reverse-transcriptase polymerase chain reaction (RT–PCR) is today considered the reference test for diagnosis of influenza because of its high sensitivity and specificity, as well as its rapid turnaround time. In contrast, conventional tube culture, shell-vial culture, and rapid antigen detection have multiple limitations. Culture tests are slow and labor-intensive, making it poorly suited to guide the management of acutely ill patients. Numerous rapid antigen detection kits are commercially available that produce test results in <15 min. Although their quick turnaround time is appealing, widespread adoption of these kits in adults has been limited by their poor sensitivity.

14.3.5.4 Treatment

Antiviral treatment should be initiated promptly or empirically in this patient population when influenza infection is suspected. Previous studies have demonstrated that early administration of antiviral therapy has been associated with reduced risk of lower RTID, intensive care unit admission, hospitalization, and death at 6 weeks (Chemaly et al. 2012c; Choi et al. 2011). However, the beneficial effect of antiviral therapy is still observed even with a delayed start from symptom onset (Choi et al. 2011).

The two main groups of antivirals for influenza are the neuraminidase inhibitors (oseltamivir, zanamivir, and peramivir), which are active against influenza A and B and the M2 inhibitors (amantadine and rimantadine), which only act against influenza A. With the increasing resistance against M2 inhibitors, the neuraminidase inhibitors are the most widely used anti-influenza drug in these patients. Oseltamivir is administered orally. In immunocompromised patients, increased doses of oseltamivir (150 mg twice a day, adjusted to the renal function) have been used, as was recommended for patients with the H5N1 avian influenza strain. Reduced absorption due to GVHD, mucositis, and concerns about increased development of resistance due to continued viral replication in these patients (Weinstock et al. 2003; Renaud et al. 2011) motivated higher dosing. However, the benefit on clinical outcomes has not been conclusively demonstrated (Khanna et al. 2009; Casper et al. 2010; Watcharananan et al. 2010). Zanamivir is administered by inhalation or intravenously. In a phase 3, double-blind clinical trial in hospitalized patients with severe influenza, two doses of intravenous zanamivir and oral oseltamivir were compared. The results do not show superiority of intravenous zanamivir compared with oseltamivir to hospitalized patients with influenza (Marty et al. 2017). Similarly, for peramivir significant clinical benefit was not demonstrated compared with placebo in patients hospitalized with suspected influenza infections (de Jong et al. 2014).

Several new agents are currently under investigation including DAS181, favipiravir, nitazoxanide, laninamivir octanoate, pimodivir, and baloxavir for influenza treatment. Studies are needed to evaluate their efficacy in patients with HM or after HCT.

As long as no better studies are available, therapy of uncomplicated influenza infection is based on expert opinions: most authors use oseltamivir 75 mg twice daily, others suggest higher dosage (150 mg bid), with adjustment to renal function. The intravenous route for antiviral agents is preferred in patients with gastrointestinal GVHD or LRTID, on mechanical ventilation, or requiring bilevel positive airway pressure to circumvent the bioavailability issues. Concerning duration, most experts recommend continuing antiviral therapy until viral replication has ceased, which typically takes longer in this patient population than the 5 days of therapy recommended for immunocompetent patients (Casper et al. 2010).

14.3.5.5 Prevention

The updated guidelines of the American Society of Bone Marrow Transplantation recommend annual inactivated influenza vaccination before the beginning of the influenza season and before transplantation or 4–6 months following transplantation (Tomblyn et al. 2009). The vaccine should be administered prior to the onset of the influenza season to avoid new infections and related complications. The main two contraindications for influenza vaccine are febrile illness and severe allergy to eggs.

During outbreaks, daily chemoprophylaxis with strain-specific anti-influenza antiviral drug has been recommended in HCT recipients (within 24 months after transplant, with GVHD or taking immunosuppressive therapy) by the Centers for Disease Control and Prevention's Advisory Committee on Immunization Practices (Tomblyn et al. 2009; Fiore et al. 2008). However this strategy may lead to the selection of resistant influenza strains, as seen during the 2009/H1N1 pandemic (Renaud et al. 2011; Baz et al. 2009). At our institution, we perform multiplex PCR in exposed patients, and if negative, we recommend treating HCT recipients for 5 days (75 mg twice daily).

14.3.6 Rhinovirus

14.3.6.1 Epidemiology

Human rhinoviruses (HRV) are members of the *Picornaviridae* family and are classified into three species, HRV-A, -B, and -C encompassing more than 160 serotypes. There are several biologic characteristics of HRV-C that differentiate it from HRV-A and -B. HRV-C readily infects upper and lower RTI, whereas HRV-A and -B species seem to be more limited to the upper RTI (Ashraf et al. 2013; Bochkov and Gern 2012). HRV infections circulate throughout the year (Turner 2010).

Due to the development of PCR assays for viral detection, HRV have become the most frequent virus detected from respiratory specimens in HCT recipients and can account for 25–40% of cases of respiratory viral infections in this patient population (Bowden 1997; Hassan et al. 2003; Milano et al. 2010).

14.3.6.2 Clinical Presentation

HRV is the most common cause of upper RTID in immunocompetent, as well as immune suppressed patients, presenting with afebrile, self-limited syndrome characterized by rhinorrhea, malaise, mild cough, and hoarseness (Arruda et al. 1997; Johnston 1995). The incubation period has been estimated as 1.9 days (95% CI, 1.4–2.4) (Lessler et al. 2009). Asymptomatic carriage in 13% in HCT recipients and prolonged shedding over 4 weeks are frequent (Parody et al. 2007).

HRV may also be associated with exacerbations of sinusitis, bronchitis, asthma, and pneumonia (Gern et al. 1997; Jain et al. 2015). In a prospective 5-year study at the MD Anderson Cancer Center, significant morbidity and mortality was reported (Ghosh et al. 1999). All patients with pneumonia had a fatal outcome. Lung biopsies/autopsies revealed findings consistent with interstitial pneumonitis and/or acute respiratory distress syndrome. It remains unclear if pneumonia is a direct cause of viral invasion of the lung tissue or by host responses in the lung. In a recent study by Seo and colleagues, overall mortality 90 days after HCT was significantly higher for patients with lower RTID than upper RTID (41% vs. 6%). The survival rate after lower RTID was not affected by the presence of co-pathogens. Moreover, lower RTID associated with HRV led to mortality rate comparable to that of RSV, PIV, and influenza (Seo et al. 2017).

Risk factors for mortality following HRV lower RTID included bone marrow stem cell source, low monocyte count, oxygen requirement at time of diagnosis, and steroid use >1 mg/kg prior to diagnosis (Seo et al. 2017).

14.3.6.3 Diagnosis

Diagnosis largely depends on multiplex NAT by RT-PCR. There are no antigen detection kits commercially available. Culture tests are labor-intensive and therefore only performed in specialized laboratories.

14.3.6.4 Treatment

There is currently no licensed antiviral agent for the treatment of HRV. Some agents have been evaluated in immunocompetent individuals including protease inhibitors and RNA synthesis inhibitors (Rollinger and Schmidtke 2011). Given the high prevalence and the severe course of this infection, there is a great need to develop drugs for prevention and treatment of lower RTID.

14.3.7 Coronavirus

14.3.7.1 Epidemiology

Coronavirus (CoV) are divided into group 1–like (CoV-229E and -NL63) and group 2–like (CoV-OC43 and -HKU1) agents that are molecularly distinct. Two additional CoVs associated with outbreaks are the severe acute respiratory syndrome (SARS) and Middle East respiratory syndrome (MERS) coronaviruses (Self et al. 2016). A previous study has demonstrated that CoV is now the second most common virus identified from the upper respiratory tract in HCT recipients detected in 6.7–15.4%, but asymptomatic shedding may be as high as 41% (Milano et al. 2010). Cases of fatal pneumonia related to CoV without co-pathogens have also been reported mainly in HCT populations (Uhlenhaut et al. 2012; Pene et al. 2003; Oosterhof et al. 2010). CoVs occur year-round with a slight predominance in winter. Novel coronavirus (SARS-CoV-2) that causes atypical pneumonia (COVID-19) has raged in China since mid-December 2019 and spread rapidly worldwide. It has developed to be a Public Health Emergency of international concern. The genome of SARSCoV-2 is similar to that of other coronaviruses and has four genes that encode the following structural proteins—the S (spike), E (envelope), M (membrane), and N (nucleocapsid)

proteins (Wu 2020). SARS-CoV-2 is a zoonotic virus, same as SARS-COV, the etiologic agent of the 2003 SARS outbreak with likely origin in bats, and likely involvement of another (intermediate) host animal such as the pangolin (Ye et al. 2020). Human-to-human transmission of SARS-CoV-2 is primarily via respiratory droplets and by direct contact with infected people and indirect contact with contaminated surfaces and objects. The mean incubation period of SARS-CoV-2 infection varies from 5 to 6 days and the range 1–14 days (WHO 2020). All age groups of humans are susceptible to SARS-CoV-2 infection but at particularly higher risk are the aged, immunocompromised individuals, and people with chronic underlying diseases. The case fatality rate of COVID-19 has been widely variable by country —from less than 0.1% to over 25% (WHO 2020).

During the preparation of this book chapter, very limited data on disease manifestation and course were available on SARS-CoV-2 in hematological-oncological patients and stem cell recipients. In adult patients with cancer or a hematological malignancy, COVID-19 resulted a risk factor for mortality together with age, sex, comorbidities, and tumor type (Liang et al. 2020; Lee et al. 2020). Noteworthy, a retrospective observational study during the pandemic months in Italy showed that adult hematological patients had a worse outcome than both the general population with COVID-19 and the patients with hematological malignancies but without COVID-19 (Passamonti et al. 2020). This dismal outcome was not confirmed in the pediatric population observed during pandemic in Italy and Spain where incidence, morbidity, and mortality were far lower (Bisogno et al. 2020; Faura et al. 2020). A prospective observational study conducted by Infectious Disease Working Party of European Society for Blood and Marrow Transplantation found that patients who underwent stem cell transplantation with COVID-19 were at increased risk for respiratory complication, admission to ICU, and mortality, this last being significantly associated with older age and performance status (Ljungman, personal communication).

14.3.7.2 Clinical Presentation

Upper RTID with rhinitis, pharyngitis, and laryngitis is the most common manifestation. Lower RTID is uncommon: patients rarely present with bronchiolitis, bronchitis, or pneumonia. A recent study analyzed 30 HCT recipients and 7 patients with HMs with lower RTID identified over a ten-year period. Twenty-one patients (60%) required oxygen therapy at diagnosis and 19 (54%) died within 90 days of diagnosis. Respiratory co-pathogens were detected in 21 episodes (57%). Mortality rates were not different between patients with and without co-pathogens (Ogimi et al. 2017).

Symptoms and signs of SARS-CoV-2 infection appear after an incubation period of 3–9 days. Importantly, during this period the patient is contagious, and it is estimated that 44% of transmissions occur before the symptoms arises (He et al. 2020). The clinical presentation can vary from an asymptomatic status to fever, fatigue, sore throat, myalgia, dry cough, dyspnea, nausea, dizziness, and less frequently, headache, diarrhea, vomiting, abdominal cramps. Interestingly, among minor symptoms, olfactory or taste disorders are reported up to 34% of patients, and in 91% of patient with taste disorder, this was present before hospitalization (Giacomelli et al. 2020). In pediatric patients, a milder course of infection is observed with a higher rate of asymptomatic cases, but up to 9% of patients may present a Kawasaki-like syndrome (Abrams et al. 2020). The most frequent abnormalities of laboratory parameters are lymphopenia, eosinopenia, thrombocytopenia, elevated AST/ALT, LDH, D-Dimer, C-reactive protein, and troponin (Siordia 2020). Pneumonia and acute respiratory distress syndrome are the most frequent complications, progression to dyspnea, hypoxemia, and/or mechanical ventilation being of 8–10 days from the beginning of symptoms. Although lung X-ray abnormalities are present in 30–60% of patients, lung CT scan resulted more sensitive and specific (Bai et al. 2020). The initial radiologic signs are groundglass opacities distributed to lower lobes followed by their bilateral diffusion and the appearance of patchy consolidation in two or more lobes (Pan et al. 2020). Other severe complications are myocardial injuries (acute coronary syndrome, myocarditis, heart failure, severe hypotension or shock, arrhythmias, pulmonary hypertension), acute kidney injury, and coinfections (RSV, Influenza A-B, Mycoplasma, Legionella, Pseudomonas, Haemophilus, Aspergillus) (Siordia 2020; Lansbury et al. 2020). Particularly SARS-CoV-2 associated pulmonary aspergillosis has emerged as an important co-infection associated with high mortality rates (Arastehfar 2020; Hoenigl 2020; Koehler 2020). Outcome of infection is dependent on the severity of COVID-19.

Severe COVID-19 disease is defined by symptomatic infection with respiratory rate >30 min and SaO2 saturation <95%. The overall mortality of severe COVID-19 is 5.6%, but it may vary according to the country (depending on local health and economical resources) and the phase of pandemic. It is associated with a rate of intensive care admission of 11% and a need of mechanical ventilation of 7%. The main risk factors for severe COVID-19 disease are preexisting factors related to the patient such as immunosuppression, malignancy, diabetes, vascular disease or hypertension and factors related to the severity or type of the clinical manifestations such as abdominal pain, nausea, vomiting, shortness of breath, and chest pain (Li et al. 2020a, b). The case fatality rate was higher for older patients, 8% for patients aged 70–79 years, 14% or more for patients aged >80 years, while it is 1% or less for patients aged <40 years, especially for pediatric and adolescent patients where death is episodic (Siordia 2020).

14.3.7.3 Diagnosis

Diagnosis largely depends on multiplex NAT by (RT-PCR). There are no antigen detection kits commercially available. Culture tests are labor-intensive and therefore only performed in specialized laboratories.

14.3.7.4 Treatment

There is currently no licensed antiviral agent for the treatment of CoV. Oral ribavirin was evaluated in retrospective studies for the treatment of MERS-CoV in immunocompetent individuals and decreased survival was observed in one study when compared to matched controls (Omrani et al. 2014; Al-Tawfiq et al. 2014).

The treatment of COVID-19 has changed rapidly from the beginning of pandemic because no specific drug was initially available, and the pathogenesis of tissue damage was not really understood. Supportive therapy has a key role to treat symptoms, to prevent respiratory or other organ failures, pulmonary thromboembolism, and coinfections, and it is based on the use of oxygen, noninvasive ventilation, mechanical ventilation, fluids, diuretics, inotropes, anticoagulants, and antibiotics. No specific antivirals are available for SARS-CoV-2. Remdesivir, an adenosine analog drug studied for Ebola, reduced the time to recovery and mortality, this last in a nonsignificant way, in a preliminary report from a double-blind randomized controlled trial although (Beigel et al. 2020). To reduce the inflammatory response and the tissue damage by a dysregulated cytokine secretion, corticosteroids, especially dexamethasone, IL-6 receptor antagonists, and IL-beta antagonists have been used (Lan et al 2020). The best evidence has been demonstrated for dexamethasone resulting in lower 28-day mortality among those who were receiving either invasive mechanical ventilation or oxygen alone at randomization but not among those receiving no respiratory support (Recovery 2020 https://www.nejm.org/doi/full/10.1056/NEJMoa2021436, https://www.recoverytrial.net/; WHO Rapid Evidence Appraisal for COVID-19 Therapies (REACT) Working Group et al. 2020). The use of convalescent plasma collected from SARS-CoV-2-recovered patients and administered early after the start of clinical symptoms has showed promising results (Li et al. 2020a, b; Farhat et al. 2020), and it is under investigation in several clinical trials.

At the time of publication of this book, no vaccine was available, but several types of vaccine were rapidly developing and assessed in phase I studies on volunteers (Marian 2020) as well as phase II and III studies and expected to become available to the public in 2021.

Current recommendation for prevention of spread of SARS-CoV-2 in HM and patients after HCT are based on guidelines, policies, and procedures decided by national authorities as well as local and institutional policies since the COVID-19 situation varies substantially between and within countries. Avoiding exposure by adhering to recommended hygiene procedures, isolation of SARS-CoV-2-infected individuals, and social or physical distancing especially for risk groups are currently the main prevention strategies utilized in most European countries (Ljungman et al. 2020).

References

Abrams JY, Godfred-Cato SE, Oster ME et al (2020.;[published online ahead of print, 2020 Aug 5] S0022-3476) Multisystem inflammatory syndrome in children (MIS-C) associated with SARS-CoV-2: a systematic review. J Pediatr (20):30985–30989. https://doi.org/10.1016/j.jpeds.2020.08.003

Al-Tawfiq JA, Momattin H, Dib J, Memish ZA (2014) Ribavirin and interferon therapy in patients infected with the Middle East respiratory syndrome coronavirus: an observational study. Int J Infect Dis 20: 42–46

Alymova IV, Taylor G, Takimoto T, Lin TH, Chand P, Babu YS et al (2004) Efficacy of novel hemagglutinin-neuraminidase inhibitors BCX 2798 and BCX 2855 against human parainfluenza viruses in vitro and in vivo. Antimicrob Agents Chemother 48:1495–1502

Apperley JF, Rice SJ, Bishop JA, Chia YC, Krausz T, Gardner SD et al (1987) Late-onset hemorrhagic cystitis associated with urinary excretion of polyomaviruses after bone marrow transplantation. Transplantation 43:108–112

Arastehfar A, Carvalho A, van de Veerdonk FL, Jenks JD, Koehler P, Krause R, et al (2020) COVID-19 associated pulmonary aspergillosis (CAPA)-from immunology to treatment. Fungi (Basel). 6(2):91. https://doi.org/10.3390/jof6020091

Arruda E, Pitkaranta A, Witek TJ Jr, Doyle CA, Hayden FG (1997) Frequency and natural history of rhinovirus infections in adults during autumn. J Clin Microbiol 35:2864–2868

Arthur RR, Shah KV, Baust SJ, Santos GW, Saral R (1986) Association of BK viruria with hemorrhagic cystitis in recipients of bone marrow transplants. N Engl J Med 315:230–234

Aschermann S, Lux A, Baerenwaldt A, Biburger M, Nimmerjahn F (2010) The other side of immunoglobulin G: suppressor of inflammation. Clin Exp Immunol 160:161–167

Ashraf S, Brockman-Schneider R, Bochkov YA, Pasic TR, Gern JE (2013) Biological characteristics and propagation of human rhinovirus-C in differentiated sinus epithelial cells. Virology 436:143–149

Averbuch D, Tridello G, Hoek J, Mikulska M, Akan H, Yanez San Segundo L et al (2017) Antimicrobial resistance in gram-negative rods causing bacteremia in hematopoietic stem cell transplant recipients:

intercontinental prospective study of the infectious diseases working party of the European bone marrow transplantation group. Clin Infect Dis 65:1819–1828

Avetisyan G, Mattsson J, Sparrelid E, Ljungman P (2009) Respiratory syncytial virus infection in recipients of allogeneic stem-cell transplantation: a retrospective study of the incidence, clinical features, and outcome. Transplantation 88:1222–1226

Avivi I, Wittmann T, Henig I, Kra-Oz Z, Szwarcwort Cohen M, Zuckerman T et al (2014) Development of multifocal leukoencephalopathy in patients undergoing allogeneic stem cell transplantation-can preemptive detection of John Cunningham virus be useful? Int J Infect Dis 26:107–109

Bai HX, Hsieh B, Xiong Z et al (2020) Performance of radiologists in differentiating COVID-19 from non-COVID-19 viral pneumonia at chest CT. Radiology 296(2):E46–E54. https://doi.org/10.1148/radiol.2020200823

Balduzzi A, Lucchini G, Hirsch HH, Basso S, Cioni M, Rovelli A et al (2011) Polyomavirus JC-targeted T-cell therapy for progressive multiple leukoencephalopathy in a hematopoietic cell transplantation recipient. Bone Marrow Transplant 46:987–992

Baugh KA, Tzannou I, Leen AM (2018) Infusion of cytotoxic T lymphocytes for the treatment of viral infections in hematopoetic stem cell transplant patients. Curr Opin Infect Dis 31:292–300

Baz M, Abed Y, Papenburg J, Bouhy X, Hamelin ME, Boivin G (2009) Emergence of oseltamivir-resistant pandemic H1N1 virus during prophylaxis. N Engl J Med 361:2296–2297

Beigel JH, Tomashek KM, Dodd LE et al (2020) Remdesivir for the treatment of Covid-19—preliminary report. N Engl J Med:NEJMoa2007764. https://doi.org/10.1056/NEJMoa2007764. [published online ahead of print, 2020 May 22]

Binet I, Nickeleit V, Hirsch HH, Prince O, Dalquen P, Gudat F et al (1999) Polyomavirus disease under new immunosuppressive drugs: a cause of renal graft dysfunction and graft loss. Transplantation 67:918–922

Bisogno G, Provenzi M, Zama D et al (2020) Clinical characteristics and outcome of SARS-CoV-2 infection in Italian pediatric oncology patients: a study from the Infectious Diseases Working Group of the AIEOP. J Pediatric Infect Dis Soc. https://doi.org/10.1093/jpids/piaa088. piaa088 [published online ahead of print, 2020 Jul 11]

Bochkov YA, Gern JE (2012) Clinical and molecular features of human rhinovirus C. Microbes Infect 14:485–494

Boeckh M (2008) The challenge of respiratory virus infections in hematopoietic cell transplant recipients. Br J Haematol 143:455–467

Bogdanovic G, Priftakis P, Giraud G, Kuzniar M, Ferraldeschi R, Kokhaei P et al (2004) Association between a high BK virus load in urine samples of patients with graft-versus-host disease and development of hemorrhagic cystitis after hematopoietic stem cell transplantation. J Clin Microbiol 42:5394–5396

Bollard CM, Heslop HE (2016) T cells for viral infections after allogeneic hematopoietic stem cell transplant. Blood 127:3331–3340

Bowden RA (1997) Respiratory virus infections after marrow transplant: the Fred Hutchinson Cancer Research Center experience. Am J Med 102:27–30. discussion 42-3

Bowden RA, Ljungman P, Snydman DR (2010) Transplant infections, 3rd edn. Lippincott Williams and Wilkins, Philadelphia, PA

Campbell AP, Chien JW, Kuypers J, Englund JA, Wald A, Guthrie KA et al (2010) Respiratory virus pneumonia after hematopoietic cell transplantation (HCT): associations between viral load in bronchoalveolar lavage samples, viral RNA detection in serum samples, and clinical outcomes of HCT. J Infect Dis 201:1404–1413

Calvignac-Spencer S, Feltkamp MC, Daugherty MD, Moens U, Ramqvist T et al (2016) Polyomaviridae Study Group of the International Committee on Taxonomy of Viruses, A taxonomy update for the family Polyomaviridae. Arch Virol. 161:1739–1750

Casper C, Englund J, Boeckh M (2010) How I treat influenza in patients with hematologic malignancies. Blood 115:1331–1342

Cesaro S, Hirsch HH, Faraci M, Owoc-Lempach J, Beltrame A, Tendas A et al (2009) Cidofovir for BK virus-associated hemorrhagic cystitis: a retrospective study. Clin Infect Dis 49:233–240

Cesaro S, Tridello G, Pillon M, Calore E, Abate D, Tumino M et al (2015) A prospective study on the predictive value of plasma BK virus-DNA load for hemorrhagic cystitis in pediatric patients after stem cell transplantation. J Pediatric Infect Dis Soc 4:134–142

Cesaro S, Dalianis T, Hanssen Rinaldo C, Koskenvuo M, Pegoraro A, Einsele H et al (2018a) ECIL guidelines for the prevention, diagnosis and treatment of BK polyomavirus-associated haemorrhagic cystitis in haematopoietic stem cell transplant recipients. J Antimicrob Chemother 73:12–21

Cesaro S, Berger M, Tridello G, Mikulska M, Ward KN, Ljungman P et al (2018b) A survey on incidence and management of adenovirus infection after allogeneic HSCT. Bone Marrow Transplant

Chakrabarti S, Mautner V, Osman H, Collingham KE, Fegan CD, Klapper PE et al (2002) Adenovirus infections following allogeneic stem cell transplantation: incidence and outcome in relation to graft manipulation, immunosuppression, and immune recovery. Blood 100:1619–1627

Chartrand C, Leeflang MM, Minion J, Brewer T, Pai M (2012) Accuracy of rapid influenza diagnostic tests: a meta-analysis. Ann Intern Med 156:500–511

Chatzis O, Darbre S, Pasquier J, Meylan P, Manuel O, Aubert JD et al (2018) Burden of severe RSV disease among immunocompromised children and adults: a 10 year retrospective study. BMC Infect Dis 18:111

Chemaly RF, Ghosh S, Bodey GP, Rohatgi N, Safdar A, Keating MJ et al (2006) Respiratory viral infections in adults with hematologic malignancies and human stem cell transplantation recipients: a retrospective study at a major cancer center. Medicine (Baltimore) 85:278–287

Chemaly RF, Torres HA, Munsell MF, Shah DP, Rathod DB, Bodey GP et al (2012a) An adaptive randomized trial of an intermittent dosing schedule of aerosolized ribavirin in patients with cancer and respiratory syncytial virus infection. J Infect Dis 206:1367–1371

Chemaly RF, Hanmod SS, Rathod DB, Ghantoji SS, Jiang Y, Doshi A et al (2012b) The characteristics and outcomes of parainfluenza virus infections in 200 patients with leukemia or recipients of hematopoietic stem cell transplantation. Blood 119:2738–2745. quiz 969

Chemaly RF, Vigil KJ, Saad M, Vilar-Compte D, Cornejo-Juarez P, Perez-Jimenez C et al (2012c) A multicenter study of pandemic influenza a (H1N1) infection in patients with solid tumors in 3 countries: early therapy improves outcomes. Cancer 118:4627–4633

Chemaly RF, Shah DP, Boeckh MJ (2014) Management of respiratory viral infections in hematopoietic cell transplant recipients and patients with hematologic malignancies. Clin Infect Dis 59(Suppl 5): S344–S351

Chen YB, Driscoll JP, McAfee SL, Spitzer TR, Rosenberg ES, Sanders R et al (2011) Treatment of parainfluenza 3 infection with DAS181 in a patient after allogeneic stem cell transplantation. Clin Infect Dis 53:e77–e80

Choi SM, Boudreault AA, Xie H, Englund JA, Corey L, Boeckh M (2011) Differences in clinical outcomes after 2009 influenza a/H1N1 and seasonal influenza among hematopoietic cell transplant recipients. Blood 117:5050–5056

Chu HY, Englund JA, Podczervinski S, Kuypers J, Campbell AP, Boeckh M et al (2014) Nosocomial transmission of respiratory syncytial virus in an outpatient cancer center. Biol Blood Marrow Transplant 20:844–851

Couch RB, Englund JA, Whimbey E (1997) Respiratory viral infections in immunocompetent and immunocompromised persons. Am J Med 102:2–9. discussion 25-6

Dalianis T, Hirsch HH (2013) Human polyomaviruses in disease and cancer. Virology 437:63–72

Debur MC, Vidal LR, Stroparo E, Nogueira MB, Almeida SM, Takahashi GA et al (2010) Human metapneumovirus infection in hematopoietic stem cell transplant recipients. Transpl Infect Dis 12:173–179

DeVincenzo JP, Whitley RJ, Mackman RL, Scaglioni-Weinlich C, Harrison L, Farrell E et al (2014) Oral GS-5806 activity in a respiratory syncytial virus challenge study. N Engl J Med 371:711–722

Dykewicz CA, National Center for Infectious Diseases CfDC, Prevention, Infectious Diseases Society of A, American Society for B, Marrow T (2001) Guidelines for preventing opportunistic infections among hematopoietic stem cell transplant recipients: focus on community respiratory virus infections. Biol Blood Marrow Transplant 7 Suppl:19S–22S

Ebner K, Rauch M, Preuner S, Lion T (2006) Typing of human adenoviruses in specimens from immunosuppressed patients by PCR-fragment length analysis and real-time quantitative PCR. J Clin Microbiol 44:2808–2815

Egli A, Infanti L, Dumoulin A, Buser A, Samaridis J, Stebler C et al (2009) Prevalence of polyomavirus BK and JC infection and replication in 400 healthy blood donors. J Infect Dis 199:837–846

Englund JA, Sullivan CJ, Jordan MC, Dehner LP, Vercellotti GM, Balfour HH Jr (1988) Respiratory syncytial virus infection in immunocompromised adults. Ann Intern Med 109:203–208

Englund JA, Whimbey E, Atmar RL (1999) Diagnosis of respiratory viruses in cancer and transplant patients. Curr Clin Top Infect Dis 19:30–59

Erard V, Kim HW, Corey L, Limaye A, Huang ML, Myerson D et al (2005) BK DNA viral load in plasma: evidence for an association with hemorrhagic cystitis in allogeneic hematopoietic cell transplant recipients. Blood 106:1130–1132

Erard V, Chien JW, Kim HW, Nichols WG, Flowers ME, Martin PJ et al (2006) Airflow decline after myeloablative allogeneic hematopoietic cell transplantation: the role of community respiratory viruses. J Infect Dis 193:1619–1625

Falsey AR, Koval C, DeVincenzo JP, Walsh EE (2017) Compassionate use experience with high-titer respiratory syncytical virus (RSV) immunoglobulin in RSV-infected immunocompromised persons. Transpl Infect Dis 19

Fan J, Henrickson KJ (1996) Rapid diagnosis of human parainfluenza virus type 1 infection by quantitative reverse transcription-PCR-enzyme hybridization assay. J Clin Microbiol 34:1914–1917

Farhat RM, Mousa MA, Daas EJ, Glassberg MK (2020) Treatment of COVID-19: perspective on convalescent plasma transfusion. Front Med 7:435. Published 2020 Jul 28. https://doi.org/10.3389/fmed.2020.00435

Faura A, Rives S, Lassaletta Á et al (2020) Initial report on Spanish pediatric oncologic, hematologic, and post stem cell transplantation patients during SARS-CoV-2 pandemic. Pediatr Blood Cancer 67(9):e28557. https://doi.org/10.1002/pbc.28557. [published online ahead of print, 2020 Jul 16]

Feucht J, Opherk K, Lang P, Kayser S, Hartl L, Bethge W et al (2015) Adoptive T-cell therapy with hexon-specific Th1 cells as a treatment of refractory adenovirus infection after HSCT. Blood 125:1986–1994

Feuchtinger T, Lang P, Handgretinger R (2007) Adenovirus infection after allogeneic stem cell transplantation. Leuk Lymphoma 48:244–255

Feuchtinger T, Richard C, Joachim S, Scheible MH, Schumm M, Hamprecht K et al (2008) Clinical grade generation of hexon-specific T cells for adoptive T-cell transfer as a treatment of adenovirus infection after allogeneic stem cell transplantation. J Immunother 31:199–206

Filipovich AH, Weisdorf D, Pavletic S, Socie G, Wingard JR, Lee SJ et al (2005) National Institutes of Health consensus development project on criteria for clinical trials in chronic graft-versus-host disease: I. diagnosis and staging working group report. Biol Blood Marrow Transplant 11:945–956

Fiore AE, Shay DK, Broder K, Iskander JK, Uyeki TM, Mootrey G et al (2008) Prevention and control of influenza: recommendations of the advisory committee on immunization practices (ACIP), 2008. MMWR Recomm Rep 57:1–60

Fry AM, Curns AT, Harbour K, Hutwagner L, Holman RC, Anderson LJ (2006) Seasonal trends of human parainfluenza viral infections: United States, 1990-2004. Clin Infect Dis 43:1016–1022

Gardner SD, Field AM, Coleman DV, Hulme B (1971) New human papovavirus (B.K.) isolated from urine after renal transplantation. Lancet 1:1253–1257

Gasparetto EL, Escuissato DL (2004) Marchiori E, Ono S, Frare e Silva RL, Muller NL. High-resolution CT findings of respiratory syncytial virus pneumonia after bone marrow transplantation. AJR Am J Roentgenol 182:1133–1137

Gaziev J, Paba P, Miano R, Germani S, Sodani P, Bove P et al (2010) Late-onset hemorrhagic cystitis in children after hematopoietic stem cell transplantation for thalassemia and sickle cell anemia: a prospective evaluation of polyoma (BK) virus infection and treatment with cidofovir. Biol Blood Marrow Transplant 16:662–671

Gern JE, Galagan DM, Jarjour NN, Dick EC, Busse WW (1997) Detection of rhinovirus RNA in lower airway cells during experimentally induced infection. Am J Respir Crit Care Med 155:1159–1161

Ghosh S, Champlin R, Couch R, Englund J, Raad I, Malik S et al (1999) Rhinovirus infections in myelosuppressed adult blood and marrow transplant recipients. Clin Infect Dis 29:528–532

Giacomelli A, Pezzati L, Conti F et al (2020) Self-reported olfactory and taste disorders in patients with severe acute respiratory coronavirus 2 infection: a cross-sectional study. Clin Infect Dis 71(15):889–890. https://doi.org/10.1093/cid/ciaa330

Gilis L, Morisset S, Billaud G, Ducastelle-Lepretre S, Labussiere-Wallet H, Nicolini FE et al (2014) High burden of BK virus-associated hemorrhagic cystitis in patients undergoing allogeneic hematopoietic stem cell transplantation. Bone Marrow Transplant 49:664–670

Giraud G, Bogdanovic G, Priftakis P, Remberger M, Svahn BM, Barkholt L et al (2006) The incidence of hemorrhagic cystitis and BK-viruria in allogeneic hematopoietic stem cell recipients according to intensity of the conditioning regimen. Haematologica 91:401–404

Giraud G, Priftakis P, Bogdanovic G, Remberger M, Dubrulle M, Hau A et al (2008) BK-viruria and haemorrhagic cystitis are more frequent in allogeneic haematopoietic stem cell transplant patients receiving full conditioning and unrelated-HLA-mismatched grafts. Bone Marrow Transplant 41:737–742

Grimley MS, Chemaly RF, Englund JA, Kurtzberg J, Chittick G, Brundage TM et al (2017) Brincidofovir for asymptomatic adenovirus Viremia in pediatric and adult allogeneic hematopoietic cell transplant recipients: a randomized placebo-controlled phase II trial. Biol Blood Marrow Transplant 23:512–521

Guerin-El Khourouj V, Dalle JH, Pedron B, Yakouben K, Bensoussan D, Cordeiro DJ et al (2011) Quantitative and qualitative CD4 T cell immune responses related to adenovirus DNAemia in hematopoietic stem cell transplantation. Biol Blood Marrow Transplant 17:476–485

Guzman-Suarez BB, Buckley MW, Gilmore ET, Vocca E, Moss R, Marty FM et al (2012) Clinical potential of DAS181 for treatment of parainfluenza-3 infections in transplant recipients. Transpl Infect Dis 14:427–433

Hall CB, Douglas RG Jr, Schnabel KC, Geiman JM (1981) Infectivity of respiratory syncytial virus by various routes of inoculation. Infect Immun 33:779–783

Hall CB, Long CE, Schnabel KC (2001) Respiratory syncytial virus infections in previously healthy working adults. Clin Infect Dis 33:792–796

Hamelin ME, Prince GA, Boivin G (2006) Effect of ribavirin and glucocorticoid treatment in a mouse model of human metapneumovirus infection. Antimicrob Agents Chemother 50:774–777

Harrington RD, Hooton TM, Hackman RC, Storch GA, Osborne B, Gleaves CA et al (1992) An outbreak of respiratory syncytial virus in a bone marrow transplant center. J Infect Dis 165:987–993

Hassan IA, Chopra R, Swindell R, Mutton KJ (2003) Respiratory viral infections after bone marrow/peripheral stem-cell transplantation: the Christie hospital experience. Bone Marrow Transplant 32:73–77

Hayden RT, Gu Z, Liu W, Lovins R, Kasow K, Woodard P et al (2015) Risk factors for hemorrhagic cystitis in pediatric allogeneic hematopoietic stem cell transplant recipients. Transpl Infect Dis 17:234–241

He X, Lau EHY, Wu P et al (2020) Temporal dynamics in viral shedding and transmissibility of COVID-19. Nat Med. 26(5):672–675. https://doi.org/10.1038/s41591-020-0869-5. [published correction appears in Nat Med. 2020 Aug 7]

Hertz MI, Englund JA, Snover D, Bitterman PB, McGlave PB (1989) Respiratory syncytial virus-induced acute lung injury in adult patients with bone marrow transplants: a clinical approach and review of the literature. Medicine (Baltimore) 68:269–281

Hirsch HH, Steiger J (2003) Polyomavirus BK. Lancet Infect Dis 3:611–623

Hirsch HH, Martino R, Ward KN, Boeckh M, Einsele H, Ljungman P (2013) Fourth European conference on infections in Leukaemia (ECIL-4): guidelines for diagnosis and treatment of human respiratory syncytial virus, parainfluenza virus, metapneumovirus, rhinovirus, and coronavirus. Clin Infect Dis 56:258–266

Hiwarkar P, Amrolia P, Sivaprakasam P, Lum SH, Doss H, O'Rafferty C et al (2017) Brincidofovir is highly efficacious in controlling adenoviremia in pediatric recipients of hematopoietic cell transplant. Blood 129:2033–2037

Hiwarkar P, Kosulin K, Cesaro S, Mikulska M, Styczynski J, Wynn R et al (2018) Management of adenovirus infection in patients after haematopoietic stem cell transplantation: state-of-the-art and real-life current approach: a position statement on behalf of the infectious diseases working Party of the European Society of blood and marrow transplantation. Rev Med Virol 28:e1980

Hodson A, Kasliwal M, Streetly M, MacMahon E, Raj K (2011) A parainfluenza-3 outbreak in a SCT unit: sepsis with multi-organ failure and multiple co-pathogens are associated with increased mortality. Bone Marrow Transplant 46:1545–1550

Hoenigl M (2020) Invasive fungal disease complicating COVID-19: when it rains it pours. Clin Infect Dis. ciaa1342. https://doi.org/10.1093/cid/ciaa1342. Online ahead of print

Huang ML, Nguy L, Ferrenberg J, Boeckh M, Cent A, Corey L (2008) Development of multiplexed real-time quantitative polymerase chain reaction assay for detecting human adenoviruses. Diagn Microbiol Infect Dis 62:263–271

Hum RM, Deambrosis D, Lum SH, Davies E, Bonney D, Guiver M et al (2018) Molecular monitoring of adenovirus reactivation in faeces after haematopoietic stem-cell transplantation to predict systemic infection: a retrospective cohort study. Lancet Haematol 5:e422–e4e9

Ison MG (2007) Respiratory viral infections in transplant recipients. Antivir Ther 12:627–638

Jain S, Self WH, Wunderink RG, Fakhran S, Balk R, Bramley AM et al (2015) Community-acquired pneumonia requiring hospitalization among U.S. adults. N Engl J Med 373:415–427

Johnston SL (1995) Natural and experimental rhinovirus infections of the lower respiratory tract. Am J Respir Crit Care Med 152:S46–S52

Johny AA, Clark A, Price N, Carrington D, Oakhill A, Marks DI (2002) The use of zanamivir to treat influenza a and B infection after allogeneic stem cell transplantation. Bone Marrow Transplant 29:113–115

de Jong MD, Ison MG, Monto AS, Metev H, Clark C, O'Neil B et al (2014) Evaluation of intravenous peramivir for treatment of influenza in hospitalized patients. Clin Infect Dis 59:e172–e185

Kassis C, Champlin RE, Hachem RY, Hosing C, Tarrand JJ, Perego CA et al (2010) Detection and control of a nosocomial respiratory syncytial virus outbreak in a stem cell transplantation unit: the role of palivizumab. Biol Blood Marrow Transplant 16:1265–1271

Keib A, Mei YF, Cicin-Sain L, Busch DH, Dennehy KM (2019) Measuring antiviral capacity of T cell responses to adenovirus. J Immunol 202:618–624

Khanna N, Widmer AF, Decker M, Steffen I, Halter J, Heim D et al (2008) Respiratory syncytial virus infection in patients with hematological diseases: single-center study and review of the literature. Clin Infect Dis 46:402–412

Khanna N, Steffen I, Studt JD, Schreiber A, Lehmann T, Weisser M et al (2009) Outcome of influenza infections in outpatients after allogeneic hematopoietic stem cell transplantation. Transpl Infect Dis 11:100–105

Kharfan-Dabaja MA, Ayala E, Greene J, Rojiani A, Murtagh FR, Anasetti C (2007) Two cases of progressive multifocal leukoencephalopathy after allogeneic hematopoietic cell transplantation and a review of the literature. Bone Marrow Transplant 39:101–107

Kmeid J, Vanichanan J, Shah DP, El Chaer F, Azzi J, Ariza-Heredia EJ et al (2016) Outcomes of influenza infections in hematopoietic cell transplant recipients: application of an immunodeficiency scoring index. Biol Blood Marrow Transplant 22:542–548

Koehler P, Cornely OA, Böttiger BW, Dusse F, Eichenauer DA, Fuchs F et al (2020) COVID-19 associated pulmonary aspergillosis. Mycoses. https://doi.org/10.1111/myc.13096

Koskenvuo M, Dumoulin A, Lautenschlager I, Auvinen E, Mannonen L, Anttila VJ et al (2013) BK polyomavirus-associated hemorrhagic cystitis among pediatric allogeneic bone marrow transplant recipients: treatment response and evidence for nosocomial transmission. J Clin Virol 56:77–81

Kosulin K, Berkowitsch B, Matthes S, Pichler H, Lawitschka A, Potschger U et al (2018) Intestinal adenovirus shedding before allogeneic stem cell transplantation is a risk factor for invasive infection post-transplant. EBioMedicine 28:114–119

La Rosa AM, Champlin RE, Mirza N, Gajewski J, Giralt S, Rolston KV et al (2001) Adenovirus infections in adult recipients of blood and marrow transplants. Clin Infect Dis 32:871–876

Lan SH, Lai CC, Huang HT, Chang SP, Lu LC, Hsueh PR (2020) Tocilizumab for severe COVID-19: a systematic review and meta-analysis. Int J Antimicrob Agents 56(3):106103. https://doi.org/10.1016/j.ijantimicag.2020.106103

Lansbury L, Lim B, Baskaran V, Lim WS (2020) Co-infections in people with COVID-19: a systematic review and meta-analysis. J Infect 81(2):266–275. https://doi.org/10.1016/j.jinf.2020.05.046

Laskin BL, Denburg M, Furth S, Diorio D, Goebel J, Davies SM et al (2013) BK viremia precedes hemorrhagic cystitis in children undergoing allogeneic hematopoietic stem cell transplantation. Biol Blood Marrow Transplant 19:1175–1182

Layman CP, Gordon SM, Elegino-Steffens DU, Agee W, Barnhill J, Hsue G (2013) Rapid multiplex PCR assay to identify respiratory viral pathogens: moving forward diagnosing the common cold. Hawaii J Med Public Health 72:24–26

Lee YJ, Huang YT, Kim SJ, Maloy M, Tamari R, Giralt SA et al (2016) Adenovirus Viremia in adult CD34(+) selected hematopoietic cell transplant recipients: low incidence and high clinical impact. Biol Blood Marrow Transplant 22:174–178

Lee YJ, Prockop SE, Papanicolaou GA (2017) Approach to adenovirus infections in the setting of hematopoietic cell transplantation. Curr Opin Infect Dis 30:377–387

Lee LYW, Cazier JB, Starkey T et al (2020.;[published online ahead of print, 2020 Aug 24]) COVID-19 prevalence and mortality in patients with cancer and the effect of primary tumour subtype and patient demographics: a prospective cohort study. Lancet Oncol. https://doi.org/10.1016/S1470-2045(20)30442-3

Leen AM, Myers GD, Sili U, Huls MH, Weiss H, Leung KS et al (2006) Monoculture-derived T lymphocytes specific for multiple viruses expand and produce clinically relevant effects in immunocompromised individuals. Nat Med 12:1160–1166

Leen AM, Bollard CM, Mendizabal AM, Shpall EJ, Szabolcs P, Antin JH et al (2013) Multicenter study of banked third-party virus-specific T cells to treat severe viral infections after hematopoietic stem cell transplantation. Blood 121:5113–5123

Lessler J, Reich NG, Brookmeyer R, Perl TM, Nelson KE, Cummings DA (2009) Incubation periods of acute respiratory viral infections: a systematic review. Lancet Infect Dis 9:291–300

Li LQ, Huang T, Wang YQ et al (2020a) COVID-19 patients' clinical characteristics, discharge rate, and fatality rate of meta-analysis. J Med Virol 92(6):577–583. https://doi.org/10.1002/jmv.25757

Li L, Zhang W, Hu Y et al (2020b) Effect of convalescent plasma therapy on time to clinical improvement in patients with severe and life-threatening covid-19: a randomized clinical trial. JAMA 324(5):460–470. https://doi.org/10.1001/jama.2020.10044. [published correction appears in JAMA. 2020 Aug 4;324(5):519]

Liang W, Guan W, Chen R et al (2020) Cancer patients in SARS-CoV-2 infection: a nationwide analysis in China. Lancet Oncol 21(3):335–337. https://doi.org/10.1016/S1470-2045(20)30096-6

Lindemans CA, Leen AM, Boelens JJ (2010) How I treat adenovirus in hematopoietic stem cell transplant recipients. Blood 116:5476–5485

Lion T (2014) Adenovirus infections in immunocompetent and immunocompromised patients. Clin Microbiol Rev 27:441–462

Lion T, Baumgartinger R, Watzinger F, Matthes-Martin S, Suda M, Preuner S et al (2003) Molecular monitoring of adenovirus in peripheral blood after allogeneic bone marrow transplantation permits early diagnosis of disseminated disease. Blood 102:1114–1120

Lion T, Kosulin K, Landlinger C, Rauch M, Preuner S, Jugovic D et al (2010) Monitoring of adenovirus load in stool by real-time PCR permits early detection of impending invasive infection in patients after allogeneic stem cell transplantation. Leukemia 24:706–714

Ljungman P (2001) Respiratory virus infections in stem cell transplant patients: the European experience. Biol Blood Marrow Transplant 7(Suppl):5S–7S

Ljungman P, de la Camara R, Perez-Bercoff L, Abecasis M, Nieto Campuzano JB, Cannata-Ortiz MJ et al (2011) Outcome of pandemic H1N1 infections in hematopoietic stem cell transplant recipients. Haematologica 96:1231–1235

Ljungman P, Mikulska M, de la Camara R et al (2020) The challenge of COVID-19 and hematopoietic cell transplantation; EBMT recommendations for management of hematopoietic cell transplant recipients, their donors, and patients undergoing CAR T-cell therapy. Bone Marrow Transplant:1–6. https://doi.org/10.1038/s41409-020-0919-0. [published online ahead of print, 2020 May 13] [published correction appears in Bone Marrow Transplant. 2020 Jun 8]

Marcolini JA, Malik S, Suki D, Whimbey E, Bodey GP (2003) Respiratory disease due to parainfluenza virus in adult leukemia patients. Eur J Clin Microbiol Infect Dis 22:79–84

Marian AJ (2020) Current state of vaccine development and targeted therapies for COVID-19: impact of basic science discoveries. Cardiovasc Pathol 107278. https://doi.org/10.1016/j.carpath.2020.107278. [published online ahead of print, 2020 Sep 1]

Martino R, Porras RP, Rabella N, Williams JV, Ramila E, Margall N et al (2005) Prospective study of the incidence, clinical features, and outcome of symptomatic upper and lower respiratory tract infections by respiratory viruses in adult recipients of hematopoietic stem cell transplants for hematologic malignancies. Biol Blood Marrow Transplant 11:781–796

Marty FM, Vidal-Puigserver J, Clark C, Gupta SK, Merino E, Garot D et al (2017) Intravenous zanamivir or oral oseltamivir for hospitalised patients with influenza: an international, randomised, double-blind, double-dummy, phase 3 trial. Lancet Respir Med 5:135–146

Matthes-Martin S, Feuchtinger T, Shaw PJ, Engelhard D, Hirsch HH, Cordonnier C et al (2012) European guidelines for diagnosis and treatment of adenovirus infection in leukemia and stem cell transplantation: summary of ECIL-4 (2011). Transpl Infect Dis 14:555–563

Milano F, Campbell AP, Guthrie KA, Kuypers J, Englund JA, Corey L et al (2010) Human rhinovirus and coronavirus detection among allogeneic hematopoietic stem cell transplantation recipients. Blood 115:2088–2094

Minnema BJ, Husain S, Mazzulli T, Hosseini-Mogaddam SM, Patel M, Brandwein J et al (2013) Clinical characteristics and outcome associated with pandemic (2009) H1N1 influenza infection in patients with hematologic malignancies: a retrospective cohort study. Leuk Lymphoma 54:1250–1255

Molinos-Quintana A, Perez-de Soto C, Gomez-Rosa M, Perez-Simon JA, Perez-Hurtado JM (2013) Intravenous ribavirin for respiratory syncytial viral infections in pediatric hematopoietic SCT recipients. Bone Marrow Transplant 48:265–268

Moscona A, Porotto M, Palmer S, Tai C, Aschenbrenner L, Triana-Baltzer G et al (2010) A recombinant sialidase fusion protein effectively inhibits human parainfluenza viral infection in vitro and in vivo. J Infect Dis 202:234–241

Muftuoglu M, Olson A, Marin D, Ahmed S, Mulanovich V, Tummala S et al (2018) Allogeneic BK virus-specific T cells for progressive multifocal Leukoencephalopathy. N Engl J Med 379:1443–1451

Mynarek M, Ganzenmueller T, Mueller-Heine A, Mielke C, Gonnermann A, Beier R et al (2014) Patient, virus, and treatment-related risk factors in pediatric adenovirus infection after stem cell transplantation: results of a routine monitoring program. Biol Blood Marrow Transplant 20:250–256

Newton AH, Cardani A, Braciale TJ (2016) The host immune response in respiratory virus infection: balancing virus clearance and immunopathology. Semin Immunopathol 38:471–482

Nichols WG, Corey L, Gooley T, Davis C, Boeckh M (2001a) Parainfluenza virus infections after hematopoietic stem cell transplantation: risk factors, response to antiviral therapy, and effect on transplant outcome. Blood 98:573–578

Nichols WG, Gooley T, Boeckh M (2001b) Community-acquired respiratory syncytial virus and parainfluenza virus infections after hematopoietic stem cell transplantation: the Fred Hutchinson Cancer Research Center experience. Biol Blood Marrow Transplant 7(Suppl):11S–15S

Nichols WG, Guthrie KA, Corey L, Boeckh M (2004) Influenza infections after hematopoietic stem cell transplantation: risk factors, mortality, and the effect of antiviral therapy. Clin Infect Dis 39:1300–1306

Obando-Pacheco P, Justicia-Grande AJ, Rivero-Calle I, Rodriguez-Tenreiro C, Sly P, Ramilo O et al (2018) Respiratory syncytial virus seasonality: a global overview. J Infect Dis 217:1356–1364

Ogimi C, Waghmare AA, Kuypers JM, Xie H, Yeung CC, Leisenring WM et al (2017) Clinical significance of human coronavirus in Bronchoalveolar lavage samples from hematopoietic cell transplant recipients and patients with hematologic malignancies. Clin Infect Dis 64:1532–1539

Ohm-Smith MJ, Nassos PS, Haller BL (2004) Evaluation of the Binax NOW, BD Directigen, and BD Directigen EZ assays for detection of respiratory syncytial virus. J Clin Microbiol 42:2996–2999

Oliveira R, Machado A, Tateno A, Boas LV, Pannuti C, Machado C (2008) Frequency of human metapneumovirus infection in hematopoietic SCT recipients during 3 consecutive years. Bone Marrow Transplant 42:265–269

Omrani AS, Saad MM, Baig K, Bahloul A, Abdul-Matin M, Alaidaroos AY et al (2014) Ribavirin and interferon alfa-2a for severe Middle East respiratory syndrome coronavirus infection: a retrospective cohort study. Lancet Infect Dis 14:1090–1095

Oosterhof L, Christensen CB, Sengelov H (2010) Fatal lower respiratory tract disease with human corona virus NL63 in an adult haematopoietic cell transplant recipient. Bone Marrow Transplant 45:1115–1116

Padgett BL, Walker DL, ZuRhein GM, Eckroade RJ, Dessel BH (1971) Cultivation of papova-like virus from human brain with progressive multifocal leucoencephalopathy. Lancet 1:1257–1260

Pan F, Ye T, Sun P et al (2020) Time course of lung changes at chest CT during recovery from coronavirus disease 2019 (COVID-19). Radiology 295(3):715–721

de Pagter AP, Haveman LM, Schuurman R, Schutten M, Bierings M, Boelens JJ (2009) Adenovirus DNA positivity in nasopharyngeal aspirate preceding hematopoietic stem cell transplantation: a very strong risk factor for adenovirus DNAemia in pediatric patients. Clin Infect Dis 49:1536–1539

Parody R, Rabella N, Martino R, Otegui M, del Cuerpo M, Coll P et al (2007) Upper and lower respiratory tract infections by human enterovirus and rhinovirus in adult patients with hematological malignancies. Am J Hematol 82:807–811

Passamonti F, Cattaneo C, Arcaini L et al (2020) Clinical characteristics and risk factors associated with COVID-19 severity in patients with haematological malignancies in Italy: a retrospective, multicentre, cohort study. [published online ahead of print, 2020 Aug 13]. Lancet Haematol. https://doi.org/10.1016/S2352-3026(20)30251-9

Pavlovic D, Patera AC, Nyberg F, Gerber M, Liu M (2015) Progressive multifocal Leukeoncephalopathy C. progressive multifocal leukoencephalopathy: current treatment options and future perspectives. Ther Adv Neurol Disord 8:255–273

Pavlovic D, Patel MA, Patera AC, Peterson I (2018) Progressive multifocal Leukoencephalopathy C. T cell deficiencies as a common risk factor for drug associated progressive multifocal leukoencephalopathy. Immunobiology 223:508–517

Peck AJ, Englund JA, Kuypers J, Guthrie KA, Corey L, Morrow R et al (2007) Respiratory virus infection among hematopoietic cell transplant recipients: evidence for asymptomatic parainfluenza virus infection. Blood 110:1681–1688

Peinemann F, de Villiers EM, Dorries K, Adams O, Vogeli TA, Burdach S (2000) Clinical course and treatment of haemorrhagic cystitis associated with BK type of human polyomavirus in nine paediatric recipients of allogeneic bone marrow transplants. Eur J Pediatr 159:182–188

Pelosini M, Focosi D, Rita F, Galimberti S, Caracciolo F, Benedetti E et al (2008) Progressive multifocal leukoencephalopathy: report of three cases in HIV-negative hematological patients and review of literature. Ann Hematol 87:405–412

Pene F, Merlat A, Vabret A, Rozenberg F, Buzyn A, Dreyfus F et al (2003) Coronavirus 229E-related pneumonia in immunocompromised patients. Clin Infect Dis 37:929–932

Protheroe RE, Kirkland KE, Pearce RM, Kaminaris K, Bloor A, Potter MN et al (2012) The clinical features and outcome of 2009 H1N1 influenza infection in Allo-SCT patients: a British Society of Blood and Marrow Transplantation study. Bone Marrow Transplant 47:88–94

Raboni SM, Nogueira MB, Tsuchiya LR, Takahashi GA, Pereira LA, Pasquini R et al (2003) Respiratory tract viral infections in bone marrow transplant patients. Transplantation 76:142–146

Randhawa PS, Finkelstein S, Scantlebury V, Shapiro R, Vivas C, Jordan M et al (1999) Human polyoma virus-associated interstitial nephritis in the allograft kidney. Transplantation 67:103–109

Renaud C, Campbell AP (2011) Changing epidemiology of respiratory viral infections in hematopoietic cell transplant recipients and solid organ transplant recipients. Curr Opin Infect Dis 24:333–343

Renaud C, Boudreault AA, Kuypers J, Lofy KH, Corey L, Boeckh MJ et al (2011) H275Y mutant pandemic (H1N1) 2009 virus in immunocompromised patients. Emerg Infect Dis 17:653–660. quiz 765

Renaud C, Xie H, Seo S, Kuypers J, Cent A, Corey L et al (2013) Mortality rates of human metapneumovirus and respiratory syncytial virus lower respiratory tract infections in hematopoietic cell transplantation recipients. Biol Blood Marrow Transplant 19:1220–1226

Rollinger JM, Schmidtke M (2011) The human rhinovirus: human-pathological impact, mechanisms of anti-rhinoviral agents, and strategies for their discovery. Med Res Rev 31:42–92

Rorije NM, Shea MM, Satyanarayana G, Hammond SP, Ho VT, Baden LR et al (2014) BK virus disease after allogeneic stem cell transplantation: a cohort analysis. Biol Blood Marrow Transplant 20:564–570

Safdar A, Rodriguez GH, Mihu CN, Mora-Ramos L, Mulanovich V, Chemaly RF et al (2010) Infections in non-myeloablative hematopoietic stem cell transplantation patients with lymphoid malignancies: spectrum of infections, predictors of outcome and proposed guidelines for fungal infection prevention. Bone Marrow Transplant 45:339–347

Schiffer JT, Kirby K, Sandmaier B, Storb R, Corey L, Boeckh M (2009) Timing and severity of community acquired respiratory virus infections after myeloablative versus non-myeloablative hematopoietic stem cell transplantation. Haematologica 94:1101–1108

Schulze M, Beck R, Igney A, Vogel M, Maksimovic O, Claussen CD et al (2008) Computed tomography findings of human polyomavirus BK (BKV)-associated cystitis in allogeneic hematopoietic stem cell transplant recipients. Acta Radiol 49:1187–1194

Sedlacek P, Petterson T, Robin M, Sivaprakasam P, Vainorius E, Brundage T et al (2018) Incidence of adenovirus infection in hematopoietic stem cell transplantation recipients: findings from the AdVance study. Biol Blood Marrow Transplant

Self WH, Williams DJ, Zhu Y, Ampofo K, Pavia AT, Chappell JD et al (2016) Respiratory viral detection in children and adults: comparing asymptomatic controls and patients with community-acquired pneumonia. J Infect Dis 213:584–591

Seo S, Campbell AP, Xie H, Chien JW, Leisenring WM, Englund JA et al (2013) Outcome of respiratory syncytial virus lower respiratory tract disease in hematopoietic cell transplant recipients receiving aerosolized ribavirin: significance of stem cell source and oxygen requirement. Biol Blood Marrow Transplant 19:589–596

Seo S, Xie H, Campbell AP, Kuypers JM, Leisenring WM, Englund JA et al (2014) Parainfluenza virus lower respiratory tract disease after hematopoietic cell transplant: viral detection in the lung predicts outcome. Clin Infect Dis 58:1357–1368

Seo S, Gooley TA, Kuypers JM, Stednick Z, Jerome KR, Englund JA et al (2016) Human Metapneumovirus infections following hematopoietic cell transplantation: factors associated with disease progression. Clin Infect Dis 63:178–185

Seo S, Waghmare A, Scott EM, Xie H, Kuypers JM, Hackman RC et al (2017) Human rhinovirus detection in the lower respiratory tract of hematopoietic cell transplant recipients: association with mortality. Haematologica 102:1120–1130

Shah JN, Chemaly RF (2011) Management of RSV infections in adult recipients of hematopoietic stem cell transplantation. Blood 117:2755–2763

Shah DP, Ghantoji SS, Shah JN, El Taoum KK, Jiang Y, Popat U et al (2013) Impact of aerosolized ribavirin on mortality in 280 allogeneic haematopoietic stem cell transplant recipients with respiratory syncytial virus infections. J Antimicrob Chemother 68:1872–1880

Shah DP, Ghantoji SS, Ariza-Heredia EJ, Shah JN, El Taoum KK, Shah PK et al (2014) Immunodeficiency scoring index to predict poor outcomes in hematopoietic cell transplant recipients with RSV infections. Blood 123:3263–3268

Shah DP, Shah PK, Azzi JM, El Chaer F, Chemaly RF (2016) Human metapneumovirus infections in hematopoietic cell transplant recipients and hematologic malignancy patients: a systematic review. Cancer Lett 379:100–106

Siordia JA Jr (2020) Epidemiology and clinical features of COVID-19: a review of current literature. J Clin Virol 127:104357. https://doi.org/10.1016/j.jcv.2020.104357

Spahr Y, Tschudin-Sutter S, Baettig V, Compagno F, Tamm M, Halter J et al (2018) Community-acquired respiratory Paramyxovirus infection after allogeneic hematopoietic cell transplantation: a single-center experience. Open Forum Infect Dis 5:ofy077

Srinivasan A, Wang C, Yang J, Shenep JL, Leung WH, Hayden RT (2011) Symptomatic parainfluenza virus infections in children undergoing hematopoietic stem cell transplantation. Biol Blood Marrow Transplant 17:1520–1527

Team RSVOI (2014) Contributing and terminating factors of a large RSV outbreak in an adult hematology and transplant unit. PLoS Curr 6

Tirindelli MC, Flammia GP, Bove P, Cerretti R, Cudillo L, De Angelis G et al (2014) Fibrin glue therapy for severe hemorrhagic cystitis after allogeneic hematopoietic stem cell transplantation. Biol Blood Marrow Transplant 20:1612–1617

Tomblyn M, Chiller T, Einsele H, Gress R, Sepkowitz K, Storek J et al (2009) Guidelines for preventing infectious complications among hematopoietic cell transplantation recipients: a global perspective. Biol Blood Marrow Transplant 15:1143–1238

Trang TP, Whalen M, Hilts-Horeczko A, Doernberg SB, Liu C (2018) Comparative effectiveness of aerosolized versus oral ribavirin for the treatment of respiratory syncytial virus infections: a single-center retrospective cohort study and review of the literature. Transpl Infect Dis 20:e12844

Turner RB (2010) Upper respiratory tract infections section B. In: DaBs M (ed) Principles and practice of infectious diseases, 7th edn. Elsevier, Philadelphia, pp 809–813

Tylden GD, Hirsch HH, Rinaldo CH (2015) Brincidofovir (CMX001) inhibits BK polyomavirus replication in primary human urothelial cells. Antimicrob Agents Chemother 59:3306–3316

Tzannou I, Papadopoulou A, Naik S, Leung K, Martinez CA, Ramos CA et al (2017) Off-the-shelf virus-specific T cells to treat BK virus, human Herpesvirus 6, cytomegalovirus, Epstein Barr virus, and adenovirus infections after allogeneic hematopoietic stem-cell transplantation. J Clin Oncol 35:3547–3557

Uhlenhaut C, Cohen JI, Pavletic S, Illei G, Gea-Banacloche JC, Abu-Asab M et al (2012) Use of a novel virus detection assay to identify coronavirus HKU1 in the lungs of a hematopoietic stem cell transplant recipient with fatal pneumonia. Transpl Infect Dis 14:79–85

Ustun C, Slaby J, Shanley RM, Vydra J, Smith AR, Wagner JE et al (2012) Human parainfluenza virus infection after hematopoietic stem cell transplantation: risk factors, management, mortality, and changes over time. Biol Blood Marrow Transplant 18:1580–1588

Walsh EE, McConnochie KM, Long CE, Hall CB (1997) Severity of respiratory syncytial virus infection is related to virus strain. J Infect Dis 175:814–820

Walsh EE, Peterson DR, Kalkanoglu AE, Lee FE, Falsey AR (2013) Viral shedding and immune responses to respiratory syncytial virus infection in older adults. J Infect Dis 207:1424–1432

Watcharananan SP, Suwatanapongched T, Wacharawanichkul P, Chantratitaya W, Mavichak V, Mossad SB (2010) Influenza a/H1N1 2009 pneumonia in kidney transplant recipients: characteristics and outcomes following high-dose oseltamivir exposure. Transpl Infect Dis 12:127–131

Weinstock DM, Gubareva LV, Zuccotti G (2003) Prolonged shedding of multidrug-resistant influenza a virus in an immunocompromised patient. N Engl J Med 348:867–868

Wendt CH, Weisdorf DJ, Jordan MC, Balfour HH Jr, Hertz MI (1992) Parainfluenza virus respiratory infection after bone marrow transplantation. N Engl J Med 326:921–926

Whimbey E, Champlin RE, Couch RB, Englund JA, Goodrich JM, Raad I et al (1996) Community respiratory virus infections among hospitalized adult bone marrow transplant recipients. Clin Infect Dis 22:778–782

WHO (2020) WHO Estimated mortality from COVID-19. https://www.who.int/news-room/commentaries/detail/estimating-mortality-from-covid-19

WHO Rapid Evidence Appraisal for COVID-19 Therapies (REACT) Working Group, JAC S, Murthy S et al (2020) Association between administration of systemic corticosteroids and mortality among critically Ill Patients With COVID-19: A Meta-analysis. [published online ahead of print, 2020 Sep 2]. JAMA. https://doi.org/10.1001/jama.2020.17023. Recovery, NEJM 2020;

Williams JV, Martino R, Rabella N, Otegui M, Parody R, Heck JM et al (2005) A prospective study comparing human metapneumovirus with other respiratory viruses in adults with hematologic malignancies and respiratory tract infections. J Infect Dis 192:1061–1065

World Health Organization (WHO) Report of the WHO-China Joint Mission on coronavirus disease 2019 (COVID 19) 2020. https://www.who.int/docs/default-source/coronaviruse/who-china-joint-mission-on-covid-19-final-report.pdf Accessed 12 May 2020.

Wu C, Liu Y, Yang Y et al (2020) Analysis of therapeutic targets for SARS-CoV-2 and discovery of potential drugs by computational methods. Acta Pharm Sin B 10(5):766–788. https://doi.org/10.1016/j.apsb.2020.02.008

Wyde PR, Chetty SN, Jewell AM, Boivin G, Piedra PA (2003) Comparison of the inhibition of human metapneumovirus and respiratory syncytial virus by ribavirin and immune serum globulin in vitro. Antivir Res 60:51–59

Xing Y, Proesmans M (2019) New therapies for acute RSV infections: where are we? Eur J Pediatr 178:131–138

Ye ZW, Yuan S, Yuen KS, Fung SY, Chan CP, Jin DY (2020) Zoonotic origins of human coronaviruses. Int J Biol Sci 16(10):1686–1697. Published 2020 Mar 15. https://doi.org/10.7150/ijbs.45472

Yoshihara S, Yanik G, Cooke KR, Mineishi S (2007) Bronchiolitis obliterans syndrome (BOS), bronchiolitis obliterans organizing pneumonia (BOOP), and other late-onset noninfectious pulmonary complications following allogeneic hematopoietic stem cell transplantation. Biol Blood Marrow Transplant 13:749–759

Zama D, Masetti R, Vendemini F, Di Donato F, Morelli A, Prete A et al (2013) Clinical effectiveness of early treatment with hyperbaric oxygen therapy for severe late-onset hemorrhagic cystitis after hematopoietic stem cell transplantation in pediatric patients. Pediatr Transplant 17:86–91

Zandvliet ML, Falkenburg JH, van Liempt E, Veltrop-Duits LA, Lankester AC, Kalpoe JS et al (2010) Combined CD8+ and CD4+ adenovirus hexon-specific T cells associated with viral clearance after stem cell transplantation as treatment for adenovirus infection. Haematologica 95:1943–1951

Zecca M, Wynn R, Dalle JH, Feuchtinger T, Vainorius E, Brundage TM et al (2019) Association between adenovirus viral load and mortality in pediatric Allo-HCT recipients: the multinational AdVance study. Bone Marrow Transplant

Zhao X, Sullender WM (2005) In vivo selection of respiratory syncytial viruses resistant to palivizumab. J Virol 79:3962–3968

Yeast Infections

15

Alexandre Alanio and Sharon C. -A. Chen

15.1 Introduction

Invasive fungal disease (IFD) caused by yeasts and yeast-like pathogens are important infection-related complications in patients with underlying haematological malignancy, specifically after both autologous and allogeneic hematopoietic stem cell transplantation (HSCT). Donor sources such as the umbilical cord or mismatched unrelated donors have expanded HSCT availability but with increased risk of IFD (Kontoyiannis et al. 2010). The epidemiology of yeast infections varies with antifungal prophylaxis practices and varies by geographical region. Nonetheless, bloodstream *Candida* infections (candidaemia) and other forms of invasive candidiasis (IC) remain the most common IFD (Kontoyiannis et al. 2010; Cornely et al. 2015). *Cryptococcus* and more uncommon pathogens such as *Trichosporon*, *Geotrichum*-like, *Rhodotorula*, *Saccharomyces cerevisiae* or *Malassezia* and species also cause serious infections (Kontoyiannis et al. 2010; Chitasombat et al. 2012; Chaaban et al. 2014). Accurate diagnosis will assist with selection of best practice antifungal therapy and other treatment. In this chapter, we focus on the management of yeast infections in haematological malignancy. The aetiology, risk factors and diagnostic approaches are also briefly discussed.

15.2 *Candida* Infections

15.2.1 Epidemiology, Risk Factors and Clinical Features

IC in the setting of haematology and HSCT carries with it both high mortality ($\approx 40\%$) and excess hospital-related costs (Ananda-Rajah et al. 2012; Cornely et al. 2015). Its occurrence has long been substantively reduced by widespread use of azole prophylaxis in cancer chemotherapy and in HSCT conditioning regimens

A. Alanio (✉)
Institut Pasteur, Molecular Mycology Unit, CNRS UMR2000, Laboratoire de Parasitologie-Mycologie, Hôpital Saint-Louis, Groupe Hospitalier Lariboisière, Saint-Louis, Fernand Widal, Assistance Publique-Hôpitaux de Paris (AP-HP), Université Paris Diderot, Sorbonne Paris Cité, Paris, France

Department of Molecular Microbiology and Immunology, Johns Hopkins Bloomberg School of Public Health, Baltimore, MD, USA
e-mail: alexandre.alanio@pasteur.fr

S. C. -A. Chen (✉)
Centre for Infectious Diseases and Microbiology, Westmead Hospital and New South Wales Health Pathology, The University of Sydney, Sydney, Australia

Marie Bashir Institute for Infectious Diseases and Biosecurity, The University of Sydney, Sydney, Australia
e-mail: sharon.chen@health.nsw.gov.au

© Springer Nature Switzerland AG 2021
O. A. Cornely, M. Hoenigl (eds.), *Infection Management in Hematology*, Hematologic Malignancies, https://doi.org/10.1007/978-3-030-57317-1_15

(Slavin et al. 1995). Estimates from after 2010 indicate an incidence of IC in patients with underlying haematological malignancy of 1.4 cases/1000 admissions in one study (Gamaletsou et al. 2014) with the Transplant Associated Infections Surveillance Network (TRANNET) noting an incidence of 1% and 1.1% at 6 and 12 months, respectively, after HSCT (Kontoyiannis et al. 2010). An incidence of fungaemia of 1.55% in HSCT was reported in Europe with 90% of such infections due to *Candida* spp. (Cornely et al. 2015). Variation in IC rates depends on differences in local practices and transplant conditioning regimens.

Risk factors for IC in patients with haematological malignancy are well known. Especially pertinent are status of underlying cancer, neutropenia, older age, corticosteroid use, recent HSCT (<6 months), recent broad-spectrum antibiotic use, total parenteral nutrition (TPN) and intensive care unit (ICU) admission (Slavin et al. 2010; Hoenigl et al. 2012; Hsu et al. 2015). Established candidaemia risk factors including disruption of the gastrointestinal mucosa after chemotherapy, radiotherapy or surgery also apply to haematology patients as does placement of a central venous access device (CVAD) (Slavin et al. 2010; Andes et al. 2012). The shift in epidemiology from *Candida albicans* to non-*albicans Candida* spp. is particularly well manifested. Specifically, *Candida glabrata*, *Candida krusei* and other non-*albicans Candida* spp. are more common in

HSCT patients compared with, e.g. solid organ transplant recipients (Lockhart et al. 2011). *C. glabrata* is associated not only with traditional candidaemia risk factors but also with prior azole exposure (Alexander et al. 2005; Trubiano et al. 2015). This species is not only less susceptible to azole antifungals but, in some countries, associated with both echinocandin and multi-drug resistance (Alexander et al. 2013; Wang et al. 2015; McCarty et al. 2018)), which impacts the choice of treatment (**see below**). Clinicians should also be alert to previously rare but emerging species, most recently *Candida auris* with its associated multidrug-drug resistant characteristics (reviewed in (Forsberg et al. 2019).

Clinical features of IC and non-*Candida* yeast infections in haematology patients are summarized in Table 15.1. Clinical presentation as candidaemia remains the most common. As patients are often receiving antifungal prophylaxis, candidaemia is typically occurring as "breakthrough" infection accounting for up to 50% of IFD in HSCT patients (Slavin et al. 2010; Cornely et al. 2015) and may be associated with resistance to one (most often the azoles) or more classes of antifungal drugs (Alexander et al. 2013). IC per se has been reported as an independent predictor of death in HSCT (Falagas et al. 2006; Hsu et al. 2015).

Other clinical syndromes include disseminated IC, which is now uncommon. Patients may present with persistent fever after neutrophil

Table 15.1 Clinical syndromes of yeast and yeast-like pathogens in haematological malignancy and hematopoietic stem cell recipients

Pathogen	Clinical syndrome							
	Fungaemia	Lung	Abdominal disease	Skin/soft tissue	CNS	Eye	Cardiac	Hepato-splenic
Candida spp.	+++	+[a]	+++	+	+	++	+	+++
Cryptococcus spp.	+	+++	+	+	+++	+	+	+
Trichosporon spp.	+++	+[a]	++	++	+	+	+	++
Geotrichum-like spp.	+++	+[a]	++	++	+	+	+	++
Rhodotorula spp.	+++	+[a]	+	+	+	+	+	+
Saccharomyces spp.	+++	+[a]	+	+	+	+	+	+
Malassezia spp.	+++	+[a]	+	+++	+	+	+	+

Abbreviations: *CNS*, central nervous system
+, relatively uncommon; ++, common; +++, very common
[a]Lesions occurring by haematogenous dissemination responsible for bilateral nodular lesions

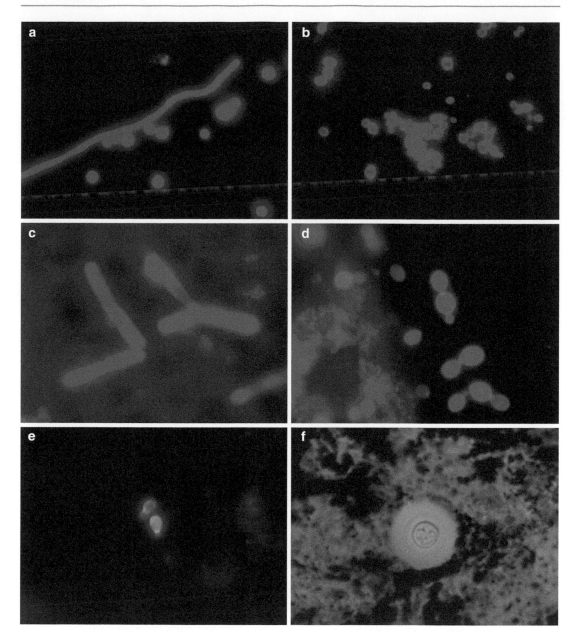

Fig. 15.1 Microscopic examination of *Candida* and non-*Candida* yeasts responsible for infections in haematology. (**a**) *Candida albicans* from a blood culture (x400 magnification, calcofluor staining), (**b**) *Candida glabrata* from a blood culture (x400 magnification, calcofluor staining), (**c**) *Saprochaete clavata* from a blood culture (x400 magnification, calcofluor staining), (**d**) *Rhodotorula mucilaginosa* from a blood culture (x1000 magnification, calcofluor staining), (**e**) *Malassezia pachydermatis* from a sinus aspirate (×400 magnification, calcofluor staining), (**f**) *Cryptococcus neoformans* from a bronchoalveolar lavage (×400 magnification, India ink examination)

recovery, accompanied by lesions (abscesses) in the kidneys, liver, spleen and lungs. A subset of patients may have hepato-splenic candidiasis, with lesions confined to the liver and spleen (Rammaert et al. 2012). Culture of affected tissue is often negative although yeasts and granulomatous changes are a clue for histopathological examination (Fig. 15.1).

15.2.2 Diagnostic Approaches

Diagnosis of IC still mostly relies on culture-based approaches. For candidaemia, blood cultures are the cornerstone of diagnosis and allow an isolate for antifungal susceptibility testing (Arendrup et al. 2012). Blood cultures for IC, although specific, lack sensitivity (<50%), and all forms of IC are limited by delayed time to positivity of result (2–3 days) (Clancy and Nguyen 2013).

Hence, non-culture-based methods are often used to assist with diagnosis. Of these, the serum beta-D-glucan (BDG) test can be a useful adjunctive tool in haematologic malignancy and other patients. However, in general and encompassing all haematologic patient groups, its widespread use is limited by variable sensitivity (50–100%) and specificity (45–100%) as well as negative predictive value (NPV; 73–100%). Specificity can be improved by obtaining two consecutive BDG results but at the expense of sensitivity. Importantly, more extensive studies of its utility in the haematology setting are required. While meta-analyses clearly point out very high sensitivity and specificity of the test for diagnosing IC, the test may be less sensitive in certain settings, with only 36% of candidaemia detected at the time of diagnosis in one study (Angebault et al. 2016). In another study of haematology patients, serum BDG testing had insufficient sensitivity for detecting breakthrough candidaemia (Abe et al. 2014). In part, the wide range of performance may be explained by difficulties of performing the test, which is prone to contamination. Since BDG is a panfungal biomarker, a positive test should prompt investigations for other IFDs, such as invasive aspergillosis or pneumocystosis (Karageorgopoulos et al. 2011). A detailed discussion of the serum BDG test is beyond the scope of this chapter and information relating to its incorporation into diagnostic algorithms are found in the Infectious Diseases Society of America guidelines for managing candidiasis (Pappas et al. 2016) and in one meta-analysis (Karageorgopoulos et al. 2011). For the present, where employed, serial testing is recommended with interpretation of results in conjunction with clinical and laboratory parameters.

Molecular methods to detect *Candida* in blood or blood cultures have likewise been developed but methodologies are not standardized, limiting their routine use. Data to support its routine use in HSCT are also lacking. Nguyen et al. found that PCR was more sensitive than blood cultures for diagnosis of intra-abdominal candidiasis, although there were no haematology/HSCT patients included in that study (Nguyen et al. 2012). Also, one FDA-approved assay, the T2 magnetic resonance (T2MR) assay, is available in the USA and Europe, which has the advantage of detecting *Candida* in whole blood specimens as opposed to blood cultures. A multicentre study, which included HSCT recipients (43% of study patients), showed a sensitivity of 91%, specificity of 98% and NPV of 99% for *Candida* spp. with time to negativity reduced to 4.4 hours (cf. 2–5 days (Mylonakis et al. 2015). However, test sensitivity was much lower in other real-life studies (Muñoz et al. 2018; White et al. 2018). Hence, whilst holding promise, experience with this new method is limited and results should be interpreted in a clinical context.

15.2.3 Treatment

The treatment principles for IC and candidaemia in the haematology and HSCT setting are similar to those provided in clinical practice guidelines for other populations (Cornely et al. 2012; Chen et al. 2014; Pappas et al. 2016).

15.2.3.1 Empirical Antifungal Treatment and General Practice Considerations

Empirical therapy should be tailored to local epidemiology and *Candida* species distribution. In addition, the site of infection, patient's clinical status and history of antifungal exposure and—if known—*Candida* colonization status may assist in the choice of antifungal agent. Although the value of empirical therapy is debated, it is clear that delay in appropriate antifungal treatment is associated with poor outcomes (Taur et al. 2010). Hence, it is reasonable for patients at high risk for IC with no explanation for fever or clinical symptoms to be treated with antifungal drugs on an empirical basis.

For candidaemia, treatment recommendations for patients who are neutropenic, or who are hemodynamically unstable, or who have had recent azole exposure (e.g. as antifungal prophylaxis) include an echinocandin (micafungin, caspofungin or anidulafungin) or a lipid formulation of amphotericin B (e.g. liposomal amphotericin B [L-AMB]) as primary treatment; however, voriconazole can be used in situations in which additional mould coverage is required (Chen et al. 2014; Pappas et al. 2016). Should the patient be non-neutropenic and haemodynamically stable, treatment with fluconazole is an acceptable alternative to the above (Cornely et al. 2012; Pappas et al. 2016). If a patient was recently colonized with *Candida* spp., consideration of the relevant species-specific susceptibility profiles is recommended. If recent echinocandin exposure has occurred/there are concerns about echinocandin resistance, the empirical use of L-AMB or voriconazole is recommended (Pappas et al. 2016). That said, available data do not indicate less favourable outcomes associated with empiric fluconazole and voriconazole, compared with lipid amphotericin formulations or an echinocandin; however, many experts favour the latter, which are fungicidal and sometimes better tolerated, as first-line agents in neutropenic patients (Pappas et al. 2016). Doses of antifungals commonly used to treat IC are shown in Table 15.2; isavuconazole use is not included in the table but briefly discussed (in Sect. X 1.4). Removal of CVADs as early as possible is strongly recommended (Andes et al. 2012). When this is not possible, an echinocandin is preferred for its anti-biofilm activity (Pappas et al. 2016).

For all cases of IC, screening for involvement of the eye, heart, abdomen and other organs is indicated. The incidence of ocular candidiasis in patients with candidaemia is estimated at 12.5–26% and if there is retinal disease at diagnosis, an echinocandin should not be used alone as this drug class does not achieve therapeutic levels in vitreous fluid in contrast to azoles (Khalid et al. 2014; Pappas et al. 2016). Antifungals excreted through the renal tract, e.g. fluconazole and 5-flucytosine, are more effective in *Candida* pyelonephritis, cystitis and fungal balls. Intra-abdominal candidiasis may be difficult to diagnose and should be suspected at least, particularly in the event of major gastrointestinal surgery. Repeat blood cultures to ensure that fungaemia has cleared during antifungal therapy should be performed. In general, the duration of therapy for candidaemia without metastatic complications is 2 weeks after established clearance of *Candida* from the bloodstream and with resolution of clinical symptoms attributable to candidaemia (Pappas et al. 2016).

The frequency of *Candida* endocarditis is difficult to estimate due to differences in clinical practice and differential use of transthoracic vs. transoesophageal echocardiography but varies between 4.2 and 17% (Lefort et al. 2012; Fernández-Cruz et al. 2015). Echocardiography is strongly recommended, especially in the presence of prosthetic cardiac valves.

15.2.3.2 Targeted Antifungal Treatment and Treatment of Invasive Candidiasis Conditions

For candidaemia, antifungal therapy should be modified according to the causative pathogen and its antifungal susceptibility profile with targeted "step-down" therapy. In the event of infections due to an azole-susceptible isolate, fluconazole (12 mg/kg loading dose then 6 mg/kg daily) can be used for step-down therapy even if the patient is neutropenic but clinically stable and, for example, has documented bloodstream clearance; voriconazole (see Table 15.2 for doses) may also be used (Pappas et al. 2016). Other azoles, e.g. posaconazole or isavuconazole, are alternatives in this context but historically there is far less (although growing) experience with their use in IC. The choice of azole should always be guided by the organism's susceptibility profile. Where the isolate is not azole-susceptible, then echinocandin or lipid amphotericin B therapy should be continued.

Table 15.3 summarizes the various forms of the suggested treatment for non-candidaemia IC including ocular candidiasis, central nervous

Table 15.2 Doses of commonly used antifungal agents in the treatment of invasive candidiasis in adults and children

Antifungal agent	Route	Recommended dose (adults)	Recommended dose (children)
Amphotericin B deoxycholate	IV	0.6–1 mg/kg daily	0.7–1 mg/kg daily
Liposomal amphotericin B	IV	3 mg/kg daily	3 mg/kg daily
5-flucytosine[a,b]	IV or oral	25 mg/kg 6 hourly	25 mg/kg 6 hourly
Fluconazole[b]	IV or oral	Loading: 12 mg/kg (single dose) Maintenance: 6–12 mg/kg daily	12 mg/kg daily
Voriconazole[c]	IV or oral	Loading: 6 mg/kg twice daily (2 doses) Maintenance: 4 mg/kg twice daily	Loading: 9 mg/kg twice daily (2 doses) Maintenance: 8 mg/kg twice daily
Caspofungin	IV	Loading: 70 mg daily (single dose) Maintenance: 50 mg daily	50 m/m² daily
Anidulafungin	IV	Loading: 200 mg daily (single dose) Maintenance: 100 mg daily	Loading: 3 mg/kg (single dose) Maintenance: 1.5 mg/kg daily
Micafungin	IV	Loading: Not required Maintenance:100 mg daily	Loading: Not required Maintenance: 2–4 mg/kg daily

Adapted from Chen et al. (2014). Also see full approved Product Information for individual antifungal agents
Abbreviations: *IV*, intravenous
[a]Trough levels required to achieve clinical efficacy (>25 mg/L) and peak levels to avoid toxicity (<100 mg/L)
[b]Require dose adjustment in renal impairment
[c]Therapeutic drug monitoring is required with trough levels to achieve clinical efficacy and peak levels to avoid toxicity (lower and upper limits vary with laboratory and should be individualized to patient)

system (CNS) disease, endocarditis and urinary tract candidiasis. Where appropriate, e.g. in endocarditis, combined antifungal therapy and surgery is the optimal treatment and should be employed. In cases of chorioretinitis with vitritis, vitrectomy has the advantage of reducing fungal burden and draining fungal microabscesses (Pappas et al. 2016). In *Candida* endocarditis, although there are some reports of successful outcomes with medical treatment alone, consensus expert opinion is to always consider early cardiac surgery (Lefort et al. 2012). Echinocandins have a central role in treating *Candida* endocarditis because of their good biofilm penetration (Fiori et al. 2011).

For initial antifungal therapy of hepatosplenic candidiasis or disseminated infection, the IDSA guidelines (Pappas et al. 2016) recommend the use of a lipid amphotericin formulation or an echinocandin followed by step-down therapy with an azole, preferably fluconazole (Table 15.3). The Australia and New Zealand Mycoses Interest Group recommendations (Chen et al. 2014) also provide the option of using an azole (fluconazole) up front if the isolate is fluconazole-susceptible.

The role of voriconazole, posaconazole and isavuconazole (see later) as initial therapy in treating this entity is uncertain. Hepatosplenic disease often requires prolonged treatment and may be accompanied by persistent fever, which may also be caused by immune reconstitution inflammatory syndrome (IRIS) and some authors have advised the short term (1–2 weeks) in certain clinical settings (Rammaert et al. 2012; Pappas et al. 2016).

The identification and management of end-organ complications of IC are important to maximize the long-term treatment success. Where neutropenia is expected to resolve, granulocyte infusions have been used to bridge a period of profound neutropenia but in the absence of RCTs, their efficacy is uncertain (Safdar et al. 2004).

15.2.3.3 Candida Auris

C. auris has emerged as a cause of nosocomial candidaemia and IC, with high mortality rates (reviewed in (Forsberg et al. 2019)). Infections occur in all patient populations, including in the setting of haematological malignancies. This species is typically resistant to fluconazole, and variably susceptible to other azoles, amphotericin and

Table 15.3 Summary of recommendations for treatment of *Candida* infections other than candidaemia in haematological malignancy

Clinical entity	Preferred agents	Alternative agents	Minimum duration	Comments
Ocular candidiasis (endophthalmitis)	c-AMB (0.7–1 mg/kg daily) or L-AMB (3–5 mg/kg/ daily) plus 5-FC (25 mg/kg 4 times daily) for fluconazole-resistant isolates *OR* Fluconazole (12 mg/kg loading dose then 6–12 mg/kg daily) for fluconazole-susceptible isolates	Voriconazole 6 mg/kg loading dose twice daily for 2 doses then 4 mg/kg twice daily	Four to six weeks and until ocular lesions have resolved	1. If vitritis, add either intravitreal c-AMB (5–10 ug/0.1 mL sterile water) or voriconazole, 100 ug/0.1 mL sterile water 2. Consider vitrectomy 3. Echinocandins are not recommended as single agents due to poor ocular penetration but have been used in combination with lipid formulations of amphotericin B
Endocarditis	Lipid amphotericin B formulations (3–5 mg/kg daily) f ± 5-FC (25 mg/kg 4 times daily) *OR* High-dose echinocandin (caspofungin 150 mg daily or micafungin 150 mg daily or anidulafungin 200 mg daily)	Step-down therapy to fluconazole (12 mg/kg loading dose then 6–12 mg/kg daily) for isolates that are fluconazole-susceptible *OR* Voriconazole (6 mg/kg loading dose for 2 doses then 4 mg/kg twice daily) or posaconazole[a], for isolates susceptible to these agents and non-susceptible to fluconazole	Six weeks	1. For all patients, valve replacement is recommended; treatment should be continued for at least 6 weeks after surgery. 2. If surgery is not possible, long-term suppressive therapy with fluconazole or an alternate azole. 3. For prosthetic valve endocarditis, long-term suppressive fluconazole (6–12 mg/kg daily) is recommended (fluconazole-susceptible isolates).
Hepatosplenic (chronic disseminated candidiasis)	Lipid formulation of AMB 3–5 mg/kg daily followed by an azole (fluconazole 6 mg/kg daily is preferred, if isolate is fluconazole-susceptible).	An echinocandin followed by an azole (fluconazole 6 mg/kg daily is preferred, if isolate is fluconazole-susceptible).	Several weeks of initial therapy followed by typically several months of azole therapy.	Therapy should continue until lesions resolve on repeat imaging, which is usually several months.

(continued)

Table 15.3 (continued)

Clinical entity	Preferred agents	Alternative agents	Minimum duration	Comments
CNS (meningitis/brain abscess)	L-AMB 3–5 mg/kg daily ± 5FC 25 mg/kg four times daily followed by fluconazole 12 mg/kg loading dose, then 6–12 mg/kg daily	Fluconazole 12 mg/kg loading dose, then 6–12 mg/kg daily	Until resolution of all neurological symptoms and radiological abnormalities	Infected devices, e.g. drains, shunts, should be removed if possible; if dev ices cannot be removed, c-AMB could be administered through the device into the ventricles (0.01–0.5 mg in 2 mL 5% dextrose in water). There are limited data for the use of posaconazole, voriconazole or the echinocandins for CNS candidiasis (Lutsar et al. 2003; Kang et al. 2009). Echinocandin and posaconazole penetrate poorly into the CNS
Candida osteomyelitis	Fluconazole 6 mg/kg daily) *OR* An echinocandin (caspofungin 50 mg daily or micafungin 100 mg daily or anidulafungin 100 mg daily) for at least 2 weeks followed by fluconazole 6 mg/kg daily	Lipid formulation of AMB 3–5 mg/kg/daily for at least 2 weeks followed by fluconazole 6 mg/kg daily	Six to 12 months	Surgical debridement in selected cases of osteomyelitis
Candida septic arthritis	Fluconazole 6 mg/kg/daily OR An echinocandin (as for "*Candida* osteomyelitis" for 23 weeks followed by fluconazole 6 mg/kg daily for 4 weeks	A lipid formulation of AMB 3–5 mg/kg/daily for 2 weeks followed by fluconazole 6 mg/kg daily for 4 weeks	Six weeks	Surgical drainage in all cases of septic arthritis Removal of infected joint prosthesis. If not possible, long-term suppressive therapy is recommended (fluconazole is preferred, if the isolate is fluconazole-susceptible).
Candida cystitis (symptomatic) or pyelonephritis	Fluconazole 3–6 mg/kg day if isolate is fluconazole-susceptible c-AMB 0.3–0.6 mg/kg daily ± 5FC (25 mg/kg 4 times daily for 1–7 days if fluconazole-resistant	Echinocandins are reserved for instances of drug resistance or drug intolerance	If fluconazole: 2 weeks If c-AMB ± 5FC: 1–7 days	AMB bladder irrigation is uncommonly used.

(continued)

Table 15.3 (continued)

Clinical entity	Preferred agents	Alternative agents	Minimum duration	Comments
Candida urinary tract fungal ball	As for *Candida* cystis and pyelonephritis	–	As for *Candida* cystis and pyelonephritis	Surgery is usually required ± local irrigation of c-AMB 25–50 mg in 200–500 sterile water via endoscopic methods
Intra-abdominal candidiasis[b]	Echinocandin (caspofungin 70 mg loading dose, then 50 mg daily; micafungin 100 mg daily; anidulafungin 200 mg loading dose, then 100 mg daily)	Fluconazole 12 mg/kg loading dose, then 6 mg/kg daily *OR* Amphotericin B lipid formulation 3–5 mg/kg daily) *OR* Voriconazole 6 mg/kg loading dose for 2 doses then 4 mg/kg twice daily	Duration of therapy should be individualized according to source control and clinical response	Choice of antifungal agent should be the same as for candidaemia and be guided by drug susceptibility results. Surgical drainage of abscess and debridement of necrotic tissue is recommended.

Adapted from Cornely et al. 2012; Chen et al. 2014; Pappas et al. 2016)
Abbreviations: *5-FC*, 5-flucytosine; *AMB*, amphotericin B; *c-AMB*, amphotericin B deoxycholate; *CNS*, central nervous system; *L-AMB*, liposomal amphotericin B
[a]Suggested dose is posaconazole slow release tablets; 300 mg daily with TDM
[b]excluding hepatosplenic candidiasis

the echinocandins. Lockhart et al. reported on 54 isolates in a US study; 93% were fluconazole-resistant, 35% were amphotericin B-resistant, 7% were echinocandin-resistant, with 41% of isolates being resistant to two drug classes (Lockhart et al. 2017). At present, although some isolates have elevated minimal inhibitory concentrations (MICs) to echinocandins, this drug class remains the first-line antifungal therapy for *C. auris* candidaemia (Chowdhary et al. 2017). Following susceptibility testing, treatment should be adapted if necessary. The recommended duration of antifungal therapy for IC is similar to that for *Candida* spp. and where indicated, CVADs should be removed (Vallabhaneni et al. 2015). As *C. auris* can persist in the environment, aggressive infection control measures are recommended (Biswal et al. 2017).

15.2.4 New Drugs for Treatment of Candidiasis

Several agents including compounds with novel mechanisms of action are under clinical evaluation or development for treatment of candidiasis

to address the limitations of drug resistance in certain *Candida* species and adverse effects of current antifungals. A detailed discussion is found in recent reviews (Wiederhold 2017; Gonzalez-Lara et al. 2017).

Current evidence for the most recently marketed triazole drug, isavuconazole, in the treatment of candidiasis has not provided data as robust as that obtained for this agent's place in the treatment of mucormycosis or aspergillosis. The ACTIVE study compared the efficacy of isavuconazole with that of caspofungin and the results failed to meet criteria for non-inferiority of isavuconazole (summarized in (Wilson et al. 2016)). Based on these data, it is not possible to position isavuconazole as initial treatment for IC but it may be reasonably used as an oral option for step-down in patients who cannot receive another azole due to tolerability or spectrum of activity limitations (Astellas Pharma US, Inc., Available from https://newsroom.astellas.us/news-releases. Accessed 01/2019).

Drugs undergoing evaluation for treatment of candidiasis include rezafungin (Cidara Therapeutics, San Diego, USA), a long-acting echinocandin with potent in vitro activity against *Candida* spp. and which is associated with low frequency of development of mutations in hot spot regions of the *Candida FKS1* and *FKS2* genes (Wiederhold 2017). A phase 2 randomized double-blind study is in progress comparing the efficacy of rezafungin with caspofungin (± fluconazole step-down therapy) in patients with candidaemia (summarized in Gonzalez-Lara et al. 2017). Ibrexafungerp (Scynexis Inc., Jersey City, NJ) is another glucan synthase inhibitor, which can be administered orally and exhibits potent activity against *Candida* spp. including azole- and echinocandin-resistant isolates, and also inhibits the biofilms of *C. auris* (Larkin et al. 2017; Schell et al. 2017). Results of a phase 2 study for treatment of IC are pending. The tetrazole compounds, inclusive of VT-1161 and VT-1598, are fungal-specific inhibitors of cyp51 also with good in vitro activity against *Candida* spp. Larger-scale data on their efficacy in IC in humans are pending (Wiederhold 2017).

15.3   Non-*Candida* Infections

Large surveillance studies have shown that non-*Candida* fungaemia accounted for 1.1% (out of 4000 fungaemia cases) in Denmark to 5.1% (of 3668 fungaemia cases) in France (Arendrup et al. 2014). Indeed, the proportion of non-*Candida* infections varies between countries and centres ranging from 2.3% in India to up to 24.9% in Thailand. Frequencies are higher in tropical areas such as Mexico, Brazil and Asia (Lin et al. 2018). In a recent report from Asia analysing 1 year of

yeast isolates in blood (total 2155 isolates) from 25 centres, non-*Candida* isolates represented 8.1% of the total (Lin et al. 2018), which included 5.1% of *Cryptococcus*, 1.1% of *Trichosporon*, 0.5% of *Rhodotorula*, 0.3% of *Kodamaea ohmeri* and 0.2% of *Malassezia* species.

Recommended antifungal treatments for non-*Candida* yeast infections in haematology patients are summarized in Table 15.4.

15.3.1   *Cryptococcus* Infections

Cryptococcus are encapsulated basidiomycetous yeasts. More than 70 species have been described but only few are associated with human infections including the two major species *Cryptococcus neoformans* and *C. gattii*. Cryptococcosis used to be typically observed in HIV-positive patients with CD4 counts below 200/mm3. However, cryptococcosis in immunocompromised non-HIV-infected patients is an increasingly reported entity parallel to a decrease in incidence of cryptococcosis in HIV-positive patients in the presence of highly effective antiretroviral treatment (O'Halloran et al. 2017). However, cryptococcosis seems to be relatively uncommon in haematology patients. In one study, underlying leukaemia was present in 2% of HIV-negative patients with cryptococcosis (Baddley et al. 2008). In a more recent study in California and Florida, describing prevalence of cryptococcosis over a 7-year period, non-HIV non-transplant cases of cryptococcosis represented 39.4% of the total cases (George et al. 2018), with 8.2% of the cases occurring in the setting of

Table 15.4 Therapeutic options for cryptococcosis and rare yeast infections in patients with haematological malignancies

Organism	First line	Other option
Cryptococcus spp.	AmB + 5FC	AmB + fluconazole
Trichosporon spp.	Voriconazole	Fluconazole
M. capitatus/S. clavata	AmB ± 5FC	Voriconazole + caspofungin
Rhodotorula spp.	AmB ± 5FC	/
Saccharomyces spp.	AmB ± 5FC	Fluconazole
Malassezia spp.	AmB	Fluconazole

Lipid formulations of amphotericin B (AmB) are preferred due to renal toxicity of deoxycholate amphotericin B. 5-FC, 5-flucytosine is myelotoxic and should be considered carefully in haematology patients haematological malignancy. Mortality is higher in non-HIV patients than in HIV patients (Bitar et al. 2014; George et al. 2018). Among haematology patients, acute leukaemia (50%) and non-Hodgkin's lymphoma (17.8%) were the most prevalent underlying diseases (Pagano et al. 2004). The administration of corticosteroids and the presence of diabetes mellitus seem to be strong risk factors (Pagano et al. 2004). Clinical presentation can vary from isolated pulmonary infection to cryptococcal meningitis and/or dissemination with fungaemia (Dromer et al. 2007). In HIV-negative patients, pulmonary localization was present in half of the patients, meningoencephalitis in 70% of the patients and dissemination in 38% of the patients (Dromer et al. 2007).

Diagnosis of cryptococcosis relies on direct examination, culture of clinical specimens and *Cryptococcus* antigen detection. Direct examination with India ink wet mount allows visualization of yeasts with their surrounding capsules (Arendrup et al. 2012). Culture can be performed on Sabouraud dextrose agar, but differentiation from ascomycetous yeasts can be difficult although *Cryptococcus* colonies tend to be more mucous. Identification can be done by subculture onto canavanin-glycine-bromothymol (CGB) medium (to differentiate between *C. neoformans* and *C. gattii*) (Kwon-Chung et al. 1982) and species identification can either be achieved accurately by Maldi-tof mass spectroscopy analysis (McTaggart et al. 2011; Firacative et al. 2012) or by molecular identification (Diaz et al. 2005). Culture may be negative in those prior exposed to antifungal drugs and culture plates should be incubated for up to 3 weeks at 30 °C. Another way to diagnose cryptococcosis is to detect soluble *Cryptococcus* antigen (glucuronoxylomannan) in biological fluids (whole blood, plasma, serum) or CSF. Antigen detection in serum is presumptive of active infection and in CSF of cryptococcal meningitis (Temstet et al. 1992). Different methods exist for detection of the antigen including latex agglutination, enzyme-linked immunosorbent assays (ELISA) and most recently a lateral flow assay (LFA). In HIV-negative patients, the LFA has been evaluated in comparison to the latex agglutination test with 100% sensitivity (Jitmuang et al. 2016). A high antigen titre (>1/512) in blood has been correlated with disease severity in CNS infections (Dromer et al. 2007; Perfect et al. 2010).

Cryptococcus spp. are intrinsically resistant to echinocandins but susceptible to amphotericin B, 5-flucytosine and fluconazole. Although fluconazole is frequently used to treat cryptococcosis, at present, antifungal susceptibility testing is not recommended on the initial isolate (Perfect et al. 2010). A recent study suggests that there is no correlation between fluconazole MICs and patient outcome upon fluconazole treatment (Vena et al. 2018).

In non-HIV non-transplant patients with meningoencephalitis or disseminated infection, the latest guidelines recommend the use of a combination of amphotericin B deoxycholate plus 5-flucytosine for more than 4 weeks (induction therapy) followed by fluconazole 400–800 mg/d for 8 weeks (consolidation therapy) and then fluconazole 200 mg/d for 6–12 months (Perfect et al. 2010). Lipid formulations of amphotericin B should be used in place of amphotericin B deoxycholate, if available. The myelotoxicity of 5-flucytosine is often a major concern in haematology patients. Therapeutic drug monitoring of 5-flucytosine should be performed to prevent drug toxicity. In non-HIV immunosuppressed patients with *Cryptococcus* infection in whom meningitis and dissemination have been ruled out, fluconazole (400 mg/d) for 6–12 weeks is recommended (Perfect et al. 2010).

15.3.2 *Trichosporon* Infections

Trichosporon spp. are basidiomycetous yeasts that are able to produce arthroconidia, blastoconidia, hyphae and pseudohyphae. These organisms are part of the normal flora on skin, respiratory tract or, uncommonly, the GI tract (Chagas-Neto et al. 2008). At least eight species are known to be associated with infection in humans out of 38 species described to date belonging to five clades (Chagas-Neto et al. 2008). The pathogenic species including *T. asahii, T. mucoides, T. cutaneum, T. asteroides, T.*

mucoides, T. inkin, T. ovoides, T. domesticum and *T. montevideense. Trichosporon* spp. can be identified using mycological culture and with phenotypic identification methods including urease testing on the colony (urease will be positive). Maldi-tof MS identification of *Trichosporon* spp. is accurate with most (>98%) of the tested strains representing 14 to 16 species correctly identified (Kolecka et al. 2013; de Almeida Júnior et al. 2014). Molecular identification using sequencing and comparison to public database can be performed accurately using the intragenic spacer (IGS) region (Sugita et al. 2002; Rodriguez-Tudela et al. 2005).

Cancer patients and more specifically patients with haematological malignancies largely comprise those at risk of trichosporonosis, with haematology patients representing more than 60% of cases reported in literature (Kontoyiannis et al. 2004; Girmenia et al. 2005). More specifically, patients most at risk were those with profound neutropenia (≤100/mmc) and/or those treated with chemotherapy for acute myeloid leukaemia. The outcome of trichosporonosis is poor, with crude mortality reported between 53 and 77% (Kontoyiannis et al. 2004; Girmenia et al. 2005; Suzuki et al. 2010). Negative outcome is associated with antibacterial use, bacterial bloodstream infection or coinfection, prophylactic/empirical antifungal therapy, admission to an intensive care unit, high APACHE II score and high dose of corticosteroid use (Kontoyiannis et al. 2004; Liao et al. 2015). A better outcome is associated with neutropenia recovery and removal of a CVAD when present (Liao et al. 2015). Fungaemia and or disseminated infection represent the main clinical presentations. *Trichosporon* infection has been associated with cross-reactions with *Aspergillus* galactomannan testing (Fekkar et al. 2009) and *Cryptococcus* antigen detection (Lyman et al. 1995; Liao et al. 2012). BDG detection have been associated with a low sensitivity with a maximum of 50% sensitivity in haematology patients with trichosporonosis, and rarely before positive blood cultures (Nakase et al. 2012).

All *Trichosporon* species share an intrinsic resistance to echinocandin drugs and *T. asahii* specifically is known to have increased MICs to amphotericin B and fluconazole (Rodriguez-Tudela et al. 2005). Triazole drugs are considered as the most effective drugs for *Trichosporon* infections (Arendrup et al. 2014). Specifically, voriconazole is considered as the most effective antifungal drug with a longer survival rate in patients (Kontoyiannis et al. 2004; Suzuki et al. 2010; Liao et al. 2015). Indeed, voriconazole displays a good in vitro activity against the most common *Trichosporon* species and a good outcome in animal models (Arendrup et al. 2014).

15.3.3 *Geotrichum*-like Infections

Geotrichum-like infections are due to few species including *Galactomyces candidus* (formerly known as *Geotrichum candidum*), *Magnusiomyces capitatus* (formerly known as *Trichosporon capitatum, Geotrichum capitatum* and *Blastoschizomyces capitatus*) and *Saprochaete clavata* (formerly known as *Geotrichum clavata*). All are ascomycetous urease-negative yeasts producing arthroconidia and hyphae. These organisms are considered part of the normal human mycobiome.

Galactomyces candidus has rarely been reported in haematology patients. On the other hand, *M. capitatus* and *S. clavata* infections are classically reported in patients with haematological malignancies with acute leukaemia as the main underlying disease (Girmenia et al. 2005; Vaux et al. 2014). Typically, patients develop fungaemia or disseminated disease (Girmenia et al. 2005; Arendrup et al. 2014). Identification is based on culture and identification of colonies using Maldi-tof mass spectrometry (Kolecka et al. 2013; Desnos-Ollivier et al. 2014) or by molecular approaches. *S. clavata* can be differentiated from *M. capitatus* using Maldi-tof (Kolecka et al. 2013; Desnos-Ollivier et al. 2014) and by ITS sequencing with a 96% similarity between both species (de Hoog and Smith n.d.). *S. clavata* infections have been probably underestimated because of easy misidentifications with *M. capitatus* (Desnos-Ollivier et al. 2014). *S. clavata* has been responsible for a nationwide outbreak in France mostly in haematology patients with profound neutropenia. More than 60% of the patients were pre-exposed to echinocandins (Vaux et al. 2014). CVADs have been reported as a possible source of infection due to *M. capitatus* (Martino et al. 2004). Mortality is reported to be around 60% (Martino et al. 2004; Girmenia et al. 2005) to 70% (Vaux et al. 2014).

Galactomannan detection may be a useful adjunctive diagnostic tool in *M. capitatus* infections (Bonini et al. 2008), and serum BDG detection in *S. clavata* (Del Principe et al. 2016) or *M. capitatus* (Oya and Muta 2018) infections.

M. capitatus may have elevated MICs to fluconazole and to amphotericin B (Girmenia et al. 2003), is considered as susceptible to 5-flucytosine, itraconazole, voriconazole and posaconazole but is intrinsically resistant to the echinocandins (Vaux et al. 2014; Arendrup et al. 2014). Although no therapeutic strategy has been systematically compared, recommendations are to use amphotericin B with or without 5-flucytosine together with early catheter removal. Voriconazole could be a good alternative (Arendrup et al. 2014). Colony-stimulating factors, Interferon-gamma and granulocyte transfusions as adjuvant therapies have been successfully used (Arendrup et al. 2014).

15.3.4 *Rhodotorula* Infections

Rhodotorula spp. are basidiomycetous yeasts containing red pigment. Although the genus contains up to 46 species, only three have been associated rarely with human infections, *R. mucilaginosa*, *R. glutinis,* and *R. minuta* (De Almeida et al. 2008; Tuon and Costa 2008). These organisms have been described as part of the normal microbiota. Infections to *Rhodotorula* seem to occur more frequently in tropical areas than in northern countries (Arendrup et al. 2014). Although rare in haematological malignancies, *Rhodotorula* spp. are increasingly recognized as emerging pathogens (De Almeida et al. 2008). In haematology, acute leukaemia and allogeneic HSCT are the main underlying diseases (García-Suárez et al. 2011; Potenza et al. 2018) with neu-

tropenia as an important risk factor. Specifically, all cases were also associated with the presence of a CVAD. The presence of CVAD was also the main risk factor for *Rhodotorula* infection in two other case series (Kiehn et al. 1992; Zaas et al. 2003; Tuon et al. 2007). Numerous cases of breakthrough infection following fluconazole, posaconazole or echinocandins treatments have been reported (Arendrup et al. 2014; Potenza et al. 2018). These infections present mainly as fungaemia. Mortality has been reported to be 15–20% (De Almeida et al. 2008; García-Suárez et al. 2011; Potenza et al. 2018). In one study, mortality in haematology patients ranged from 0% in patients with lymphoma to 15.7% in acute leukaemia (De Almeida et al. 2008). Fungal culture is the main method of detecting and identifying this pathogen. Colonies are orange to salmon coloured, which make *Rhodotorula* spp. easily recognizable although other fungi such as *Sporobolomyces* spp. can also be orange coloured. Species identification relies on sequence analysis of the D1–D2 region of the 28S rDNA and of the ITS loci (Arendrup et al. 2014). Galactomannan testing has been shown to cross-react with *Rhodotorula* (Kappe and Schulze-Berge 1993).

Rhodotorula spp. are considered as resistant to the triazoles (fluconazole, voriconazole, posaconazole, itraconazole) and to echinocandins as MICs are especially high for these drugs. The MICs to amphotericin B and 5-flucytosine are low. Consequently, the treatment of choice will be any formulation of amphotericin B with or without 5-flucytosine. CVADs should be removed promptly.

15.3.5 *Saccharomyces* Infections

Saccharomyces cerevisiae is another ascomycetous yeast also known as "baker's yeast." It has low pathogenicity and is part of the normal gut flora. A genetically close-related species, *Saccharomyces boulardii*, is used in probiotic preparations for the prevention and treatment of diarrhoea in various settings. This organism is also closely related to *C. glabrata* and shares with it some phenotypic traits.

Saccharomyces fungaemia is rare but can be observed mainly in immunocompromised patients who have taken probiotic therapy (Arendrup et al. 2014). Out of 92 cases reported in the literature, fungaemia was the main clinical presentation and predisposing factors were similar to other *Candida* infections including the presence of a CVAD, and prior antibiotic therapy. *S. boulardii* infections accounted for half of all *Saccharomyces* infections and were exclusively fungaemia. These cases were mostly observed in non-immunocompromised hosts and were associated with better outcomes (Enache-Angoulvant and Hennequin 2005). Global mortality was 38%. Diagnosis is based on classical culture procedures. There are not enough data to put forward any recommendations on the use of fungal biomarkers to detect *Saccharomyces* infection but BDG may have utility as a biomarker (Yoshida et al. 1997).

Saccharomyces harbours intrinsically high MICs to amphotericin B and fluconazole. Treatment with fluconazole or amphotericin B has given favourable outcomes for 60% and 77% of cases, respectively (Arendrup et al. 2014). Amphotericin B with or without 5-flucytosine can be considered as the treatment of choice. *S. boulardii* probiotic treatments should also be stopped and CVAD removal discussed.

15.3.6 *Malassezia* Infections

Malassezia spp. are basidiomycetous lipid-dependent and lipophilic yeasts. These organisms are part of the normal microbiota specifically on skin. Fourteen species have been identified so far (Velegraki et al. 2015) with the four species, *M. globosa*, *M. restricta*, *M. pachydermatis* and *M. furfur* associated frequently with human infections. *M. pachydermatis* is the only *Malassezia* species that is not dependent on lipids to grow. It is able to grow on classical media like Sabouraud dextrose agar. *Malassezia* spp. are associated with a variety of skin diseases including pythiriasis versicolor, seborrhoeic dermatitis, dandruff, atopic eczema and folliculitis and, less commonly, onychomycosis (Gaitanis et al. 2012).

Systemic infections have been described mainly in infants treated with parenteral nutrition (Gueho et al. 1987) and in infants or adults with various types of immunosuppression (Gaitanis et al. 2012). Patients, specifically those with in situ CVADs, are at risk of fungaemia (Morrison and Weisdorf 2000; Tragiannidis et al. 2010). Diagnosis relies on culture with the limitation that only *M. pachydermatis* can grow on classical media. For the other species, addition of lipid is required. The modified Dixon Agar is one specific medium that can be used in case of suspicion of *Malassezia* infection. Blood cultures are not optimized for *Malassezia* recovery except for the Isolator 10 system with subculture on lipid-containing media (Arendrup et al. 2014). Once grown, *Malassezia* species can be identified by Maldi-tof MS (Kolecka et al. 2014) and molecular tools (Velegraki et al. 2015). As these organisms are difficult to grow and require specific media, susceptibility testing has not been standardized and MICs are difficult to interpret. Fluconazole and amphotericin B are the preferred agents for treating *Malassezia* infections and where there is the most clinical experience. 5-Flucytosine and the echinocandins are inactive against *Malassezia* spp. and should not be used. CVAD removal and discontinuation of lipid-containing parenteral nutrition are part of the treatment of systemic infections (Arendrup et al. 2014).

15.4   Conclusion

Despite the use of prophylactic strategies in haematology, yeast infections remain the most prevalent invasive fungal infections in haematological malignancies. The use of these drugs impacts patients' ecology and is one of the possible reasons to explain the emergence of non-*Candida* infections due to organisms carrying intrinsic resistance to some of those antifungal drugs. These yeast infections are still associated with a high mortality rates (15 to 70% depending on the organism and the underlying disease), reinforcing that there is still room for improvement of prophylaxis, diagnostic and therapeutic strategies.

References

Abe M, Kimura M, Araoka H et al (2014) Serum (1,3)-beta-D-glucan is an inefficient marker of breakthrough candidemia. Med Mycol 52:835–840. https://doi.org/10.1093/mmy/myu066

Alexander BD, Schell WA, Miller JL et al (2005) Candida glabrata fungemia in transplant patients receiving voriconazole after fluconazole. Transplantation 80:868–871

Alexander BD, Johnson MD, Pfeiffer CD et al (2013) Increasing Echinocandin resistance in Candida glabrata: clinical failure correlates with presence of FKS mutations and elevated minimum inhibitory concentrations. Clin Infect Dis 56:1724–1732. https://doi.org/10.1093/cid/cit136

de Almeida Júnior JN, Figueiredo DSY, Toubas D et al (2014) Usefulness of matrix-assisted laser desorption ionisation-time-of-flight mass spectrometry for identifying clinical Trichosporon isolates. Clin Microbiol Infect 20:784–790. https://doi.org/10.1111/1469-0691.12502

Ananda-Rajah MR, Grigg A, Downey MT et al (2012) Comparative clinical effectiveness of prophylactic voriconazole/posaconazole to fluconazole/itraconazole in patients with acute myeloid leukemia/myelodysplastic syndrome undergoing cytotoxic chemotherapy over a 12-year period. J Antimicrob Chemother 97:459–463. https://doi.org/10.3324/haematol.2011.051995

Andes DR, Safdar N, Baddley JW et al (2012) Impact of treatment strategy on outcomes in patients with candidemia and other forms of invasive candidiasis: a patient-level quantitative review of randomized trials. Clin Infect Dis 54:1110–1122. https://doi.org/10.1093/cid/cis021

Angebault C, Lanternier F, Dalle F et al (2016) Prospective evaluation of serum β-Glucan testing in patients with probable or proven fungal diseases. Open forum. Infect Dis 3:ofw128. https://doi.org/10.1093/ofid/ofw128

Arendrup MC, Bille J, Dannaoui E et al (2012) ECIL-3 classical diagnostic procedures for the diagnosis of invasive fungal diseases in patients with leukaemia. Bone Marrow Transplant 47:1030–1045. https://doi.org/10.1038/bmt.2011.246

Arendrup MC, Boekhout T, Akova M et al (2014) ESCMID and ECMM joint clinical guidelines for the diagnosis and management of rare invasive yeast infections. Clin Microbiol Infect 20(Suppl 3):76–98. https://doi.org/10.1111/1469-0691.12360

Baddley JW, Perfect JR, Oster RA et al (2008) Pulmonary cryptococcosis in patients without HIV infection: factors associated with disseminated disease. Eur J Clin Microbiol Infect Dis 27:937–943. https://doi.org/10.1007/s10096-008-0529-z

Biswal M, Rudramurthy SM, Jain N et al (2017) Controlling a possible outbreak of Candida auris infection: lessons learnt from multiple interventions.

J Hosp Infect 97:363–370. https://doi.org/10.1016/j.jhin.2017.09.009

Bitar D, Lortholary O, Le Strat Y et al (2014) Population-based analysis of invasive fungal infections, France, 2001–2010. Emerg Infect Dis 20:1163–1169. https://doi.org/10.3201/eid2007.140087

Bonini A, Capatti C, Parmeggiani M et al (2008) Galactomannan detection in Geotrichum capitatum invasive infections: report of 2 new cases and review of diagnostic options. Diagn Microbiol Infect Dis 62:450–452. https://doi.org/10.1016/j.diagmicrobio.2008.08.008

Chaaban S, Wheat LJ, Assi M (2014) Cryptococcal meningitis post autologous stem cell transplantation. Transpl Infect Dis 16:473–476. https://doi.org/10.1111/tid.12216

Chagas-Neto TC, Chaves GM, Colombo AL (2008) Update on the genus Trichosporon. Mycopathologia 166:121–132. https://doi.org/10.1007/s11046-008-9136-x

Chen SC, Sorrell TC, Chang CC et al (2014) Consensus guidelines for the treatment of yeast infections in the haematology, oncology and intensive care setting, 2014. Intern Med J 44:1315–1332. https://doi.org/10.1111/imj.12597

Chitasombat MN, Kofteridis DP, Jiang Y et al (2012) Rare opportunistic (non-Candida, non-Cryptococcus) yeast bloodstream infections in patients with cancer. J Infect 64:68–75. https://doi.org/10.1016/j.jinf.2011.11.002

Chowdhary A, Sharma C, Meis JF (2017) Candida auris: a rapidly emerging cause of hospital-acquired multidrug-resistant fungal infections globally. PLoS Pathog 13:e1006290. https://doi.org/10.1371/journal.ppat.1006290

Clancy CJ, Nguyen MH (2013) Finding the "missing 50%" of invasive candidiasis: how nonculture diagnostics will improve understanding of disease spectrum and transform patient care. Clin Infect Dis 56:1284–1292. https://doi.org/10.1093/cid/cit006

Cornely OA, Bassetti M, Calandra T et al (2012) ESCMID* guideline for the diagnosis and management of Candida diseases 2012: non-neutropenic adult patients. Clin Microbiol Infect 18:19–37. https://doi.org/10.1111/1469-0691.12039

Cornely OA, Gachot B, Akan H et al (2015) Epidemiology and outcome of fungemia in a cancer cohort of the infectious diseases group (IDG) of the European Organization for Research and Treatment of Cancer (EORTC 65031). Clin Infect Dis 61:324–331. https://doi.org/10.1093/cid/civ293

De Almeida GMD, Costa SF, Melhem M et al (2008) Rhodotorula spp. isolated from blood cultures: clinical and microbiological aspects. Med Mycol 46:547–556. https://doi.org/10.1080/13693780801972490

Del Principe MI, Sarmati L, Cefalo M et al (2016) A cluster of Geotrichum clavatum (Saprochaete clavata) infection in haematological patients: a first Italian report and review of literature. Mycoses 59:594–601. https://doi.org/10.1111/myc.12508

Desnos-Ollivier M, Blanc C, Garcia-Hermoso D et al (2014) Misidentification of Saprochaete clavata as

Magnusiomyces capitatus in clinical isolates: utility of internal transcribed spacer sequencing and matrix-assisted laser desorption ionization-time of flight mass spectrometry and importance of reliable databases. J Clin Microbiol 52:2196–2198. https://doi.org/10.1128/JCM.00039-14

Diaz M, Boekhout T, Kiesling T, Fell J (2005) Comparative analysis of the intergenic spacer regions and population structure of the species complex of the pathogenic yeast. FEMS Yeast Res 5:1129–1140. https://doi.org/10.1016/j.femsyr.2005.05.005

Dromer F, Mathoulin-Pélissier S, Launay O et al (2007) Determinants of disease presentation and outcome during cryptococcosis: the CryptoA/D study. PLoS Med 4:e21. https://doi.org/10.1371/journal.pmed.0040021

Enache-Angoulvant A, Hennequin C (2005) Invasive Saccharomyces infection: a comprehensive review. Clin Infect Dis 41:1559–1568. https://doi.org/10.1086/497832

Falagas ME, Apostolou KE, Pappas VD (2006) Attributable mortality of candidemia: a systematic review of matched cohort and case-control studies. Eur J Clin Microbiol Infect Dis 25:419–425. https://doi.org/10.1007/s10096-006-0159-2

Fekkar A, Brun S, D'Ussel M et al (2009) Serum cross-reactivity with Aspergillus galactomannan and cryptococcal antigen during fatal disseminated Trichosporon dermatis infection. Clin Infect Dis 49:1457–1458. https://doi.org/10.1086/644499

Fernández-Cruz A, Cruz Menárguez M, Munoz P et al (2015) The search for endocarditis in patients with candidemia: a systematic recommendation for echocardiography? A prospective cohort. Eur J Clin Microbiol Infect Dis 34:1543–1549. https://doi.org/10.1007/s10096-015-2384-z

Fiori B, Posteraro B, Torelli R et al (2011) In vitro activities of anidulafungin and other antifungal agents against biofilms formed by clinical isolates of different Candida and Aspergillus species. Antimicrob Agents Chemother 55:3031–3035. https://doi.org/10.1128/AAC.01569-10

Firacative C, Trilles L, Meyer W (2012) MALDI-TOF MS enables the rapid identification of the major molecular types within the Cryptococcus neoformans/C. gattii species complex. PLoS One 7:e37566. https://doi.org/10.1371/journal.pone.0037566.t001

Forsberg K, Woodworth K, Walters M et al (2019) Candida auris: the recent emergence of a multidrug-resistant fungal pathogen. Med Mycol 57:1–12. https://doi.org/10.1093/mmy/myy054

Gaitanis G, Magiatis P, Hantschke M et al (2012) The Malassezia genus in skin and systemic diseases. Clin Microbiol Rev 25:106–141. https://doi.org/10.1128/CMR.00021-11

Gamaletsou MN, Walsh TJ, Zaoutis T et al (2014) A prospective, cohort, multicentre study of candidaemia in hospitalized adult patients with haematological malignancies. Clin Microbiol Infect 20:O50–O57. https://doi.org/10.1111/1469-0691.12312

García-Suárez J, Gómez-Herruz P, Cuadros JA, Burgaleta C (2011) Epidemiology and out-come of Rhodotorula infection in haematological patients. Mycoses 54:318–324. https://doi.org/10.1111/j.1439-0507.2010.01868.x

George IA, Spec A, Powderly WG, Santos CAQ (2018) Comparative epidemiology and outcomes of human immunodeficiency virus (HIV), non-HIV non-transplant, and solid organ transplant associated Cryptococcosis: a population-based study. Clin Infect Dis 66:608–611. https://doi.org/10.1093/cid/cix867

Girmenia C, Pizzarelli G, D'Antonio D et al (2003) In vitro susceptibility testing of Geotrichum capitatum: comparison of the E-test, disk diffusion, and Sensititre colorimetric methods with the NCCLS M27-A2 broth microdilution reference method. Antimicrob Agents Chemother 47:3985–3988

Girmenia C, Pagano L, Martino B et al (2005) Invasive infections caused by Trichosporon species and Geotrichum capitatum in patients with hematological malignancies: a retrospective multicenter study from Italy and review of the literature. J Clin Microbiol 43:1818–1828. https://doi.org/10.1128/JCM.43.4.1818-1828.2005

Gonzalez-Lara MF, Sifuentes-Osornio J, Ostrosky-Zeichner L (2017) Drugs in clinical development for fungal infections. Drugs 77:1505–1518. https://doi.org/10.1007/s40265-017-0805-2

Gueho E, Simmons RB, Pruitt WR et al (1987) Association of Malassezia pachydermatis with systemic infections of humans. J Clin Microbiol 25:1789–1790

Hoenigl M, Strenger V, Buzina W et al (2012) European Organization for the Research and Treatment of Cancer/mycoses study group (EORTC/MSG) host factors and invasive fungal infections in patients with haematological malignancies. J Antimicrob Chemother 67:2029–2033. https://doi.org/10.1093/jac/dks155

de Hoog GS, Smith M (n.d.) Ribosomal gene phylogeny and species delimitation in Geotrichum and its teleomorphs. Stud Mycol:489–515

Hsu LY, Lee DG, Yeh SP et al (2015) Epidemiology of invasive fungal diseases among patients with haematological disorders in the Asia-Pacific: a prospective observational study. Clin Microbiol Infect 21:594.e7–594.11. https://doi.org/10.1016/j.cmi.2015.02.019

Jitmuang A, Panackal AA, Williamson PR et al (2016) Performance of the Cryptococcal antigen lateral flow assay in non-HIV-related Cryptococcosis. J Clin Microbiol 54:460–463. https://doi.org/10.1128/JCM.02223-15

Kang C-I, Rouse MS, Mandrekar JN et al (2009) Anidulafungin treatment of candidal central nervous system infection in a murine model. Antimicrob Agents Chemother 53:3576–3578. https://doi.org/10.1128/AAC.00646-09

Kappe R, Schulze-Berge A (1993) New cause for false-positive results with the Pastorex Aspergillus antigen latex agglutination test. J Clin Microbiol 31:2489–2490

Karageorgopoulos DE, Vouloumanou EK, Ntziora F et al (2011) β-D-glucan assay for the diagnosis of invasive fungal infections: a meta-analysis. Clin Infect Dis 52:750–770. https://doi.org/10.1093/cid/ciq206

Khalid A, Clough LA, Symons RCA et al (2014) Incidence and clinical predictors of ocular candidiasis in patients with Candida fungemia. Interdisciplinary perspectives on infectious diseases. 2014:650235. https://doi.org/10.1155/2014/650235

Kiehn TE, Gorey E, Brown AE et al (1992) Sepsis due to Rhodotorula related to use of indwelling central venous catheters. Clin Infect Dis 14:841–846

Kolecka A, Khayhan K, Groenewald M et al (2013) Identification of medically relevant species of arthroconidial yeasts by use of matrix-assisted laser desorption ionization-time of flight mass spectrometry. J Clin Microbiol 51:2491–2500. https://doi.org/10.1128/JCM.00470-13

Kolecka A, Khayhan K, Arabatzis M et al (2014) Efficient identification of Malassezia yeasts by matrix-assisted laser desorption ionization-time of flight mass spectrometry (MALDI-TOF MS). Br J Dermatol 170:332–341. https://doi.org/10.1111/bjd.12680

Kontoyiannis DP, Torres HA, Chagua M et al (2004) Trichosporonosis in a tertiary care cancer center: risk factors, changing spectrum and determinants of outcome. Scand J Infect Dis 36:564–569. https://doi.org/10.1080/00365540410017563

Kontoyiannis DP, Marr KA, Park BJ et al (2010) Prospective surveillance for invasive fungal infections in hematopoietic stem cell transplant recipients, 2001-2006: overview of the transplant-associated infection surveillance network (TRANSNET) database. Clin Infect Dis 50:1091–1100. https://doi.org/10.1086/651263

Kwon-Chung KJ, Polacheck I, Bennett JE (1982) Improved diagnostic medium for separation of Cryptococcus neoformans var. neoformans (serotypes a and D) and Cryptococcus neoformans var. gattii (serotypes B and C). J Clin Microbiol 15:535–537

Larkin E, Hager C, Chandra J et al (2017) The emerging pathogen Candida auris: growth phenotype, virulence factors, activity of antifungals, and effect of SCY-078, a novel Glucan synthesis inhibitor, on growth morphology and biofilm formation. Antimicrob Agents Chemother 61:e02396–e02316. https://doi.org/10.1128/AAC.02396-16

Lefort A, Chartier L, Sendid B et al (2012) Diagnosis, management and outcome of Candida endocarditis. Clin Microbiol Infect 18:E99–E109. https://doi.org/10.1111/j.1469-0691.2012.03764.x

Liao Y, Hartmann T, Ao J-H, Yang R-Y (2012) Serum glucuronoxylomannan may be more appropriate for the diagnosis and therapeutic monitoring of Trichosporon fungemia than serum β-D-glucan. Int J Infect Dis 16:e638. https://doi.org/10.1016/j.ijid.2012.03.009

Liao Y, Lu X, Yang S et al (2015) Epidemiology and outcome of Trichosporon Fungemia: a review of 185 reported cases from 1975 to 2014. Open Forum Infect Dis 2:ofv141. https://doi.org/10.1093/ofid/ofv141

Lin S-Y, Lu P-L, Tan BH et al (2018) The epidemiology of non-Candida yeast isolated from blood: the Asia surveillance study. Mycoses. https://doi.org/10.1111/myc.12852

Lockhart SR, Wagner D, Iqbal N et al (2011) Comparison of in vitro susceptibility characteristics of Candida species from cases of invasive candidiasis in solid organ and stem cell transplant recipients: transplant-associated infections surveillance network (TRANSNET), 2001 to 2006. J Clin Microbiol 49:2404–2410. https://doi.org/10.1128/JCM.02474-10

Lockhart SR, Etienne KA, Vallabhaneni S et al (2017) Simultaneous emergence of multidrug-resistant Candida auris on 3 continents confirmed by whole-genome sequencing and epidemiological analyses. Clin Infect Dis 64:134–140. https://doi.org/10.1093/cid/ciw691

Lutsar I, Roffey S, Troke P (2003) Voriconazole concentrations in the cerebrospinal fluid and brain tissue of Guinea pigs and immunocompromised patients. Clin Infect Dis 37:728–732. https://doi.org/10.1086/377131

Lyman CA, Devi SJ, Nathanson J et al (1995) Detection and quantitation of the glucuronoxylomannan-like polysaccharide antigen from clinical and nonclinical isolates of Trichosporon beigelii and implications for pathogenicity. J Clin Microbiol 33:126–130

Martino R, Salavert M, Parody R et al (2004) Blastoschizomyces capitatus infection in patients with leukemia: report of 26 cases. Clin Infect Dis 38:335–341. https://doi.org/10.1086/380643

McCarty TP, Lockhart SR, Moser SA et al (2018) Echinocandin resistance among Candida isolates at an academic medical Centre 2005-15: analysis of trends and outcomes. J Antimicrob Chemother 73:1677–1680. https://doi.org/10.1093/jac/dky059

McTaggart LR, Lei E, Richardson SE et al (2011) Rapid identification of Cryptococcus neoformans and Cryptococcus gattii by matrix-assisted laser desorption ionization-time of flight mass spectrometry. J Clin Microbiol 49:3050–3053. https://doi.org/10.1128/JCM.00651-11

Morrison VA, Weisdorf DJ (2000) The spectrum of Malassezia infections in the bone marrow transplant population. Bone Marrow Transplant 26:645–648. https://doi.org/10.1038/sj.bmt.1702566

Muñoz P, Vena A, Machado M et al (2018) T2Candida MR as a predictor of outcome in patients with suspected invasive candidiasis starting empirical antifungal treatment: a prospective pilot study. J Antimicrob Chemother 73:iv6–iv12. https://doi.org/10.1093/jac/dky047

Mylonakis E, Clancy CJ, Ostrosky-Zeichner L et al (2015) T2 magnetic resonance assay for the rapid diagnosis of candidemia in whole blood: a clinical trial. Clin Infect Dis 60:892–899. https://doi.org/10.1093/cid/ciu959

Nakase K, Suzuki K, Kyo T et al (2012) Is elevation of the serum β-d-glucan level a paradoxical sign for trichosporon fungemia in patients with hematologic disorders? Int J Infect Dis 16:e2–e4. https://doi.org/10.1016/j.ijid.2011.09.017

Nguyen MH, Wissel MC, Shields RK et al (2012) Performance of Candida real-time polymerase chain reaction, β-D-Glucan assay, and blood cultures in the diagnosis of invasive candidiasis. Clin Infect Dis 54:1240–1248. https://doi.org/10.1093/cid/cis200

O'Halloran JA, Powderly WG, Spec A (2017) Cryptococcosis today: it is not all about HIV infection. Curr Clin Microbiol Rep 4:88–95. https://doi.org/10.1007/s40588-017-0064-8

Oya S, Muta T (2018) Breakthrough infection of Geotrichum capitatum during empirical caspofungin therapy after umbilical cord blood transplantation. Int J Hematol 108:558–563. https://doi.org/10.1007/s12185-018-2481-8

Pagano L, Fianchi L, Caramatti C et al (2004) Cryptococcosis in patients with hematologic malignancies. A report from GIMEMA-infection. J Antimicrob Chemother 89:852–856

Pappas PG, Kauffman CA, Andes DR et al (2016) Clinical practice guideline for the Management of Candidiasis: 2016 update by the Infectious Diseases Society of America. Clin Infect Dis 62:e1–e50

Perfect JR, Dismukes WE, Dromer F et al (2010) Clinical practice guidelines for the management of cryptococcal disease: 2010 update by the infectious diseases society of america. Clin Infect Dis 50:291–322

Potenza L, Chitasombat MN, Klimko N et al (2018) Rhodotorula infection in haematological patient: risk factors and outcome. Mycoses. https://doi.org/10.1111/myc.12875

Rammaert B, Desjardins A, Lortholary O (2012) New insights into hepatosplenic candidosis, a manifestation of chronic disseminated candidosis. Mycoses 55:e74–e84. https://doi.org/10.1111/j.1439-0507.2012.02182.x

Rodriguez-Tudela JL, Diaz-Guerra TM, Mellado E et al (2005) Susceptibility patterns and molecular identification of Trichosporon species. Antimicrob Agents Chemother 49:4026–4034. https://doi.org/10.1128/AAC.49.10.4026-4034.2005

Safdar A, Hanna HA, Boktour M et al (2004) Impact of high-dose granulocyte transfusions in patients with cancer with candidemia: retrospective case-control analysis of 491 episodes of Candida species bloodstream infections. Cancer 101:2859–2865. https://doi.org/10.1002/cncr.20710

Schell WA, Jones AM, Borroto-Esoda K, Alexander BD (2017) Antifungal activity of SCY-078 and standard antifungal agents against 178 clinical isolates of resistant and susceptible Candida species. Antimicrob Agents Chemother 61:e01102–e01117. https://doi.org/10.1128/AAC.01102-17

Slavin MA, Osborne B, Adams R et al (1995) Efficacy and safety of fluconazole prophylaxis for fungal infections after marrow transplantation--a prospective, randomized, double-blind study. J Infect Dis 171:1545–1552

Slavin MA, Sorrell TC, Marriott D et al (2010) Candidaemia in adult cancer patients: risks for fluconazole-resistant isolates and death. J Antimicrob Chemother 65:1042–1051. https://doi.org/10.1093/jac/dkq053

Sugita T, Nakajima M, Ikeda R et al (2002) Sequence analysis of the ribosomal DNA intergenic spacer 1 regions of Trichosporon species. J Clin Microbiol 40:1826–1830

Suzuki K, Nakase K, Kyo T et al (2010) Fatal Trichosporon fungemia in patients with hematologic malignancies. Eur J Haematol 84:441–447. https://doi.org/10.1111/j.1600-0609.2010.01410.x

Taur Y, Cohen N, Dubnow S et al (2010) Effect of antifungal therapy timing on mortality in cancer patients with candidemia. Antimicrob Agents Chemother 54:184–190. https://doi.org/10.1128/AAC.00945-09

Temstet A, Roux P, Poirot JL et al (1992) Evaluation of a monoclonal antibody-based latex agglutination test for diagnosis of cryptococcosis: comparison with two tests using polyclonal antibodies. J Clin Microbiol 30:2544–2550

Tragiannidis A, Bisping G, Koehler G, Groll AH (2010) Minireview: Malassezia infections in immunocompromised patients. Mycoses 53:187–195. https://doi.org/10.1111/j.1439-0507.2009.01814.x

Trubiano JA, Leung VKY, Worth LJ et al (2015) Candida glabrata fungaemia at an Australian cancer Centre: epidemiology, risk factors and therapy. Leuk Lymphoma 56:3442–3444. https://doi.org/10.3109/10428194.2015.1023724

Tuon FF, Costa SF (2008) Rhodotorula infection. A systematic review of 128 cases from literature. Rev Iberoam Micol 25:135–140

Tuon FF, De Almeida GMD, Costa SF (2007) Central venous catheter-associated fungemia due to Rhodotorula spp. a systematic review. Med Mycol 45:441–447. https://doi.org/10.1080/13693780701381289

Vallabhaneni S, Cleveland AA, Farley MM et al (2015) Epidemiology and risk factors for Echinocandin nonsusceptible Candida glabrata bloodstream infections: data from a large multisite population-based Candidemia surveillance program, 2008–2014. Open Forum Infect Dis 2:ofv163. https://doi.org/10.1093/ofid/ofv163

Vaux S, Criscuolo A, Desnos-Ollivier M et al (2014) Multicenter outbreak of infections by *Saprochaete clavata*, an unrecognized opportunistic fungal pathogen. MBio 5:e02309–e02314. https://doi.org/10.1128/mBio.02309-14

Velegraki A, Cafarchia C, Gaitanis G et al (2015) *Malassezia* infections in humans and animals: pathophysiology, detection, and treatment. PLoS Pathog 11:e1004523. https://doi.org/10.1371/journal.ppat.1004523

Vena A, Muñoz P, Guinea J et al (2018) Fluconazole resistance is not a predictor of poor outcome in patients with cryptococcosis. Mycoses. https://doi.org/10.1111/myc.12847

Wang E, Farmakiotis D, Yang D et al (2015) The ever-evolving landscape of candidaemia in patients with acute leukaemia: non-susceptibility to caspofungin and multidrug resistance are associated with increased mortality. J Antimicrob Chemother 70:2362–2368. https://doi.org/10.1093/jac/dkv087

White PL, Barnes RA, Gorton R et al (2018) Comment on: T2Candida MR as a predictor of outcome in patients with suspected invasive candidiasis starting empirical antifungal treatment: a prospective pilot study. J Antimicrob Chemother:iv6–iv73. https://doi.org/10.1093/jac/dky325

Wiederhold NP (2017) Antifungal resistance: current trends and future strategies to combat. Infect Drug Resist 10:249–259. https://doi.org/10.2147/IDR.S124918

Wilson DT, Dimondi VP, Johnson SW et al (2016) Role of isavuconazole in the treatment of invasive fungal infections. Ther Clin Risk Manag 12:1197–1206. https://doi.org/10.2147/TCRM.S90335

Yoshida M, Obayashi T, Iwama A et al (1997) Detection of plasma (1 --> 3)-beta-D-glucan in patients with Fusarium, Trichosporon, Saccharomyces and Acremonium fungaemias. J Med Vet Mycol 35:371–374

Zaas AK, Boyce M, Schell W et al (2003) Risk of fungemia due to Rhodotorula and antifungal susceptibility testing of Rhodotorula isolates. J Clin Microbiol 41:5233–5235. https://doi.org/10.1128/JCM.41.11.5233-5235.2003

Mould Infections

E. A. de Kort, N. M. A. Blijlevens, and K. Lagrou

16.1 Epidemiology and Background

16.1.1 Moulds in the Environment

Most human infections are caused by fungi that grow as saprophytes in the environment, meaning that they acquire nutrients from the environment and decaying organic matter. Moulds grow optimally in moist conditions and require zinc, calcium, and iron for their growth. They can be found in soil, ground, and water. Moulds are a subset of fungi, unlike yeasts they are multicellular and grow by forming filaments. They have a worldwide distribution with some moulds, mainly the dimorphic fungi, being endemic in certain geographical regions. These moulds can cause infection in immunocompetent hosts while most moulds only cause disease in the immunocompromised host.

The genus *Aspergillus* contains about 250 species divided into eight subgenera (*Aspergillus, Fumigati, Circumdati, Candidi, Terrei, Nidulantes, Warcupi,* and *Ornati*). Most invasive infections are caused by members of the *A. fumigatus* species complex, followed by *A. flavus, A. terreus,* and *A. niger* species complexes. Variations in the environmental distribution of the different species can lead to local increased occurrence of *A. flavus* and *A. terreus. Aspergillus* species are the most common cause of invasive mould disease in the hematological setting, followed by the species of Mucorales and *Fusarium* spp. *Fusarium* spp. are commonly encountered in certain geographical areas, in Brazil, they account for most of the invasive mould infections while in Europe they mainly cause disease in the Mediterranean countries.

In this chapter, we focus on disease caused by moulds, the term fungal disease will replace mould disease where appropriate for classification or literature reporting purposes. Frequent and infrequent fungi encountered in human disease are mentioned in Fig. 16.1.

E. A. de Kort (✉) · N. M. A. Blijlevens (✉)
Department of Hematology, Radboud University Medical Center, Nijmegen, The Netherlands
e-mail: Elizabeth.Dekort@Radboudumc.nl;
Nicole.Blijlevens@radboudumc.nl

K. Lagrou (✉)
Department of Microbiology and Immunology, KU Leuven, Leuven, Belgium

Clinical Department of Laboratory Medicine and National Reference Center for Mycosis, University Hospitals Leuven, Leuven, Belgium
e-mail: katrien.lagrou@uzleuven.be

16.1.2 Incidence of Invasive Mould Disease

Nearly half of all worldwide cases of invasive mould disease (IMD) occur in the hematological population with acute leukemia or recipients of

© Springer Nature Switzerland AG 2021
O. A. Cornely, M. Hoenigl (eds.), *Infection Management in Hematology*, Hematologic Malignancies, https://doi.org/10.1007/978-3-030-57317-1_16

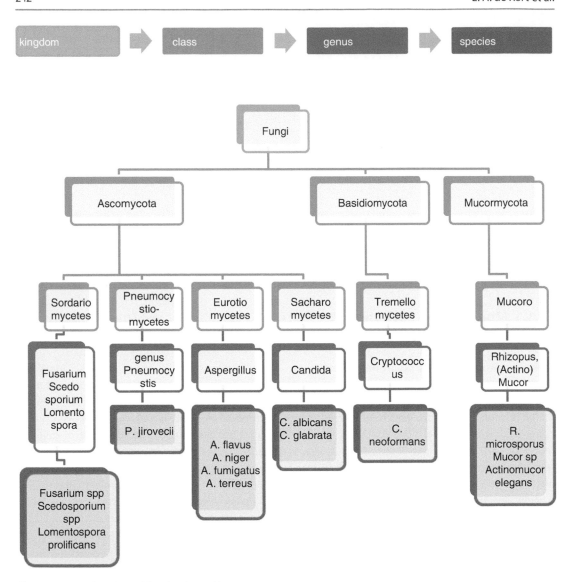

Fig. 16.1 Classification of fungi and moulds

allogeneic stem cell transplantation (HSCT). A large German multicenter prospective study in 3067 patients receiving intensive chemotherapeutic treatment for acute leukemia, reported an incidence of invasive aspergillosis of 6%, this is in line with the previous reports in Europe and USA. More than half of the patients were receiving antifungal prophylaxis at diagnosis. In the allogeneic transplantation setting, the incidence goes up to 10% in the first year following HSCT.

Recently, there have been several observations of increased incidence of invasive mould disease in hematology patients receiving immune or targeted therapy. The higher incidence of invasive aspergillosis in chronic lymphocytic leukemia (CLL) patients receiving ibrutinib has been published by independent groups, a clarifying mechanism for this association has not yet been identified.

Mortality of hematological patients with IMD is high, with 12-week mortality rates of 18% for probable/proven aspergillosis and 1-year overall survival rates limited to 20–30%. The outcome of mucormycosis infections is even more dire. A recent report from the European Confederation of Medical Mycology working group showed the mortality for 230 consecutive patients across Europe with a probable or proven mucormycosis infection. There was an overall mortality of 47%, with the lowest mortality of 6% reported in the immunocompetent patient group. In the hematological patients, mortality ranged from 52% to76%, the latter being the transplant recipients. This rate is certainly higher than one might expect following transplantation, and reflects the poor outcome associated with mucormycosis infections. The incidence of IMD differs between institutions, this is due to variable regional environmental occurrence, differences between prophylactic and treatment strategies between institutions and local implementation of early detection testing.

16.1.3 IMD in the Hematological Population

16.1.3.1 Immune Defense in the Host

Moulds are widely present in soil and organic material and they are distributed throughout the environment. On starvation, these fungi release spores (conidia) which are commonly inhaled and typically remain in a dormant state in the airways of healthy individuals. The innate immune system is a key player in controlling germination of these asexual conidia and invasion of tissues. At the sites of mould interaction with mucosal surfaces, the host immune system, via pattern recognition receptors (PRRs), can recognize molecular patterns released upon germination of conidia. Polymorphonuclear cells and macrophages respond by activating the adaptive immune system, but also by directly inhibiting the growth of hyphae by respiratory burst and ROS-independent killing mechanisms. Dendritic cells activate Th17 and CD4+ -Th1 and Th2 cells. Th1 cells produce cytokines (interferon-γ and TNF-α) and stimulate further phagocytosis at the sites of infection. The adaptive immune system, including other T-cells and NK-cells, is able to produce specific antifungal effector mechanisms. Inadequate or absent immune responses may lead to persistence of

fungi and failure of antifungal therapy. On the other hand, overzealous immune responses can lead to hyperinflammatory reactions.

16.1.3.2 Risk for IMD in the Hematological Patient

The highly immunocompromised patient receiving intensive antileukemic treatment or the recipient of allogeneic HSCT is most prone to develop IMD. In this population, and in the appropriate setting, conidia can germinate into hyphae until there is invasion of underlying structures. In the lungs, invasion of small and medium-sized pulmonary vessels causes thrombosis and subsequent ischemic necrosis of the lung parenchyma. In the sinuses, there is invasion of vessels as well as bony structures. Direct infiltration in the skin has also been described with certain moulds.

The intensity and duration of granulocytopenia are important determinants for acquiring IMD, with a duration of >7 days associated with invasive mould disease. The use of T-cell immunosuppressants during transplantation further contributes to failure of an adequate immune response to moulds. Other important risk factors for developing IMD include previous and current environmental exposure, iron overload, and prior fungal infections. A lack of effector mechanisms and mucosal damage lead to both stimulation of fungal invasion and evasion of immune response.

Some of these risk factors have been adopted as host factors in the new EORTC/MSG consensus guidelines for defining invasive fungal disease (Table 16.1). A single center retrospective case-control study (Hoenigl et al) in hematological patients with invasive fungal disease (IFD) noted a significant contribution to the risk for IFD with the following host factors: prolonged neutropenia of >10 days (OR 4.57), use of corticosteroids for more than 14 days (OR 5.35) and when more than three host factors are present (OR 3.28).

Probable IFD requires the presence of a host factor, a clinical criterion and a mycological criterion.

Possible IFD is established when cases meet the criteria for a host factor and a clinical criterion, but NOT mycological criteria.

Table 16.1 EORTC Criteria Table

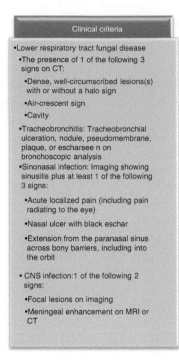

Host factors

- Recent history of neutropenia (<0.5 x 10e9 neutrophils/L [<500 neutrophils/mm3] for >10 days) temporally related to the onset of fungal disease

- Receipt of an allogeneic stem cell transplant

- Prolonged use of corticosteroids (excluding among patients with allergic bronchopulmonary aspergillosis) at a mean minimum dose of 0.3 mg/kg/day of prednisone equivalent for >3 weeks

- Treatment with other recognized T cell immunosuppressants, such as cyclosporine, TNFblockers, specific monoclonal antibodies (such as alemtuzumab), or nucleoside analogues during the past 90 days

- Inherited severe immunodeficiency (such as chronic granulomatous disease or severe combined immunodeficiency)

Clinical criteria

- Lower respiratory tract fungal disease
  - The presence of 1 of the following 3 signs on CT:
    - Dense, well-circumscribed lesions(s) with or without a halo sign
    - Air-crescent sign
    - Cavity
- Tracheobronchitis: Tracheobronchial ulceration, nodule, pseudomembrane, plaque, or escharsee n on bronchoscopic analysis
- Sinonasal infection: Imaging showing sinusitis plus at least 1 of the following 3 signs:
  - Acute localized pain (including pain radiating to the eye)
  - Nasal ulcer with black eschar
  - Extension from the paranasal sinus across bony barriers, including into the orbit
- CNS infection:1 of the following 2 signs:
  - Focal lesions on imaging
  - Meningeal enhancement on MRI or CT

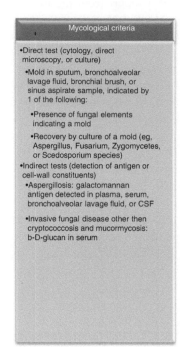

Mycological criteria

- Direct test (cytology, direct microscopy, or culture)
  - Mold in sputum, bronchoalveolar lavage fluid, bronchial brush, or sinus aspirate sample, indicated by 1 of the following:
    - Presence of fungal elements indicating a mold
    - Recovery by culture of a mold (eg, Aspergillus, Fusarium, Zygomycetes, or Scedosporium species)
- Indirect tests (detection of antigen or cell-wall constituents)
  - Aspergillosis: galactomannan antigen detected in plasma, serum, bronchoalveolar lavage fluid, or CSF
  - Invasive fungal disease other then cryptococcosis and mucormycosis: b-D-glucan in serum

Patients with intermediate or high-risk myelodysplastic syndrome, acute myeloid leukemia (especially in the refractory relapsed setting), aplastic anemia and recipients of allogeneic HSCT following a myeloablative or reduced intensity conditioning regimen, usually have a combination of these various risk factors.

The recipient of an allogeneic transplantation has a prolonged phase of vulnerability and experiences three periods of susceptibility for invasive mould disease. In the pre-engraftment phase, the risk is due to granulocytopenia, where depth and duration of granulocytopenia correspond to the risk for IMD. The second period is the early post-engraftment phase when there is depletion of T cells or blunting of T-cell response by immunosuppression. The third and possibly longest period is the late post-engraftment phase with cytomegalovirus (CMV) reactivation as a determinant of risk as well as chronic graft versus host disease, the former has adverse effects on host immunity and the latter re-introduces the need for immunosuppression. The degree of immunosuppression corresponds to the risk of invasive mould disease.

16.2 Clinical Manifestations of Disease

The first febrile episode during the neutropenic phase of intensive remission induction or conditioning regimen is almost always caused by bacterial pathogens. Defervescance usually occurs after a median 4–5 days of adequate antibiotic treatment. Clinical deterioration, persistent fever >4–5 days or new episodes of unexplained fever during granulocytopenia should prompt investigation for another source of infection such as invasive mould disease. However, mucosal barrier injury is an alternative cause of persistent fever that should be kept in mind.

The clinical pictures of aspergillosis or mucormycosis are not fundamentally different from each other. The organs that are primarily affected are the lungs (i.e., invasive pulmonary aspergillosis) and/or sinuses. Fever is commonly the only presenting symptom. As the disease progresses, other symptoms include those of sinusitis (i.e., sinus pain, epistaxis, and nasal eschars) or pneumonia including cough, sputum, hemoptysis, dyspnea, pleuritic pain, rales, and pleural friction rub. If left

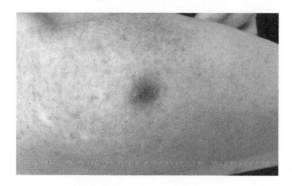

Fig 16.2 Maculo-papular skin lesions in a patient with prolonged severe neutropenia: Biopsy revealed Fusarium spp

untreated, pulmonary aspergillosis will disseminate hematogenously to all organs including skin, heart, kidneys, liver, and brain. A paranasal infection with any mould will continue to grow locally through bone and extend into cerebral tissue (rhinocerebral infection). *Fusarium* dissemination can lead to severe myalgias and skin manifestations, including multiple maculopapular lesions or ecthyma gangrenosum-like lesions (Fig. 16.2).

Thus, clinical suspicion is essential for preventing delay in diagnosis and treatment. Any delay will contribute to treatment failure and mortality. Additionally, ongoing clinical deterioration may preclude diagnostic tissue sampling and antineoplastic treatment.

16.3 Diagnostic Tools

Historically, there has always been a difference in reporting cases of IMD between clinicians and researchers. Whereas for research purposes, the certainty of the diagnosis is of utmost importance, in daily practice, missing a diagnosis can be fatal for the patient, and often a diagnosis of IMD is reported based on different criteria and devoid of histological proof. In 2002, the European Organization for Research and Treatment of Cancer (EORTC) and the Mycosis Study Group (MSG) developed the original criteria for defining opportunistic invasive fungal infections in order to standardize definitions, classify, and homogenize populations for clinical research. In summary, the diagnosis of invasive fungal disease could be made with three levels of certainty: possible, probable,

and proven IFD, with the purpose of achieving as much certainty as clinically feasible. These criteria were revised in 2008 to allow additional populations at risk to be included, redefine the category of possible IFD, and harbor the growing body of evidence for different diagnostic tests. It is important to note that not one single test reaches 100% negative- or positive predictive value; therefore, in the absence of proven IFD by histopathology, a combination of criteria is needed to establish a diagnosis with any level of certainty. The 2008 EORTC/MSG revised criteria for the diagnosis of IFD are universally applied in fungal research and they are increasingly also being used in routine clinical practice. Possible IFD is determined by a host factor (patient population at risk) and a clinical factor. Probable IFD requires the presence of a host factor, a clinical criterion (i.e., imaging) and a mycological criterion. Proven IFD requires histopathological evidence of hyphal growth in normally sterile tissues which is determined by microscopic investigation. Hyphal growth patterns are used to distinguish *Aspergillus* spp. or other invasive moulds from mucormycetes. Culture of the specific species is used for definitive diagnosis. In routine practice, the task of trying to establish proven IMD in the hematological patient may present significant difficulties to the clinician. Cytopenias and mucositis often make diagnostic sampling of deeper tissues less attractive if not impossible. Sputum cultures are neither specific nor sensitive and are therefore not discriminatory. Inconclusive results because of erroneous tissue sampling or previous antifungal treatment are also frequently encountered. Still, sufficient effort should be put into excluding other possible causes of infections in the hematological population and objectifying possible or even probable IMD. A microbiological diagnosis in the era of antifungal resistance is critical in guiding therapy.

The first step in the diagnostic workup of IMD is acquiring a CT scan of the chest or sinuses to identify lesions specific for IMD. These lesions can later on be targeted for diagnostic sampling. If available, routine blood testing for galactomannan, a polysaccharide released from hyphae during their growth phase, should be carried out to detect circulating or disseminated aspergillus. β-D-glucan is another cell wall component, present in many pathogenic yeasts and filamentous fungi. Its detection in serum can indicate fungal invasion, but it is not specific for one certain mould or yeast. It does not detect the Mucorales spp., *Cryptococcus* or *Trichosporon*. PCR assays for *Aspergillus* species have been developed, but are mostly used in combination with other diagnostic tests. These tests will be discussed in detail in the next paragraphs.

16.3.1 Imaging

High resolution CT scanning of the chest has proven to be of great importance in the early detection of IMD in the lungs, indeed, some lesions are clinical criteria in the EORTC/MSG definitions of IMD. The first detectable sign of invasive mould disease is the halo sign and its detection is an indicator of early stage invasive pulmonary aspergillosis (IPA) in the neutropenic host. The halo sign is a macronodule>1 cm in diameter with a solid nodular core surrounded (3/4) by ground-glass opacity through which lung parenchyma is still visible. Its histopathological counterpart is a nodule of angioinvasive aspergillosis with infarction and coagulative necrosis of lung parenchyma, surrounded by alveolar hemorrhage (halo of ground glass). In the severely neutropenic patient, it is highly suggestive for invasive aspergillosis as aspergillosis is more common than mucormycosis. Nevertheless, the incidence of halo sign in both groups of moulds is the same, around 21–25%. Thus, the sensitivity is low and is at least partly due to its transient properties. Most halo signs disappear within days of first clinical suspicion.

A macronodule is an ovoid soft-tissue opacity of >1 cm that fully conceals the background of underlying bronchovasculature. Most patients with IMD present with at least >1 macronodule on a chest CT (Fig. 16.3). In mucormycosis, lesions are commonly more abundant (>10) unifocal and restricted to the upper lobes.

The reverse halo sign is associated with pulmonary mucormycosis (PM). It is a focal rounded area of ground-glass opacity surrounded by a crescent or complete ring of consolidation. It represents infarcted lung tissue with more hemorrhage and inflammation at the periphery of the lesion instead of centrally. It develops early in the clinical course of the disease. Its subsequent evolution is

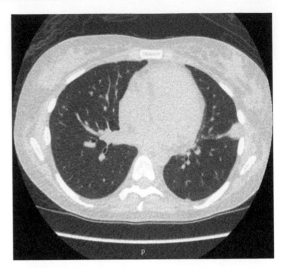

Fig 16.3 CT image of a macronodule in a patient with persistent fever during neutropenic phase of treatment

Table 16.2 Clinical implications of radiological findings of IMD

Radiological sign	Implications for clinical management
Halo sign	Early indicator of IPA: Start anti-mould treatment
Reverse halo sign	Early indicator of PM: Consider starting anti-mucor treatment
Macronodules	Not specific but can indicate IMD: Consider bronchoscopic alveolar lavage (BAL) and starting anti-mould treatment
Air-crescent sign	Late sign of IPA or other IMD. No change in treatment.

unknown and its presence has been described in other infections such as paracoccidioidomycosis.

Moulds can also cause airway disease (aside from angioinvasion) with a CT scan revealing tree-in bud, centrilobular micronodules, and bronchiolar wall destruction. Both forms can be simultaneously present in the same patient.

The air-crescent sign is a crescentic pocket of gas occupying a separation interface between a lung sequestrum attributable to necrosis and a rim of viable lung. It is a late marker of Invasive pulmonary aspergillosis and develops 1–2 weeks after the onset of clinical suspicion, as the granulocytes recover. It therefore has little impact on the treatment of the patient.

Chest CT can also be used to guide diagnostic tissue sampling toward a more suitable area

(Table 16.2). A follow-up CT scan is recommended 2 weeks after the initiation of anti-mould treatment to assess response. The size of lesions usually increases during the first week of treatment, and lesions in close proximity to pulmonary vessels may need earlier follow-up. Ideally, the CT scan should be a thin-section CT, and contrast is not routinely used.

Recently, a group from the university hospital of Bologna has published a detailed report on the use of CT-pulmonary angiogram (CTPA) in detecting early invasive pulmonary aspergillosis. CTPA was able to detect vaso-occlusion or the hypodense sign and differentiate between angioinvasive mould disease and other pulmonary consolidations on the first day of fever during the neutropenic phase of intensive chemotherapy. The sensitivity of CTPA to detect invasive pulmonary aspergillosis almost reached 100%, without sacrificing renal function. The results of this study are promising and the impact for the future of imaging is surely to be significant. However, the results still need to be validated before it makes its way into clinical practice.

Sinus disease may also be diagnosed with CT sinus or MRI to detect sinusitis and bony lesions. Sinus lesions are often unilateral and although specific for IMD, bone destruction is a relatively late occurrence. Other signs visible on CT scan are retro-antral fat pad thickening, orbital involvement and facial cellulitis. Recent retrospective studies have focused on extrasinus tissue invasion as an earlier marker and contrast enhanced MRI of the sinus may show areas of low contrast enhancement. CNS aspergillosis presents with either solitary abscess in frontal or temporal lobe by local extension or multiple abscesses at the gray-white junction resulting from hematogenous spread.

16.3.2 Tissue and Fluid Sampling

16.3.2.1   Bronchoscopy and Lavage

Flexible bronchoscopy with bronchoalveolar lavage is crucial for acquiring mycological evidence of IMD and can be useful for visualizing other signs of IMD such as tracheobronchial ulceration, pseudomembranes, or eschars in the bronchial tree. Lavage is an invasive procedure in which fluid (Normal Saline: NaCl 0.9%) is instilled in the lungs with a bronchoscope and

then re-collected for examination. In the hematological population experiencing mucositis and low platelet counts due to intensive antileukemic treatment or a conditioning regimen for transplantation, concerns about bleeding and the need for mechanical ventilation are on point. Nonetheless, even in this select population, bronchoscopy can be performed safely when appropriate precautions are taken such as platelet transfusion, ICU monitoring and noninvasive ventilation. Recent studies have not found an increased need for mechanical ventilation or increased mortality related to diagnostic bronchoscopy.

BAL fluid examination includes gross observation, cell count and microbiological culture and testing. Mycological analysis of BAL fluid includes microscopy using optical brighteners to detect branching hyphae and culture, detection of fungal antigens, that is, galactomannan, and detection of fungal DNA through polymerase chain reaction.

16.3.2.2   Lung Biopsies

Lung biopsy for the histological establishment of proven IMD is often not possible in the transplantation setting or in patients receiving intensive anti-leukemic treatment. Concomitant thrombocytopenia, mucositis, and coagulation abnormalities are often reasons to forego biopsies altogether. CT-guided lung biopsy can on the other hand be a method for increasing diagnostic yield in this population and measures to improve coagulation abnormalities and thrombocytopenia may improve the overall safety of this intervention. A retrospective study by Lass-Floerl of 168 lung biopsies in immunocompromised patients with possible IMD according to EORTC criteria, reported a diagnostic yield of 80% with a negative predictive value of 100%. This procedure was particularly useful in detecting infections with non-*Aspergillus* moulds and exclude other (also noninfectious) reasons for CT-abnormalities. CT-guided biopsy may be preferred over BAL in the setting of peripheral lesions, where performance of bronchoalveolar lavage is known to be low. Potential complications of lung biopsies are air embolism, pulmonary hemorrhage, hemoptysis, and pneumothorax. In the above series, one fatality due to air embolism was reported and two patients had major bleeding due to pulmonary hemorrhage. Overall, CT-guided lung biopsy was deemed a safe approach.

16.3.3 Laboratory Testing

Sputum cultures are neither sensitive nor specific. Negative sputum cultures are common in patients with proven invasive pulmonary aspergillosis. On the other hand, positive cultures do not necessarily imply pathogenicity, as cultures can be positive due to colonization of the respiratory tract. Cultures of bronchoalveolar lavage fluid also lack sensitivity but should always be performed when a BAL is performed.

16.3.3.1 Galactomannan

Various serological assays have been developed to overcome this diagnostic conundrum. The galactomannan (GM) assay has long made its way into clinical practice. Galactomannan is a polysaccharide present in the cell wall of *Aspergillus* spp. It is released during hyphal growth, and can be detected in patient's serum, it correlates with the growth phase of *Aspergillus*. The Platelia sandwich ELISA is the assay that has been used more extensively. Positivity is measured using the optical density index of each sample. The optimal cutoff for positivity has been set at OD of ≥ 0.5. Serial GM monitoring to detect aspergillosis has been studied in different patient groups and a meta-analysis from 27 studies showed a sensitivity of 70–82% and a specificity of 86–93% in the hematological population. The sensitivity in the non-neutropenic (hematological) patient is less than 20%. The sensitivity in the hematological population can also be significantly reduced following reduction of fungal load, for example, use of antifungal prophylaxis. The role of GM in monitoring of therapy has also been reported by Chai and colleagues, and reduction of >35% in the early phase of treatment is correlated with a positive outcome, while an increase in serum GM by as low as OD of 0.1 during therapy is associated with treatment failure. There are many reports on the correlation of GM with clinical outcome, with better survival in patients who became GM negative by 12 weeks in a prospective trial by Maertens et al. False-positives results have been seen in the past with the use of piperacillin–tazobactam, amoxicillin–clavulanate. Severe mucositis of the gastrointestinal tract can also lead to false-positive results due to translocation associated with mucosal barrier injury. GM is water-soluble and can be detected in other bodily fluids. However, the performance of this test has not been adequately investigated for all fluids.

The sensitivity for galactomannan detection in BAL fluid is 70–92% in several studies. The optimal threshold for GM positivity in the BAL has not yet been determined; most centers use a cut-off OD index of 1.0. A higher threshold for GM positivity leads to higher specificity at the expense of sensitivity. OD > 3.0 is 100% specific for proven/probable invasive aspergillosis in patients at risk for IMD. False-positive results have been reported when plasmalyte fluid is used for lavage or in airway colonization.

16.3.3.2 Beta-D-Glucan

Beta-D-glucan is another cell wall component that can be detected in serum. Contrary to galactomannan which is specific for *Aspergillus*, beta-D-glucan is a cell wall component of many yeasts and fungi including *Pneumocystis jirovecii*, making it nonspecific for moulds. It does not detect the Mucorales. The sensitivity of beta-glucan ranges from 65% to 91% and the specificity from 31% to 79%, the performance of the assay varies in different populations. False-positives are seen with several antibiotics (cephalosporins, carbapenems), contaminated blood tubing and lining, gauze, and chemotherapeutic agents such as PEG-asparginase. The negative predictive value was high in studies with patient categories with low fungal prevalence, but the low sensitivity does not allow its indiscriminate use in the hematological population where the rate of fungal infection is higher. The assay has varied sensitivity across different patient populations and its use in the hematological population remains limited due to its low specificity.

16.3.3.3 Polymerase Chain Reaction

PCR testing is currently being validated as a new method for detecting *Aspergillus* spp. and other moulds. Ribosomal fungal DNA is the most frequently used target. During the last 5–10 years, important steps forward were made regarding the standardization of PCR-based tests. Commercial as well as in-house PCR assays have been developed and are available for the diagnosis of specific fungal infection such as aspergillosis or for the detection of a broad range of fungi. *Aspergillus* PCR has been validated on serum as well as BAL fluid and can detect *Aspergillus* to the species level in different specimens. There is a proposal for it to be included as a fungal criterion in the upcoming revision of the EORTC/MSG criteria. An additional advantage of PCR assays is that some can also detect azole-resistant *Aspergillus* strains. As a screening method, blood samples provide a sensitivity of 84–88% and specificity of 75%. Specificity improves to 95% when two positive samples are required to define PCR positivity. *Aspergillus* PCR has also demonstrated a good diagnostic accuracy in BAL fluid, with sensitivity of 91% and specificity of 92% according to one meta-analysis.

16.3.3.4   Lateral Flow Device Assays

An important downside of the galactomannan ELISA assay is that it is a high-volume assay, and that only centralized centers offer the test. This leads to diagnostic delay. The *Aspergillus*-specific lateral flow device (LFD, OLM diagnostics) consists of a self-contained immuno-chromatographic assay for the detection of an extracellular glycoprotein produced by *Aspergillus* during active growth. Because of its single-test design and the minimal preparation required, this assay has the potential to be used for local or point-of-care testing. Several manuscripts evaluating this assay were published, but this test was recently reformatted and the diagnostic performance of this assay is still being studied. A LFD for the detection of *Aspergillus* Galactomannan LFA (IMMY) was recently commercialized, and studies of this assay in the hematological patient population are currently ongoing.

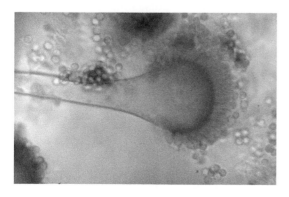

Picture of Aspergillus fumigatus. Courtesy of Marc Lontie

16.3.4   Clinical Impact

None of the above described biomarkers can be used alone to detect or rule out IMD, however, the diagnostic performance of biomarkers can be improved by combining them. Botch et al. recently studied several combinations of markers in blood and BAL samples, integrating them in a diagnostic approach in the immunocompromised population. The diagnostic performance for probable and proven invasive *aspergillosis* in their patient population was acceptable, with sensitivities ranging from 54% to 97% and specificities approaching 100% when using different combinations of diagnostic tests.

16.4   Management

As indicated before, diagnosing invasive mould disease can be a difficult undertaking. In high-risk hematology patients, many clinicians opt for primary mould active antifungal prophylaxis for which we refer the readers to Chap. 4. In centers where no antifungal prophylaxis is given, clinicians often decide to start antifungal treatment if fever persists despite proper antibiotic treatment (empirical approach). Some centers have adopted a preemptive or diagnostic-driven approach and have a strategy set in place for rapid decision-making following results of diagnostic testing for IMD. Preference for either approach depends on the local incidence of mould infections, use of primary anti-mould prophylaxis and the specific capabilities of different institutions to perform serial serological testing, CT scanning, and bronchoalveolar lavage on demand.

16.4.1   Empirical Approach

The basis for empirical treatment was laid in the 1980s, when two pivotal trials demonstrated the effectiveness of (conventional) amphotericin B deoxycholate in reducing mortality in neutropenic patients were already on broad-spectrum antibiotics. In later randomized controlled trials, Walsh and colleagues reported the same effectiveness for liposomal amphotericin B and caspofungin in neutropenic patients and showed noninferiority for voriconazole when compared to L-AmB for empirical treatments in patients at high risk for IFD. Because of the increased resis- tance to voriconazole and its lack of effect on the Mucorales spp., some centers still choose to start with liposomal amphotericin B for pan-mould coverage.

Resolution of fever is the maindriver

	Liposomal Amphotericin B (N=343)		Conventional Amphotericin B (N=344)	
	No of patients	Success rate (95% CI)	No of patients	Success rate (95% CI)
Overall success	172	50.1	170	49.4
Fever resolved during neutropenic period	199	58.0	200	58.1
No breakthrough fungal infection	309	90.1	307	89.2
Baseline fungal infection cured	9	81.8	8	72.7
Survived 7 days after initiation of study drug	318	92.7	308	89.5
Study drug not prematurely discontinued because of toxicity or lack of efficacy	294	85.7	280	81.4

16.4.2 Diagnostic-Driven Approach

As our diagnostic strategies for invasive mould infections evolve, certain centers have moved away from the empirical approach based on neu- tropenic fever and have adopted a diagnostic or goal-driven approach based on the presence of cri- teria suggestive of invasive mould disease. Indeed, Maertens et al. demonstrated the effectiveness and safety of such an approach in their prospective fea- sibility trial of leukemia patients with neutropenic fever. Serum GM and CT scans were used to detect IMD. This strategy reduced the use of antifungal therapy by 78%, but missed one case of zygomy- cosis. Importantly, 10 (7% of total) cases of IA were diagnosed in the absence of fever and would have been missed by the empirical approach to treatment. In a subsequent randomized trial in Australia which included 240 patients with leuke- mia or allogeneic transplantation, survival was similar in the diagnostic-driven versus empirical therapy group. Based on serum GM, PCR screen- ing and high resolution CT (HRCT) scan, 18% of patients received antifungal treatment versus 36% in the empirical therapy group. Half of the cases of probable/prove aspergillosis were established in the absence of fever by the diagnostic-driven approach and thus would have been missed with empiric treatment. Of note, this approach is mostly of value in patients not receiving primary antifun- gal prophylaxis, as antifungal therapy decreases GM sensitivity to values as low as 20%.

One example of a diagnostic-driven treatment algorithm is given below (Fig. 16.4) and is based on serial galactomannan assays in combination with CT scanning. In this approach, no prophy- laxis with anti-mould activity is given.

Treatment is started once the criteria for pos- sible IMD have been established and the first goal is to provide coverage for *Aspergillus*, as it is the most prevalent mould recovered in hematological patients. For a detailed guide on the management, we refer the readers to ESCMID-ECMM-ERS guideline. Voriconazole is the first line fungicide

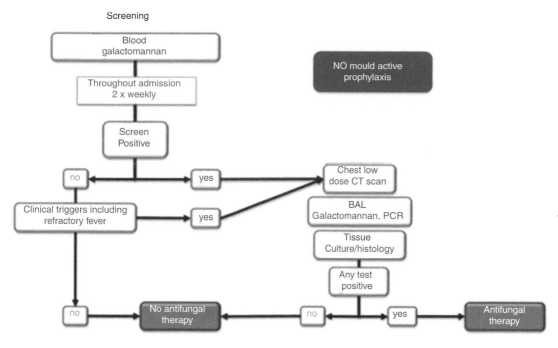

Fig 16.4 Approach to diagnostic driven management of IMD

for possible invasive aspergillosis (IA), isavuconazole is a comparable alternative. Voriconazole is considered to have activity against all common species of *Aspergillus*. It also has activity against some but not all *Scedosporium* species and *Fusarium* species. In 2002, the use of AmB deoxycholate for IA was challenged in a multicenter randomized trial by the EORTC/MSG where voriconazole proved to be superior when compared to conventional amphotericin B for the treatment of IA. Response rates were 52.8% and 31.6% respectively. Survival rate at 12 weeks after starting treatment was 70.8% in the voriconazole group versus 57.9% in the c-AmB group. There have been no trials directly comparing voriconazole to liposomal AmB for the treatment of invasive aspergillosis; however, L-Amb has been shown to be as effective as c-AmB in head-to-head comparison for the treatment of aspergillosis, with less side effects. In patients already experiencing hepatic or renal toxicity, isavuconazole is a good alternative to voriconazole. Isavuconazole was recently compared with voriconazole in a randomized trial of patients with

IMD according to EORTC criteria. The trial showed noninferiority in all cause mortality 20% versus 19%. Isavuconazole-treated patients had less hepatic side effects. More importantly, isavuconazole shows greater affinity for the fungal CYP51 protein, therefore, having activity against some resistant strains of *Aspergillus*. Isavuconazole has been approved by the EMA and the FDA for first-line therapy of invasive aspergillosis. However, its costs limit its widespread use. Although posaconazole has demonstrated its efficacy as primary prophylaxis, a study as primary therapy for invasive aspergillosis is still ongoing. It does however have a role in salvage therapy. Echinocandins act as fungistatic on *Aspergillus* and have been approved for salvage treatment.

When a non-*Aspergillus* mould is suspected or confirmed, treatment should be switched to L-AmB which is the fungicide with more extensive evidence of clinical efficacy (albeit in retrospective trials and in higher dosage) for the treatment of mucormycosis. Response rates are 50–75%. Isavuconazole has been studied for the primary treatment of invasive mucormycosis with reasonable response rates, however, the small number of patients and comparison to a historical cohort limits the level of recommendation by the EMA. It is a good alternative for patients who cannot tolerate L-AmB. Posaconazole has shown some efficacy on mucormycosis as salvage treatment in retrospective cohorts, mostly only partial responses were observed.

There should also be careful consideration given to the immunosuppressive state of the patient and whenever possible, immunosuppression should be tapered or removed. In the case of non-*Aspergillus* infection, surgical debridement should also be considered. Antifungal treatment is continued based on the results of diagnostic tests, including tissue sampling. If no fungal infection can be confirmed, antifungal therapy is stopped. In other cases, treatment should be continued for 6–12 weeks while monitoring for clinical response accompanied by imaging or galactomannan follow-up. Treatment should continue for at least 2 weeks after recovery from neutropenia. The results of antifungal susceptibility testing and therapeutic drug monitoring may redirect the initial treatment choice.

16.4.3 Secondary Prophylaxis

The relapse rate for IMD reaches 30–50%. For patients treated for IMD who remain immunosuppressed or undergo a second period of immunosuppression, maintenance treatment or secondary prophylaxis should be considered. The choice of antifungal is based on known susceptibility patterns. Data from two prospective trials showed a significant decrease in relapse rates (6.7%) in patients with IMD who receive an allogeneic transplantation after primary treatment.

16.5 Antifungal Drugs and Monitoring

Voriconazole, posaconazole and the newest compound isavuconazole are synthetic triazoles with increased anti-mould activity. They inhibit ergos-

terol biosynthesis in fungi cell wall by targeting a fungal CYP450 enzyme and arresting fungal growth. The similarity with human CYP450 is responsible for the hepatic side effects of triazoles and the interactions with other medications.

All azoles inhibit human CYP3A4 leading to significant bidirectional drug–drug interactions, especially in the transplantation setting with cyclosporine and tacrolimus and with the newer drugs, for example, Midostaurin. Significant reduction in the metabolism of these drugs can lead to important side effects. Similarly, CYP3A4 inducers can lead to an increase in the elimination of the triazoles. The extent of the drug interactions depends on whether the drugs act as a substrate and whether they act as inducer or inhibitor. Monitoring drug levels, especially in the transplantation setting can be of utmost importance. Drug monitoring hinges on three different criteria. There must be an accurate assay that will have results within days. The antifungal must have an established therapeutic range and there must be an unpredictable blood drug level. Currently, three triazoles, itraconazole, posaconazole, and voriconazole meet the criteria of drug level monitoring.

Drug monitoring has been most extensively studied in the case of voriconazole. Voriconazole has oral and intravenous formulations. Its intravenous solution contains the nephrotoxic beta-cyclodextrin. It has an oral bioavailability of >90%, but should be taken on an empty stomach. Time to steady state is 1–2 days when given a loading dose, when omitting a loading dose steady state is reached after 5 days. Voriconazole penetrates the cerebrospinal fluid and reaches concentrations of up to 50% of plasma concentrations. Its half-life is approximately 6 h. Adverse effects frequently associated with voriconazole are hepatotoxicity, encephalopathy, visual disturbances and hallucinations, and photosensitivity. The pharmacodynamic relationship, that is, the relationship between drug exposure and outcome has been previously described by Pascual and colleagues. Patients with low serum concentrations (<1 mg/L) appear to have a worse outcome than patients with higher concentrations (>1 mg/L), hepatic and cerebral toxicity appear with serum trough concentrations of >5 mg/L. But, the pharmacokinetic response for voriconazole is unpredictable. Voriconazole is primarily metabolized by CYP2C19 which is known for its extensive gene polymorphism. This can lead to relatively 'poor metabolizers' but also to 'extensive'. The inter-patient variability in response to the same dosing frequency and schedule is therefore high but the response in the same patient can also change over time. Park and colleagues showed in their RCT that voriconazole therapeutic drug monitoring (TDM) resulted in higher response rates to therapy with significantly less adverse events. Results from the Dutch ZonMw clustered randomized trial investigating the role of therapeutic monitoring on treatment outcome and toxicity are currently pending. Pending more results, drug level monitoring should be initiated 2–5 days after first administration and repeated 1–2 times weekly during therapy.

Posaconazole also has oral and iv formulations. Its oral suspension has poor bioavailability and has been almost completely replaced by tablets. Posaconazole has only minor metabolism by cytochrome 450, but is a strong CYP3A4 inhibitor, therefore raising the concentrations of other drugs, for example, calcineurin inhibitors. Hepatotoxicity is an important side effect but is not dose-related, other common side effects include nausea, vomiting, and diarrhea. It can prolong the QT interval, mostly when combined with other QT lengthening substrates. The intravenous solution should ideally be administered over a central venous line. If no central access is available, peripheral infusion should be limited to 30 min to avoid thrombophlebitis and other infusion site reactions.

For oral posaconazole drug, monitoring should be initiated within 7 days after the start of therapy and continued once weekly. A steady-state trough concentration is reached at the end of the first week. Trough levels of >1 mg/L are recommended for the treatment of *Aspergillus fumigatus* based on the prospective data from salvage therapy with posaconazole. Serum samples can be collected earlier than 7 days (before the attainment of steady state), but the use of a lower

therapeutic target of 0.35 mg/L after 48 h of therapy is appropriate (see guidelines BSMM).

Itraconazole has oral and intravenous formulations. The bioavailability for the liquid suspension is higher than that for the tablets. It is highly protein-bound (>99%) and is extensively metabolized by CYP3A4 system. Significant side effects including gastrointestinal, electrolyte disturbances and elevated transaminase levels are observed. Serious interactions with chemotherapeutic drugs, that is, vincristine and QTc-prolonging drugs are also encountered. Significant variation in pharmacokinetic response exists between patients, and therapy should be monitored within 5–7 days after initiating the treatment and trough level of 0.5–1 mg/L is recommended.

The water-soluble prodrug isavuconazonium sulfate was developed specifically to facilitate iv infusion and does not contain cyclodextrin. Isavuconazonium has an oral and an intravenous formulation. The volume of distribution is 450 L and has a half-life of 130 h. It needs a loading dose every 8 h for 2 days, then a continuous dosing schedule of once daily oral or iv solution is given. It has 98% bioavailability, not limited by food intake and has low inter-patient variability. Unlike the other azoles, isavuconazole shortens the QTc interval. Adverse effects are mostly gastrointestinal. Optimal trough levels for isavuconazole have not yet been established, but based on models target trough levels are set at 2–4 mg/L impending more studies.

Amphotericin B comes in different formulations, either conventional amphotericin B deoxycholate or several lipid formulations. There are many routes of administration. AmB induced ion channels in the fungal membrane, but can also extract ergosterol from the lipid bilayer resulting in cell death. AmB is protein-bound and distributes to kidneys and reticuloendothelial system. It has a half-life of 15 days and the elimination route is unclear. There are many known side effects including infusion reactions, phlebitis, nephrotoxicity and azotemia, and moderate-to-severe electrolyte disturbances. Lipid-based formulae display less nephrotoxicity, penetrate the CNS, but hepatic and especially electrolyte disturbances do occur. Dosing for mucormycosis ($\geq$5 mg/kg/day) is higher than that for *Aspergillus* (3 mg/kg/day).

Echinocandins are semisynthetic lipopeptide agents. They inhibit the synthesis of 1–3-beta-glucan which is a polysaccharide in the cell wall of fungi (but not the Mucorales spp). There are oral and intravenous formulations available. Echinocandins are highly protein-bound, thus do not enter the cerebrospinal fluid or urine. The half-life is >10 h with a predictable dose–response curve. There are few side effects, but caspofungin is primarily metabolized by the liver and interactions with other medications are therefore possible. There is limited data for their efficacy in the primary treatment of mould infections, and only recommended as an adjunct in salvage therapy.

16.6 Susceptibility and Resistance

Therapeutic failure is often multifactorial but an important mechanism is the resistance of fungi to antifungal drugs. Resistance can be either primary, due to intrinsic resistance of fungi to the given fungicide or secondary due to acquired resistance. *Aspergillus terreus* is intrinsically resistant to amphotericin B while some cryptic species of *Aspergillus* are less susceptible to azoles. In azole-naive patients, resistance is also seen and this is due to environmental resistance which is at least in part driven by agricultural use of fungicides. In 2015, a Dutch center published results on triazole resistance in the ICU and hematological ward, where clinical isolates of *Aspergillus fumigatus* were analyzed for MIC and resistance by genotypic analysis. Up to 20% of the patients had resistant strains to voriconazole and itraconazole, a surprising figure which cannot yet be explained.

16.6.1 Azole Resistance

Azoles are fungicidal in moulds where they target the cytochrome p450 enzyme sterol 14-alpha-demethylase, which converts lanosterol to ergosterol, the functional component of the cell wall. This enzyme is encoded by Cyp51A in moulds. Azole resistance has been found in many clinical and environmental isolates of *Aspergillus fumigatus* and follows modification of Cyp51A gene and its promoter region TR34/Leu98His: TR46/Tyr121Phe/Thr289Ala. Environmental isolates of azole-resistant *Aspergillus* have been recovered from various regions and countries, including Europe, the Americas, India, and the Middle East. As spores are able to cover thousands of miles in the air, it is not surprising that resistance could soon become a global problem.

The direct impact of antifungal resistance in daily practice is best exemplified by the recent change in the Dutch guideline for the management of invasive pulmonary aspergillosis. The high prevalence (up to 35%) of resistant strains of *Aspergillus fumigatus* recovered from the ICU patients in some parts of the Netherlands has prompted key recommendations for resistance detection as well as dual initial therapy. Similarly, an expert panel with candidates from 11 countries convened on this issue. It was recommended that all *Aspergillus fumigatus* isolates recovered by culture-based methods, be identified to the species complex level. Drug susceptibility testing should be performed on multiple colonies (as different resistance patterns might be seen in one culture) and reported within 72 h of culture positivity. Agar-based screening tests are very useful to check the isolates for triazole resistance. And as previously mentioned, there are several PCR-based methods that can detect the most important strains of azole resistance. Resistance to one azole implies resistance to all azoles. A rising galactomannan index while on azole treatment should also raise concern about resistance. For the hematology patient in the ICU, dual therapy with an azole/L-AmB or azole/echinocandin combination is recommended while awaiting susceptibility or PCR results. For the non-ICU hematological patient, initial therapy with an azole is justified pending susceptibility and PCR testing results. Considering the increased mortality rate (up to 100%) in case-series of patients infected by resistant strains of *Aspergillus fumigatus* these efforts are certainly warranted.

16.7 Future Considerations

16.7.1 Novel Host Factors

Immunotherapeutic and molecular-targeted treatments will continue to make their way into clinical practice in the coming years. These treatments are often offered to the highly pretreated hematological patient. There have been several reports of unexpected high infectious complication rates in these patients, with increasing evidence for a role of Ibrutinib in promoting invasive aspergillosis, pneumocystis, and other endemic fungi. The exact mechanism remains unknown, but the pattern of infections suggests an interplay between concurrent therapy, direct effect of Bruton kinase (BTK) inhibition on macrophages and monocytes, disease state and environmental exposure. Surveillance and reporting on these unexpected infectious complications will be of paramount importance and will likely bring new insights into the pathophysiology of invasive mould and other fungal infections.

16.7.2 Boosting the Host

As discussed in the previous paragraphs, the immune response is of vital importance for preventing and clearing mould infections. Prolonged granulocytopenia and CD4+ lymphopenia are both associated with worse outcome. Restoring immunity is therefore an important field of current and future research.

Enhancement of immunity can grossly be divided into two mechanisms, those therapies aimed at stimulating the function of immune cells and those aimed at increasing the circulating effector cells. Some of these methods have already been tested in clinical studies while others like cellular therapy are still being studied in cellular and animal models. These modes of therapy should be seen as an adjunct to treatment with fungicides and are currently not standard of care.

16.7.3 Colony Stimulating Factors

Shortening the granulocytopenic period using colony-stimulating factors has been investigated by several groups. A meta-analysis of 34 studies showed that GM-CSF could reduce the risk of documented infections after stem cell transplantation, but it had no effect on infection- or transplant-related mortality. In a prospective trial of prophylactic colony-stimulating factors in allogeneic HSCT recipients, GM-CSF but not G-CSF decreased the incidence of invasive candidiasis. There was no effect on the incidence of invasive mould disease.

16.7.4 IFN γ

IFN-y augments the antifungal activity of macrophages and neutrophils and has been shown to reduce aspergillosis burden in mouse models. In patients with chronic granulomatous disease, IFN-y treatment provided substantial protection against aspergillosis. Its application in hematological patients is limited and concerns exist for the potential of inducing or aggravating GVHD in the allogeneic transplantation recipient.

16.7.5 Granulocyte Transfusions

Granulocyte transfusions have been investigated with the purpose of increasing circulating neutrophils until bone marrow recovery. Alloimmunization leading to graft failure is a potential risk that needs to be taken into account when applying transfusion in the allogeneic transplantation setting. A randomized trial in patients with neutropenia to evaluate the efficacy of granulocyte transfusions in reducing mortality and improve clinical response to infections, failed to show success of granulocyte transfusions. The trial suffered from low accrual rate and there was a trend for superior efficacy at higher delivered doses >0.6 × 10^9 granulocytes. Further trials are needed to determine if higher doses are associated with higher efficacy. When used for antifungal purposes, it is essential to know that

AmB is associated with increased incidence of acute lung injury when combined with granulocyte transfusion. Therefore, administration of the two agents should be separated by several hours.

16.7.6 Cellular Therapy

Adoptive T-cell transfer of functionally active Aspergillus-specific TH1 cells has been shown to reduce galactomannan antigenemia and improve clinical condition in haploidentical HSCT recipients. In these patients, it was shown that transfer of donor alloantigen deleted CD4-positive TH1 cells induced high-frequency T-cell responses to pathogens in vivo, demonstrating a protective high interferon-gamma/low interleukin-10 production phenotype (i.e., TH1 response) within 3 weeks of infusion. About 9 out of 10 patients cleared the invasive *Aspergillus* infection.

Chimeric antigen receptor (CAR)-T cells are potential aids in fungal disease as well. In recent studies, the variable portion of CAR-T cell was substituted for the fungal-specific C-type lectin receptor Dectin-1, the resulting CAR-T cell was specific for beta-D-glucan and was effective in killing *Aspergillus fumigatus* in murine models. Induction of alloreactivity and cytokine storm can lead to GVHD, which have not been confirmed by studies, but is the complication most worry about.

NK cells also recognize fungal spores. Recently, the group of Ziegler identified CD 56 as a PRR which directly binds to hyphae of *Aspergillus fumigatus*. Once NK cells are activated, they confer direct lyse cells or activate other immune cells for killing. The potential for fungal-specific NK-cell therapy for *Aspergillus* and *Rhizopus* is currently under investigation. Other sources of immunogenic potential are Tregs, which can stimulate immune reconstitution while protecting against GVHD. $\gamma\delta$T cells have also been shown to produce cytokines to stimulate CD4 T cells in mice, without mediating alloreactivity. DC cells form a bridge between the innate and the adaptive immune system, upon recognition of fungal spores and hypha, they release cytokines and prime naïve T cells to induce either a TH1 or TH2 response. Cellular therapy is costly, still difficult and time-consuming to be engineered and will have to make its way into clinical trials before any recommendations can be made on their use in the clinical setting.

16.7.7 Iron Chelation

Iron chelation with deferoxamine has long been known to be a risk factor for mucormycosis caused by acting as a siderophore to enhance iron uptake by the organism and promote its growth. Deferasirox has the opposite effect and steals irons from the Mucorales. This was the basis for a randomized control trial of patients with probable or proven mucormycosis. The overall mortality was higher (82%) in deferasirox group than in the patient group not receiving deferasirox (22%).

16.7.8 Handling of Resistance

Antifungal resistance is a problem that will likely continue to rise in different parts of the world. Travel, commercial application of azoles as well as exchange of goods, plants, and animals will continue to form an obstacle in controlling the spread of resistant organisms including *Aspergillus* spp. and other moulds. It is time to establish antifungal stewardship programs to try to reduce the prophylactic and empirical use of fungicides. A diagnostic-driven approach as discussed in the previous paragraph will also help in decreasing the amount of patients exposed to antifungal drugs. A recent tool developed by Huurneman and colleagues might have a role in guiding adequate azole exposure during treatment. They established a mathematical model for voriconazole in which pharmacokinetic responses to voriconazole administration are translated into a pharmacodynamic response model based on circulating galactomannan levels for the particular patient. Similar PK-PD models are currently being tested.

16.7.9 Hospital Environmental Protection

Reduction of in-hospital mould exposure can be accomplished by protected hospital rooms, special ventilation systems (laminar flow or HEPA filtration) and dust reduction. Fresh flowers or plants and consumption of unpeeled fruits and vegetables are advised against. Most hospital outbreaks of aspergillosis have been related to facility construction and renovation. When renovations are being held it is necessary to have special measures in place, such as impermeable barriers and patient redirection routes to reduce exposure to contaminated air or dust.

When patients are not admitted, there should be inquiry about environmental exposure (smoking, gardening, and farming) and action should be taken to reduce mould exposure in the patient's surroundings.

Further Reading

1. Herbrecht R, Caillot D, Cordonnier C, Auvrignon A, Thiebaut A, Brethon B et al (2012) Indications and outcomes of antifungal therapy in French patients with haematological conditions or recipients of haematopoietic stem cell transplantation. J Antimicrob Chemother 67(11):2731–2738
2. Ashbee HR, Barnes RA, Johnson EM, Richardson MD, Gorton R, Hope WW (2014) Therapeutic drug monitoring (TDM) of antifungal agents: guidelines from the British Society for Medical Mycology. J Antimicrob Chemother 69(5):1162–1176
3. Bercusson A, Colley T, Shah A, Warris A, Armstrong-James D (2018) Ibrutinib blocks Btk-dependent NF-κB and NFAT responses in human macrophages during Aspergillus fumigatus phagocytosis. Blood 132(18):1985–1988
4. Ghez D, Calleja A, Protin C, Baron M, Ledoux M-P, Damaj G et al (2018) Early-onset invasive aspergillosis and other fungal infections in patients treated with ibrutinib. Blood 131(17):1955–1959
5. Cordonnier C, Pautas C, Maury S, Vekhoff A, Farhat H, Suarez F et al (2009) Empirical versus preemptive antifungal therapy for high-risk, febrile, neutropenic patients: a randomized, controlled trial. Clin Infect Dis 48(8):1042–1051
6. Cordonnier C, Robin C, Alanio A, Bretagne S (2014) Antifungal pre-emptive strategy for high-risk neutropenic patients: why the story is still ongoing. Clin Microbiol Infect 20(Suppl 6):27–35
7. Tissot F, Agrawal S, Pagano L, Petrikkos G, Groll AH, Skiada A et al (2017) ECIL-6 guidelines for the treatment of invasive candidiasis, aspergillosis and mucormycosis in leukemia and hematopoietic stem cell transplant patients. Haematologica 102(3):433–444
8. Maertens JA, Raad II, Marr KA, Patterson TF, Kontoyiannis DP, Cornely OA et al (2016) Isavuconazole versus voriconazole for primary treatment of invasive mould disease caused by Aspergillus and other filamentous fungi (SECURE): a phase 3, randomised-controlled, non-inferiority trial. Lancet 387(10020):760–769
9. Skiada A, Pagano L, Groll A, Zimmerli S, Dupont B, Lagrou K et al (2011) Zygomycosis in Europe: analysis of 230 cases accrued by the registry of the European Confederation of Medical Mycology (ECMM) working group on Zygomycosis between 2005 and 2007. Clin Microbiol Infect 17(12):1859–1867
10. Stanzani M, Sassi C, Lewis RE, Tolomelli G, Bazzocchi A, Cavo M et al (2015) High resolution computed tomography angiography improves the radiographic diagnosis of invasive mold disease in patients with hematological malignancies. Clin Infect Dis 60(11):1603–1610
11. Armstrong-James D, Brown GD, Netea MG, Zelante T, Gresnigt MS, van de Veerdonk FL et al (2017) Immunotherapeutic approaches to treatment of fungal diseases. Lancet Infect Dis 17(12):e393–e402
12. D'Haese J, Theunissen K, Vermeulen E, Schoemans H, De Vlieger G, Lammertijn L et al (2012) Detection of galactomannan in bronchoalveolar lavage fluid samples of patients at risk for invasive pulmonary aspergillosis: analytical and clinical validity. J Clin Microbiol 50(4):1258–1263
13. Neofytos D, Horn D, Anaissie E, Steinbach W, Olyaei A, Fishman J et al (2009) Epidemiology and outcome of invasive fungal infection in adult hematopoietic stem cell transplant recipients: analysis of multicenter prospective antifungal therapy (PATH) Alliance registry. Clin Infect Dis 48(3):265–273
14. Georgiadou SP, Sipsas NV, Marom EM, Kontoyiannis DP (2011) The diagnostic value of halo and reversed halo signs for invasive mold infections in compromised hosts. Clin Infect Dis 52(9):1144–1155
15. White PL, Wingard JR, Bretagne S, Löffler J, Patterson TF, Slavin MA et al (2015) Aspergillus polymerase chain reaction: systematic review of evidence for clinical use in comparison with antigen testing. Clin Infect Dis 61(8):1293–1303
16. Lestrade PP, van der Velden WJFM, Bouwman F, Stoop FJ, Blijlevens NMA, Melchers WJG et al (2018) Epidemiology of invasive aspergillosis and triazole-resistant Aspergillus fumigatus in patients with haematological malignancies: a single-Centre retrospective cohort study. J Antimicrob Chemother 73(5):1389–1394
17. Resendiz Sharpe A, Lagrou K, Meis JF, Chowdhary A, Lockhart SR, Verweij PE, et al. Triazole resistance surveillance in Aspergillus fumigatus. Med Mycol. 2018;56(suppl_1):83–92
18. Patterson TF, Thompson GR 3rd, Denning DW, Fishman JA, Hadley S, Herbrecht R et al (2016) Practice guidelines for the diagnosis and Management of Aspergillosis: 2016 update by the Infectious Diseases Society of America. Clin Infect Dis 63(4):e1–e60